ELEMENTARY SCHOOL
HEALTH EDUCATION

ELEMENTARY SCHOOL HEALTH EDUCATION

ECOLOGICAL PERSPECTIVES

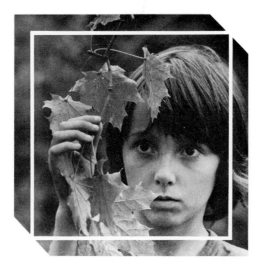

Donald B. Stone *University*
Lawrence B. O'Reilly *of*
James D. Brown *Illinois*

wcb WM. C. BROWN COMPANY PUBLISHERS

Dubuque, Iowa

Consulting Editor

Robert Kaplan
The Ohio State University

TO
SUE
SHIRLEY
AND
JUDY

FOR THEIR PATIENCE

AND
ENCOURAGEMENT
IN
MAKING
THIS
BOOK
A
REALITY

CONTENTS

SECTION TWO
PROGRAMS OF SCHOOL HEALTH

Chapter 9   Healthful School Living – 164

Chapter 10   The Health Instruction Program – 188

SECTION THREE
EFFECTIVE HEALTH INSTRUCTION

Chapter 11   Teaching and Learning: Theoretical Foundations – 205

Contents

PREFACE

This book is designed for prospective elementary and middle school teachers as well as for in-service teachers desiring to integrate the ecological approach to the study of health and safety education. There is a growing recognition among professional health educators of the need to provide students with provocative, stimulating ideas, challenging new concepts, models, and educational materials based upon the ecological approach. Concepts of teaching health education have undergone drastic reforms due to the knowledge explosion and to changes that have occurred in the behavioral and biological sciences as well as in modern educational philosophy.

In addition to the emphasis on ecology and health, we also attempted to focus on providing the teacher with (1) meaningful content derived from the physical and behavioral sciences that is necessary for understanding the health related problems of today's children; (2) an appreciation of the basic issues and concerns in the school health program; (3) an understanding of education; and (4) the basic skills and competencies for developing and implementing effective health and safety education programs.

The textbook is divided into three major sections. Section I focuses on the modern-day ecological approach to health and safety education. Section II is primarily concerned with issues and programs in school health, and Section III is devoted to making health and safety instruction more effective.

We would like to state that for succinctness masculine pronouns have been used freely and are intended to refer to both girls and boys and men and women.

We wish to express our appreciation to the many elementary teachers and undergraduate and graduate students who contributed their suggestions and comments relative to what they would like to see included in a textbook of this type. Our thanks are also extended to Edward Bowers for his editorial help in the preparation of this manuscript as well as to the staff of Wm. C. Brown Company Publishers.

Donald B. Stone
Lawrence B. O'Reilly
James D. Brown

SECTION ONE

ECOLOGY
AND
HEALTH

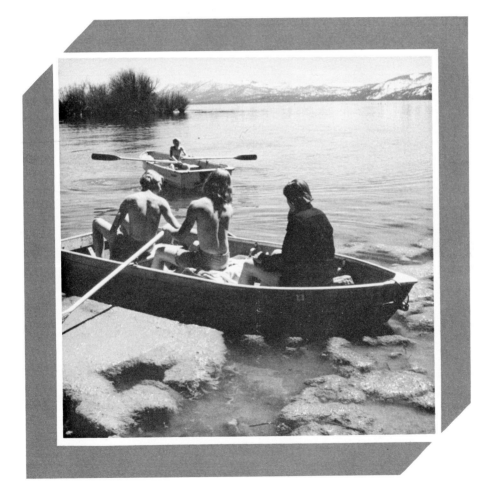

Chapter 1
ECOLOGICAL PERSPECTIVES ON HEALTH

What are some of the basic concepts of ecology?

Why is epidemiology considered a tool of ecology?

Of what significance are ecology and epidemiology in aiding medicine and science to seek solutions to some of our major health problems?

What contributions did some of the earlier concepts of disease make to our culture?

The study of the human organism as it relates to current health problems and issues cannot be accomplished through the science of biology alone. It is only through the interrelationships and the application of the physical, biological, and behavioral sciences that we can intelligently assess, utilize, and apply our scientific knowledge to ultimately improve the health of populations in the twentieth century. Today, the field of public and school health education is being nourished by the field of human ecology and epidemiology. Human health, disease, disability, aging, senescence, and death are all assumed to be dynamic, interrelated processes, not isolated static conditions. Their status is determined by multiple interacting ecological variables—hereditary, environmental, and behavioral—and not by single factors acting in isolation. Epidemiology is the study of all the factors and their interrelationships that affect the occurrence and course of health and disease in a population.

ECOLOGY DEFINED

Ecology is an organized body of knowledge that studies the interrelationships between living organisms and their environment. The term is derived from two Greek words: *ekos,* "the house," and *logus,* "knowledge of." While the observation of plants and animals has occurred for millions of years by man in search of food and clothing, the term *ecology* has been in use only since the nineteenth century.

The magnitude of modern-day health problems is somewhat staggering; however it offers a great challenge for human betterment. Progress, in both the less-developed and more-developed regions and countries, will depend upon the identification of health problems and the intelligent application of ecological principles to their solution.

An understanding of terminology employed by a discipline is a basic prerequisite to the comprehension of major concepts within any broad field of study. Certain key terms need to be emphasized before one can proceed to appreciate the tremendous potential that the fields of ecology and epidemiology offer in the possible solution and/or control of our health problems.

General ecology is a discipline that focuses on the interrelationships between organisms and their environment and their combined effect on the community and ecosystem levels of organization. Included are both plant, animal, and human ecology. Human ecology deals with the relationships of human populations to the ecosystem of which they are an integral part. It is based upon a broad multidisciplinary approach requiring the cooperative efforts of biological and physical scientists, psychologists, sociologists and anthropologists, economists, political scientists, educators, and other experts. Human ecology is based upon a unitive view of man and employs broad-based conceptual models and designs involving the use of clinical, laboratory, and epidemiological field studies. Broadly conceived, human ecology is the science that studies the relationships of man interacting with his total physical, biological, and sociocultural environment.

In ecology, a population is defined as a group of individuals of the same species of organisms—for instance, all of the human beings living in Chicago or all of the largemouth bass found in Lake Ontario. *Species* refers to a group of animals or plants exhibiting reproductive isolation in that the members of a group form an interbreeding community but do not mate outside the group, thus preserving their identity as a species. A community consists of all the individuals of different populations living in a given geographic area. Hence, a community and its nonliving physical environment is referred to as an ecosystem. The term *ecosystem* is generally employed when it is deemed desirable to emphasize the physical, chemical, and biological relationships that bind communities and their physical surroundings into more or less functional units. For example, it is generally known that phosphates promote the growth of plankton which support life in the sea. The microscopic green plants are the life-support system for billions of crustaceans which in turn are devoured by *Sagittas* (arrowworms) and by small fishes which become prey to larger fishes. Hence we see that plants and animals are inseparably bound up with other living matter as well as with their environment. Plankton could not grow properly without the aid of phosphates and phosphates could not be returned to the water to be recycled if bacteria did not decompose the bodies of dead plants and animals on the ocean floor. The ceaseless exchanges of materials and of energy between living organisms and their environment follow circular pathways that are repeated in endless cycles.

An ecosystem is shown conceptually in figure 1–1: X is an organism, and the arrows stand for mutual relationships of physical $\leftrightarrows X$, physical $\rightleftarrows$ biotic, and biotic $\leftrightarrows X$.

The ecosystems of the world are linked by movements of energy, chemicals, and organisms into one entire global ecosystem referred to as the biosphere or ecosphere. The biosphere can be thought of as a single interconnected, endlessly diversified system made up of many different types of biological communities that possess a common web in which all life is basically organized on the same fundamental principles.

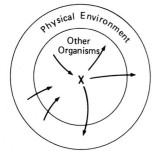

Fig. 1–1. Model of an ecosystem. (From Philip Handler, ed. *Biology and the Future of Man*, Oxford University Press, 1970, p. 432.)

In order to comprehend the concept of energy flow and material cycling in ecological systems, it is necessary to understand the importance of the food web and trophic levels.

In the oceans, energy is trapped and utilized to synthesize organic tissue through minute plants, the phytoplankton (algae, diatoms, etc.). The phytoplankton are fed upon by the zooplankton (small invertebrates) which in turn are consumed by larger invertebrates and small fish. The small fish in turn are eaten by larger fish, seals, and other predatory animals. Each link in the food chain may be thought of as a trophic level consisting of a group of organisms feeding on similar food supplies. Basically food webs represent the pathways along which energy and nutrients move, and trophic levels may be perceived as transfer points at which nutrients are broken down and used or converted into new tissue. Every biological system requires a trophic level, if it is to sustain life, that traps solar energy and synthesizes food.[1] Life itself depends upon the transformation of solar energy into the chemical energy of hydrocarbons through the process of photosynthesis.

Ecologists call organisms that carry on the photosynthesis process "producers." Animals that live off the producers either directly or indirectly are referred to as "consumers." All animals and some parasitic plants are consumers of plants and/or animals since they are unable to manufacture food from inorganic matter as the producers do. Bacteria, yeasts, molds, and other fungi that break down the bodies and execreta of organisms into simpler substances that can be converted into nitrogen compounds usable by plants for building proteins are called "decomposers." Decomposers through their function in nature permit the dead plants and animal tissue to also release carbon dioxide, phosphates, and other substances that can be reused by the plants.

Certain general principles concerning basic laws of ecology exist in the literature. Commoner, however, has in a more simplified manner organized a number of generalizations concerning the ecosphere into an informal set of "laws of ecology."[2] These are briefly presented below for purposes of clarification and discussion.

First law "Everything is connected to everything else." This concept manifests the existence of a complex network of interconnections in the ecosphere involving different organisms, populations, species, and individual organisms and their physical and chemical environments. Disturbances in the ecological balance may lead to other upsets within the system. For example, when a lake receives an inordinate increase of nutrients from sewage wastes and minerals (primarily nitrogen and phosphorous) washed in from agricultural land exposed to fertilizers, rapid acceleration of the process of eutrophication results. *Eutrophic* stems from two Greek words meaning "well fed." Ironically, the oligotrophic or poorly fed lakes are the beautiful clear lakes in which some of the most desirable fish live, whereas the eutrophic lakes are choked with algae, lack sufficient oxygen, and contain little life.

1. W. W. Murdoch, ed., *Environment: Resources, Pollution and Society* (Stanford, Conn.: Sinauer Associates, Inc., 1971), p. 5.
2. Barry Commoner, *The Closing Circle* (New York: Bantam Books, Inc., 1971), pp. 29–44.

Lake Erie provides an example of how the process of eutrophication occurs. Raw sewage, animal wastes, plastics, insecticides, detergents, fertilizers, rubbage, and other organic and inorganic wastes were dumped into the lake. Inorganic molecules were consequently released into the water through the decay of organic wastes which speed up the growth of algae. The waters that drain the farmlands in this area were also rich in nitrogen as a result of the abundant use of inorganic fertilizers. Their estimated nitrogen content is equivalent to the sewage of twenty million people or twice the total population found in the Lake Erie area.[3] As a result, the nitrogen balance of the lake has been distorted, and the oversupply of inorganic nitrates further stimulates the growth of algae. Algae spread rapidly and cover the surface of water with a thick layer. Since algae absorb the sunlight, plants submerged at lower levels within the lake cannot carry on photosynthesis and produce oxygen because they do not receive sufficient light to carry out this process. This in turn decreases the amount of oxygen found within the deeper parts of the lake. The oversupply of algae leads eventually to their destruction, and when the decay process occurs, the large masses of algae consume oxygen which further reduces the amount of oxygen available to support marine life and other organisms. Hence, human intervention was almost totally responsible for upsetting the ecological balance and creating the deterioration of Lake Erie.

Fig.1–2. Compliance with water quality standards will help prevent contamination such as this that causes eutrophication of our lakes and streams. (From U.S., Environmental Protection Agency, Office of Public Affairs, *Action for Environmental Quality*, 1973, p. 13. EPA-Documerica. Photograph by Belinda Rain.)

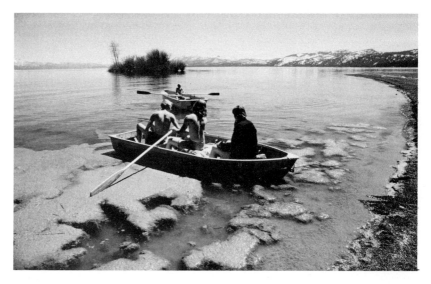

Second law "Everything must go somewhere." Inherent within this context is the fact that matter is indestructible. One organism's waste becomes another's food. Animals release carbon dioxide as a respiratory waste which is an essential nutrient for green plants; plants in turn produce oxygen that is necessary for sustaining animal life. When this concept is applied to pollution control, many of the suggested technological solutions simply shift environmental impact rather than remove it; removal of lead from gasoline has been shown to be associated with an increase in certain dangerous hydrocarbon compounds; removing ash and sulfur dioxide from power plant

3. P. Ehrlich, A. Ehrlich, and J. Holdren, *Human Ecology: Problems and Solutions* (San Francisco: W. H. Freeman & Co., 1973), p. 185.

effluent produces more solid waste to dispose of.[4] Our physical environment cannot tolerate countless tons of noxious gases and poisonous particulates because it too has a finite capacity for waste, and we may soon reach the tolerance limit.

Third law "Nature knows best." Commoner implies that for all organic substances produced by living organisms nature has created an enzyme capable of breaking that substance down, and thus recycling of by-products is enforced. However, he argues that when modern technology creates organic substances that depart significantly from types found in nature the probability exists that no degradative enzymes exist and the material may accumulate in the environment. Perhaps that is what technology and the ingenuity of man have accomplished with the creation of certain detergents, insecticides, and herbicides.

Fourth law "There is no such thing as a free lunch." Everything costs something, and payments of some kind must be paid now or in the future. In our attempts to make people more comfortable we have relied on technological methods that all too often have resulted in delayed consequences.

The direct effects of pollution on human health and on the quality of life are varied and important, but they may ultimately prove to pose a more serious threat to the ecological systems that sustain human life. The ability of an ecosystem to persist and perform its function in light of inevitable environmental change is related to the complexity of an ecosystem.

The more species that flourish and share in the energy that flows through the system, the more stable the system is likely to be and the less likelihood exists that minor changes in conditions will create major disruptions in the ecosystem. However, mankind is systematically diminishing the capacity of the environment to perform its waste and refuse disposal, nutrient cycling, and other essential roles at the same time that the growing population and increasing affluence of its citizens are creating heavier demands for these services.

Figure 1–3 underscores the facts that human beings are manipulators of the ecosystem and that understanding of ecosystems requires consideration of the interaction among the various components of the system. Ecologists are beginning to examine the complexities of ecosystems, and hopefully our understanding of these delicate ecological balances will be increased in future years. Unfortunately the present energy crisis may create ecological disasters as man seeks instant solutions to his environmental problems. The Program Area Committee on Environmental Health of the American Public Health Association has stressed that the administration of our environmental health programs has now become so complex that it must weigh, balance, and take action on situations involving in various and different proportions water pollution, air pollution, surface water and ground water disposal; food protection; solid waste collection and disposal; occupational health; radiation protection; insect and rodent control; housing conservation and rehabilitation; institutional sanitation; subdivision control; hospital sanitation; accident prevention; sanitation and safety supervision of swimming pools; planning and zoning; flood control; road networks; transportation; topography; recreation; traffic; budgeting; tax jurisdiction; and adjoining

4. Ehrlich, et al., *Human Ecology,* p. 14.

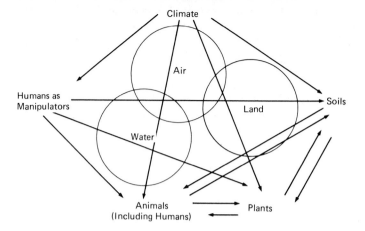

Fig. 1–3. Interactions between man, climate, soils, plants, animals, and the physical environment. (Adapted from George M. Van Dyne, *The Ecosystem Concept in Natural Resource Management,* Academic Press, 1969.)

Climate

Air

Land

Soils

Humans as Manipulators

Water

Animals (Including Humans)

Plants

communities and special areas.[5] Furthermore, agencies administering these programs need to place the political, social, economic, and legal factors in their proper perspective in relation to the technological factors that are involved in our environmental problems.

Dubos also elaborates on the complexities of seeking simple solutions to health-related problems in that "social and technological changes cannot be predicted with confidence because they have determinants peculiar to each area and to each community."[6] For example, smog differs in composition according to the climate, topography, type of technological operation, and kind of fuel used in a given geographic region. Clearly, ecologically sound solutions require programs of research and control based upon the peculiar characteristics of a specific community.

As former Secretary of Commerce Maurice Stans has pointed out, "If we try to solve our environmental problems more quickly than our technology permits, not only will we raise costs sharply and suddenly, but we will also increase the number of false steps that we take along the way."[7] Unfortunately, sometimes lack of knowledge has led to unforeseen consequences, the results of which had a greater impact on our ecosystem than that of the original threat itself. For example, detergent phosphates were quickly labeled as a leading source of pollution in our waterways. Consequently, many state and local governing bodies passed legislation banning the sale of detergents containing phosphates. In response to the challenge, industry developed and marketed alternate detergents containing substances such as nitrilotriacetate (NTA) which was later banned by the Surgeon General because of its possible long-term effects on human health and the environment. More recently other chemical substances have been found to contain caustic materials that can accidentally kill, burn, and blind human beings if improperly used. Some substitutes have also been found to wash

5. American Public Health Association Program Area Committee on Environmental Health, "Description of Environmental Health," *American Journal of Public Health,* June 1965, p. 928.

6. René J. Dubos, *Man, Medicine, and Environment* (New York: New American Library, 1968), p. 124.

7. Maurice H. Stans, "Wait a Minute. The Good Old Days That Never Were," *Vital Speeches of the Day,* 1 September 1971, p. 690.

Chapter 1

out the flameproofing protection factors that are sometimes built into clothing materials.

Our present environmental problems have not suddenly emerged but have resulted from the operation and interaction of many complex ecological forces. Such factors as the concentration of population in urban areas, technological advances, and man's exorbitant faith in his ability to absorb his own waste products coupled with his attitude of exploitative dominance of his life space have all played a part in the current ecological crisis.

Mankind must learn to make its ecological decisions more rationally based upon sound scientific principles as well as to be able to anticipate the unforeseen consequences of its actions. Ecology is still an embryonic science. However as Handler has stated, "ecology does insist on the complex interrelatedness and stability of ecosystems" and the lesson to be learned from those who hastily attempt simplistic solutions to our environmental problems is to "use well before shaking."[8]

EPIDEMIOLOGY

Epidemiology broadly defined involves the study of the determinants and distribution of disease prevalence. Consequently it possesses descriptive, analytical, and experimental components. *Descriptive* epidemiology attempts to describe the distribution of disease in terms of such factors as age, sex, race, socioeconomic status, occupation, geographic location, time, marital status, and other descriptive attributes. *Analytical* epidemiology attempts to interpret the distribution of disease in terms of possible causal factors.

In attempting to investigate the possible causal factors in disease, epidemiologists often employ two types of designs: prospective and retrospective studies. The *prospective* study involves the assessment of a specific population that is currently free of a disease and careful study of the group over a period of time—for example, study of a group of cigarette smokers and another group of nonsmokers over a period of time to determine who ultimately contract a disease. The *retrospective* study involves the utilization of a group of individuals who currently have a specific disease (e.g., lung cancer) as compared to a group free of the disease in order to assess various factors which may account for the presence or absence of disease in the respective groups. In order to test various hypotheses, data are elicited from the groups concerning their prior exposure to suspected causal factors (e.g., living habits and life-styles). *Experimental* epidemiology tests a specific hypothesis, for example, that the incidence of measles will be reduced by immunizing children with a preventive measure such as the Enders vaccine. The hypothesis is then tested by employing the experimental condition in one group of individuals (experimental) but not in another comparable group (control) and observing the effects over a certain period of time.

CONCEPTS OF DISEASE

To gain some understanding of the origin and evolution of epidemiology, it is necessary to explore briefly some of the earlier concepts of disease that dominated man's thought in his search to explain and treat disease. Man's early ideas and attitudes about illness and the disease process were a product of his interaction with the personalities and culture of his immediate en-

8. Philip Handler, "In Defense of Science: The End of the Beginning," *Vital Speeches of the Day*, 15 September 1971, p. 715.

vironment. His basic attitudes concerning disease enabled him to accept or reject certain ideas pertaining to the origin of disease. Various psychological mechanisms employed by man enabled him to treat disease in one of two ways—subjectively or objectively. In subjective analysis, his thoughts and actions became dominated by his feelings, urges, desires, hopes, and fears. He tended to perceive of disease as being due either to "spirit-like" forces or to forces that were intrapsychic (within the mind) in nature. In general, his perception of the world was distorted and his judgment was clouded by the more emotional aspects of his imagination. In essence, he reasoned that recovery followed treatment; hence the treatment method employed by the healer caused the recovery of the patient and restored him to health.

In objective analysis, phenomena such as illness, death, and life are treated and interpreted as they actually exist. Disease is due to various agents which are subject to scientific study and control. Hence, objective thinking is synonymous with the scientific method of problem solving. However, it should be pointed out that man is not entirely subjective or objective in his thinking or behavior. Most individuals tend to fall into the continuum between the two extremes in searching for causal explanations of illness and death.

CULT OF ASCLEPIUS

Asclepius, the first Greek physician, according to legendary accounts lived around the twelfth or thirteenth century B.C. and eventually was proclaimed a god sometime during the sixth century B.C. He was considered to be the chief healing god of Greece by virtue of his heavenly position, and in tribute to their god, the Greeks erected several hundred healing centers throughout their kingdom.[9]

Patients who visited the healing temples for treatment often had to travel hundreds of miles before reaching their final destination, hungry and exhausted. At the temple elaborate preparations were undertaken to prepare the patient for indoctrination into the magic-religious form of treatment. Attendants often bathed and annointed the patients with oil, prayers were offered, sacrifices were made, and the legends of the cult were explained to the weary travelers.

It was believed that during sleep the soul departed from the body and communicated with divine beings in the "spirit-like" world. However, snakes were employed as a necessary link in the communication process concerning the establishment of relationships with the earth gods. Hence, snakes were allowed to crawl among the sleeping patients at the temple in order to ensure that the proper communication system was established. Prior to this primitive treatment, patients were told to pray for the relief of their ailment with all the emotional fervor that they could gather for the occasion. As a result, the patient often dreamed of his illness and its cure and related the events to the priest-physician who interpreted the event according to his knowledge and skills. Treatment was then initiated according to the nature of the ailment and the dreams of the patient.

Historical accounts indicate that miraculous cures were obtained with patients who were blind, deaf, and paralyzed.[10] In reality, this cult was some-

9. René J. Dubos, *Mirage of Health* (New York: Doubleday & Co., 1961), p. 114.
10. Lloyd Ackerman, *Health and Hygiene* (New York: Ronald Press Co., 1943), p. 56.

what effective in treating those conditions which were of a psychosomatic nature. Modern psychiatry stresses that each of these conditions can be brought about by psychological causes (i.e., conversion neuroses) and can be treated by psychotherapy. This apparently was a crude form of shock therapy applied for treating a conversion neurosis.

The cult flourished for about ten centuries after the birth of Christ and eventually underwent several modifications and gradually became extinct. However, the symbolic remains of the cult can be seen today on the caduceus, the symbolic staff of the medical herald. The caduceus or physician's staff has two entwined snakes and two wings which are located on the top of the herald.

Asclepius is shown in most of Greek iconography with his two daughters, Hygeia and Panakeia. The goddess Panakeia symbolizes the attitude of modern medicine searching for the universal cure-all. Hygeia on the other hand was the goddess who taught the Greeks that they could be healthy if they lived according to reason, with moderation in all forms of behavior. Thus Hygeia represents the preventive aspects of medicine, while Panakeia reflects the concept of restorative medicine.

EYE OF HORUS

The Egyptians not to be outdone by the Greeks also had their god of healing. According to mythology, Horus as a child lost his vision after being shot in the eye with an arrow fired by Seth, the demon of evil. Thoth, the god of wisdom, later restored the eye to Horus who became their chief healing god.

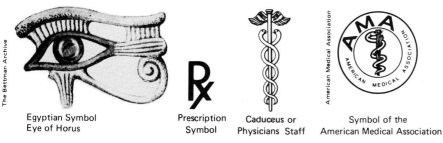

The Bettman Archive

Egyptian Symbol   Prescription   Caduceus or   Symbol of the
Eye of Horus   Symbol   Physicians Staff   American Medical Association

American Medical Association

Fig. 1–4. Origin of physician's staff and prescription symbol.

The Egyptians used a magic eye in the form of an amulet to guard against disease, suffering, and evil. Over the years the amulet gradually changed in structure and design and eventually became in symbolism the origin of the prescription symbol ℞. The imperfect R represented the eye and the diagonal slash (/), the arrow.

DEMONIAC CONCEPT

The demoniac concept probably originated in prehistoric times and has persisted throughout historic times to the present, being still practiced in remote areas of the world. Basically, the demoniac theory purports that evil demons have infested the sick man, have broken open his bones, have sucked out the marrow, and are devouring his flesh.[11] The treatment therefore necessitated that the demons be driven out of the body through various forms of treatment. Shouting, praying, dancing, beating drums, tramping on the body, and ingesting noxious potions were often employed by the local

11. Otto L. Bettmann, *A Pictorial History of Medicine* (Springfield, Ill.: Charles C Thomas, 1956), p. 3.

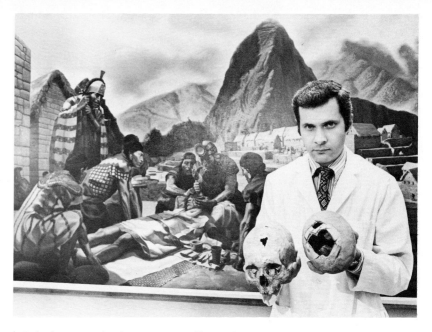

Fig. 1–5. Dr. Donald J. Ortner of the Smithsonian Institution holds Peruvian trephined skulls, with openings once the same size. New growth in skull at left shows patient lived, whereas the other patient died. (From *Medical World News* 15, no. 2 (1974):49. Photograph by George Tames.)

witch doctor or healer to scare off evil demons or spirits. If all else failed, the skull was perforated at times by crude surgical techniques (trephination) to let the evil spirits exit the body. Surprisingly, archeological evidence indicates that some individuals did survive the act of trephination.

HUMORAL CONCEPT

The origin of the humoral concept is often attributed to Hippocrates, the father of medicine, but evidence indicates that it probably was in existence long before the birth of Christ. This concept was based on the assumption that the human body is composed of four humors or liquids: blood, yellow bile, black bile, and phlegm. Disease, therefore, was due to an imbalance of the four humors, and consequently good health could be maintained through achieving the proper balance between the humors. Since sickness was due to the patient's having either too much or too little of one or more of the humors, the treatment was relatively simple; bleed the patient to restore the balance.

Physicians soon tired of such practices and delegated bloodletting to barbers. The barber, in order to advertise his trade, soaked a white cloth in blood and placed the blood-soaked cloth upon a stick in front of his establishment. Hence, we see the symbolic origin of the barbershop pole found in our culture today. A valuable contribution, however, was made by the barbers in that they began to take accurate records of their patients. Thus emerged the early beginnings of the medical case history.

A crude form of urinalysis was also used to measure the humors and establish the presence of illness.[12] If the urine sample was cloudy at the top of the urine glass, the diagnosis was head trouble; in the middle, an infection of the abdomen; and in the lower portion of the glass a leg infection. A sample that was cloudy throughout the urine glass indicated that the pa-

12. Bettmann, *Pictorial History*, p. 73.

tient was sick "all over." Bloodletting was then employed to restore the patient to health.

Even though the humoral concept appeared to contribute relatively little to the practice of medicine during man's early history, Hippocrates reasoned that the four humors were influenced by several factors. Heredity, advancing age, climate, wind velocity, soil, and rainfall were all believed to be capable of disturbing the distribution of the humors. Thus, Hippocrates was concerned with the relationship of man to his physical environment and recognized that disease was not simply a random process, but that disease occurred among different populations and also that some diseases appeared to be more prevalent during different seasons of the year. Hence, the origin of the science of epidemiology is often attributed to the father of medicine.[13]

Of all the concepts, the humoral concept perhaps survived the longest in medical history. It flourished during the Middle Ages and as is true of many health concepts soon was carried to extremes. Bloodletting began to merge with astrology, and patients could only be bled during certain time periods according to the position of the stars. However, the humoral concept still prevails today in its original form in some foreign countries. In fact, a famous Hollywood actor was bled several years ago on location in Spain when he suffered a cerebral hemorrhage. It was reported that a rural Spanish physician attributed his recovery to the bloodletting process.

MIASMATIC CONCEPT

The miasmatic concept arose during the Middle Ages when the idea of miasmas was introduced to explain the presence of disease. It was thought that disease was caused by certain poisonous odors or gases (miasmas) that originated in the earth and were carried by the wind to the susceptible host who subsequently became ill after his exposure to the foul air or gases.[14] As marshes were known to generate gas, it was logical to assume that malaria was caused by the presence of foul air. In fact, the word *malaria* comes from *mal* ('bad') and *aria* ('air'). However it was not until the end of the nineteenth century that the role of the mosquito in the spread of malaria offered a better explanation for the prevalence of malaria in certain sections of the United States. It is noteworthy to mention that once again scientific thought turned attention to the relationship of the physical environment to man's health.

GERM THEORY

Prior to the classical findings reported by Pasteur and Koch during the latter part of the nineteenth century relatively little improvement had been made in protecting man from the ravages of disease. Pasteur and Koch by virtue of their experimentation were able to reveal the true pathogenic potential of microorganisms in disease causation. Scientists accepted the validity of the microbe as the true cause of infectious disease, and the scientific world soon turned its major attention to identifying the causative agents of specific diseases as well as to directing their efforts toward the specific environmental places where bacteria might breed (i.e., food, water, air).

13. John Fox, Carrie Hall, and Lila Elveback, *Epidemiology—Man and Disease* (New York: Macmillan Co., 1970), p. 20.
14. John Cassel, "Potentialities and Limitations of Epidemiology," in *Health and the Community,* eds. A. Katz and J. Felton (New York: Free Press, 1965), p. 433.

The bacteriological era unfortunately limited man's ability to comprehend the real causes of disease because it was felt that all that was necessary to understand disease was to be able to identify the specific organism and the manner in which man contracted the disease. It was not recognized at this point in history that the presence of an infectious agent in man might be only a partial cause in the total disease process. However, the bacteriological era did contribute to the application of aseptic techniques in surgery and medicine, to the development of vaccines to prevent specific diseases, and to the purification of water supplies, pasteurization of milk, and sanitary control of man's environment.

The germ theory of disease stressed the general concept that there is a single cause or pathological agent for each specific disease found in man. For example, the cause of cholera is the cholera bacillus; tuberculosis, the presence of the tubercle bacillus; and the like. However, this theory of disease cannot account for the fact that only three out of one hundred people who are exposed to the tubercle bacillus in the United States develop tuberculosis.[15]

Obviously, there is more to consider in the disease process as it effects population groups than the mere presence of or exposure to a pathogenic organism. This is particularly noticeable with respect to the chronic diseases that afflict modern man. Specific microorganisms have been replaced by social, psychological, and genetic factors which interact upon the host to initiate the disease process.

MULTIPLE CAUSATION THEORY

The multiple causation concept of disease underscores the fact that illness is rarely the result of the impact of a single disease-causing agent such as the tubercle bacillus upon a so-called healthy individual. Instead, it implies that most of our illness is an expression of a basic imbalance in man's adaptation to multiple physical and emotional stresses that are for the most part initiated by his external environment. Disease, therefore, is viewed as one of a number of the resultant forces of ecology. Health and disease are basically expressions of a dynamic relationship that exists between three ecological factors: the agent of disease, the host that is affected, and the environment that contains the agent and the host.

Cassel reports on an experimental study involving breast cancer in mice which may be used to reflect many of the concepts inherent in the multiple causation theory.[16] Several laboratory studies have indicated that by selective inbreeding a strain of mice can be bred in which 60 to 80 percent of the female offspring will develop breast cancer, even though breast cancer occurs infrequently under normal conditions. This suggests a possible genetic factor may be involved in the causation of breast cancer. However, it has also been demonstrated that if the genetically susceptible mice do not receive milk from their mother's breast but suckle from a substitute mother of another strain they will not develop breast cancer. Apparently, the susceptible mothers excrete a virus in their milk which must be present in order for breast cancer to develop in the offspring. Thus, a virus is now a prime suspect as a causative agent in cancer of the breast.

15. Cassel, "Potentialities and Limitations," p. 435.
16. Cassel, "Potentialities and Limitations," pp 437–438.

It must also be pointed out that mice who were born from nonsusceptible mothers and who were fed milk containing the virus did not develop cancer. In addition, only the female offspring who suckled at the breast of their susceptible mothers developed breast cancer. The males did not develop cancer of the breast, only the females. However, if the female hormone estrogen is injected into the male offspring of the susceptible strain, they also will devlop the disease. Hence, a hormonal factor is now implicated as a possible causative agent.

In addition, if all three factors so far identified by scientific investigation are present, the susceptible mice will not develop cancer of the breast if they are placed on a low caloric diet. Thus, there also appears to be a dietary factor involved in the causation process. In fact, all four factors must be present for breast cancer to develop in mice under these experimental conditions. If just one factor is absent, the disease will not appear. As can be ascertained from objectively analyzing the available information on breast cancer in mice, it would indeed be erroneous to attribute a singular cause to cancer of the breast. It is evident that many factors need to be present in order for the disease to occur under experimentally controlled conditions.

In order to make the multiple causation theory applicable to man, a more relevant example employing a modern epidemiological study concerning tuberculosis will be presented in some detail. Traditionally, tuberculosis has been explained in terms of a singular cause, that is, the presence of the tubercle bacillus. However, only about three out of one hundred Americans exposed to the bacillus will develop the disease. Epidemiologists would immediately raise several basic questions such as How does the group of individuals that develop tuberculosis differ from the group that do not contract the disease even though they were also exposed?

In order to study the ecological-epidemiological aspects of tuberculosis, Holmes divided the city of Seattle into four distinct socioeconomic areas.[17] The population residing in area I was predominately male and unmarried and two-thirds of the group were thirty-five years of age or older. This area contained the worst housing facilities and the most overcrowded living conditions. Area II had the lowest proportion of males, but the environmental conditions were slightly better for most of the inhabitants even though they also exhibited overcrowded facilities. Also, area II had a substantially less concentration of older unmarried individuals. Area III was most nearly typical of the entire Seattle population in that the residents approximated the citywide mean or average with respect to age, sex, marital status, and percent of nonwhite population. Residents living in area IV had the highest property valuations and contained the wealthiest families. In addition this area had the lowest proportion of nonwhites, approximately one percent.

As was expected, the investigators found a strong correlation between place of residence and the tuberculosis attack rate. The crude attack rate or the general rate of tuberculosis regardless of age, race, and sex was 398 per 100,000 population in area I as compared to only 54 per 100,000 population in area IV. However, when the racial factor was examined, the same correla-

17. Thomas H. Holmes, "Multidiscipline Studies of Tuberculosis," in *Personality, Stress and Tuberculosis,* ed, P. Sparer (New York: International Universities Press, 1956), pp. 65–146.

tion existed for the white population, but for the nonwhites the situation was almost reversed. Both the male and female nonwhite populations had higher tuberculosis attack rates in area IV, the wealthiest part of Seattle. The nonwhites who resided in this area were for the most part business executives, lawyers, physicians, and other professional people. The lowest rate for nonwhites occurred in area II when the rates were adjusted for the different age composition of the population. The nonwhites who resided in this area were characterized as living in the more densely organized, compact, and ethnic neighborhoods. Thus, the highest tuberculosis rates for nonwhites and whites occurred in areas in which they were in the minority; that is, they resided in areas which presented or afforded little opportunity for social participation or for the development of interpersonal relationships with those of the majority group.

In addition, the researchers discovered that the tuberculosis patients were highly mobile in terms of both residential and job mobility. These patients changed job and place of residence about five times more frequently than the average person. Also, the tuberculosis patients were more likely to be single, divorced, or widowed and living alone than is true for the general population. Furthermore, an analysis of the hospital records revealed consistent patterns of poor health with respect to infectious diseases, accidents, operations, and behavior disorders.

In summary, the tubercular group were characterized as being socially isolated, highly mobile, single, divorced or widowed, living alone, and generally displaying past medical histories of poor physical and mental health.

A study by Guerrin and Borgatta concluded that the major factor involved in tuberculosis morbidity was cultural deprivation.[18] In addition, it was also observed that cultural deprivation was most closely identified with the literacy level of the inhabitants of the census tract, thus indicating that the specific environmental conditions which underlie illiteracy are also related to tuberculosis. This appears to be consistent with the idea that tuberculosis is not an immediately contagious disease, but one that originates from a history of poor environmental conditions and exposure—factors which indeed characterize the ghettos of our major cities today.

Other epidemiological studies have shown an association between a high mortality from tuberculosis and migration from rural to urban life. Dubos has observed that the peak incidence of mortality from tuberculosis occurs in a society within ten to twenty years after industrialization has been established and thereafter declines sharply.[19] The existing epidemiological evidence makes a potent case for the importance of environmental and social influences on the development of tuberculosis. Evidence has also been recently accumulating to indicate that tuberculosis patients are characterized by exhibiting extremely high stress during the two-year period that precedes the onset or relapse of the disease.[20] Although the exact role that the stress mechanism plays in the development of tuberculosis is not fully known, numerous physiological studies have demonstrated significant

18. R. F. Guerrin, and E. Borgatta, "Socio-Economic and Demographic Correlates of Tuberculosis Incidence," *Milbank Memorial Fund Quarterly* 43, no. 3 (1965): 281.

19. Dubos, *Mirage of Health*, pp. 161–162.

20. David Mechanic, *Medical Sociology—A Selective View* (New York: Free Press, 1968), p. 274.

alterations in adrenocortical function in response to a variety of emotional stresses. The very fact that alterations do occur suggests strongly that adrenocortical hormones influence resistance or susceptibility to tuberculosis and that adrenal changes are closely related to stress factors.

STRESS THEORY

Epidemiology, medicine, and psychology are giving increasing attention today to the stress mechanism as a possible contributing or initiating factor in the development of several diseases among which are included duodenal ulcer, colitis, primary hypertension, arteriosclerosis, atherosclerosis, rheumatoid arthritis, and tuberculosis. Selye's theory of stress advocates that almost any disease can be caused by various factors or agents that place the body in a state of general stress. Stress is defined as the "sum of all the nonspecific biological changes (those which can be produced by multiple agents) caused by function or damage."[21] Hence, various entities such as infection, trauma, emotion, strain, heat, cold, hemorrhaging, fasting, and overeating are thought to be stressor agents.

The mechanism of the stress reaction is quite complex and involves a whole set of different hormones of the anterior pituitary and adrenal cortex glands. Briefly, the theory maintains that whenever individuals are subject to stress, the anterior pituitary is stimulated by adrenalin or some other possible agent to release certain hormones such as adrenocorticotrophic hormone (ACTH) and somatotrophic hormone (STH). It is felt that STH aids in building up several of the body defense mechanisms such as antibodies and white blood cells. On the other hand ACTH stimulates the adrenal cortex to release the hormone cortisone and several other closely allied hormones. Cortisone and the related hormones aid the body in adapting to stress by regulating body fluids and sugar. Essentially, both the STH and ACTH hormones help the body to fight off stress.

Subsequent studies by Selye have shown that the initial reaction is the first stage of a much more prolonged general adaptation syndrome which is comprised of three distinct stages, namely:

1. Alarm reaction—this stage is the initial phase of the stress mechanism just elucidated and is put into play by the stress agent.

2. Stage of resistance—this stage involves the successful adaptation of the body to the stress agent. However, if the body cannot adapt or the defense mechanisms provoked in the alarm reaction fail to prevent the successful adaptation by overreacting, then the final stage develops.

3. Stage of exhaustion—this is the stage in which hormonal adaptation breaks down and disease or death occurs. Resistance had been previously established in the second stage but could no longer be maintained.[22]

Selye emphasizes that in tuberculosis, as in many other diseases, stress does not necessarily cause disease.[23] More specifically it is the capacity of the body to resist disease, that is, to overcome the stress component, which often means the difference between succumbing to the disease (disease of

21. Hans Selye, "Recent Progress in Stress Research with Reference to Tuberculosis," in *Personality, Stress and Tuberculosis,* ed. P. Sparer (New York: International Universities Press, 1956), p. 48.
22. Hans Selye, *The Stress of Life* (New York: McGraw-Hill Book Co., 1956), p. 31.
23. Selye, *Stress of Life,* p. 60.

Fig. 1–6. The stress theory of disease.

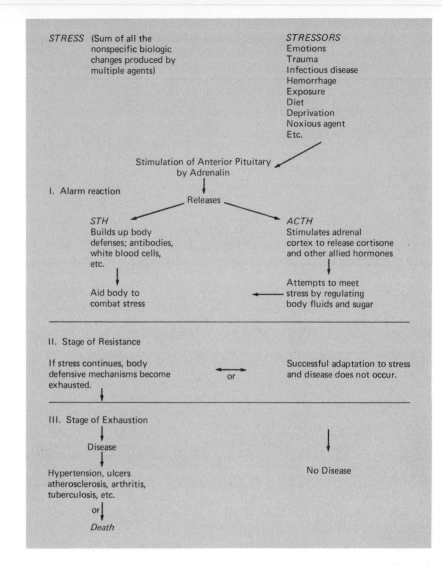

adaptation) and not getting it (physiological adaptation syndrome). Thus, it is the inherent failure of the body's response to stress (stressors) which leads to the development of the disease itself.

MODERN-DAY EPIDEMIOLOGY

Modern-day epidemiology is concerned with the study of the determinants and distribution of disease as it affects population groups. In epidemiology the central focus of study is the group rather than the individual. Specifically, what are the distinguishing characteristics of the population that are affected by the disease? How does this population group differ from groups who do not get the disease? Thus, one can see that epidemiology is concerned with the assembly and analysis of various types of information involving certain characteristics of the agent, host, and environment and in particular with the interaction effect of these factors between and within each other (see figs. 1–7, 1–8, and 1–9).

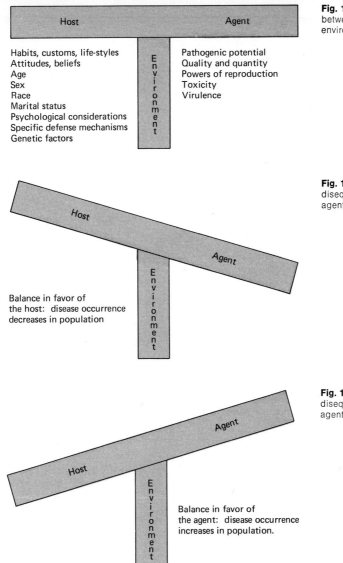

Fig. 1–7. Ecological equilibrium between host, agent, and environment.

Host   Agent

Habits, customs, life-styles   Pathogenic potential
Attitudes, beliefs   Quality and quantity
Age   Powers of reproduction
Sex   Toxicity
Race   Virulence
Marital status
Psychological considerations
Specific defense mechanisms
Genetic factors

Environment

Fig. 1–8. Ecological disequilibrium between the host, agent, and environment.

Host

Agent

Balance in favor of
the host: disease occurrence
decreases in population

Environment

Fig. 1–9. Ecological disequilibrium between the host, agent, and environment.

Agent

Host

Environment

Balance in favor of
the agent: disease occurrence
increases in population.

The agent is usually conceived of as a factor whose presence can initiate or cause the disease process to occur, although in some cases the absence of an agent may also produce disease. Such a case occurs in kwashiorkor where the individual has had an insufficient intake of protein in his dietary pattern. Characteristics of the host which determine susceptibility or resistance to an agent are multiple in nature and generally include such factors as habits, attitudes, beliefs, living conditions, age, sex, race, and occupation as well as the specific defense mechanisms contained within the host and the possible genetic influences which may operate to retard or enhance the disease process. The environment itself will also act to either suppress or enhance the spread of disease. Physical characteristics of the environment

(Pages 20–21)
Fig. 1–10. Which America do you choose? (From U.S., Department of the Interior, Office of the Secretary, *The Third Wave, Conservation Yearbook No. 3,* 1967, pp. 24–25.)

A POOR PLACE TO LIVE

Abuse of land, air, and water create problems that turn appealing areas into ghettos of ugliness and decay. The illustration immediately to the right tells the story of a watershed area where users of resources have sacrificed their environment for the quick profit—the short-term gain. Follow the keys below to conditions depicted by related keys in the illustration.

1. Lack of Water Control

A rampant stream destroys valuable land, fails to recharge ground water supplies, and jeopardizes lives. Usually it goes through periodic low-water cycles that make it an unreliable source of supply for cities. Not all streams should be dammed, of course, but some must be.

2. Ruinous Forestry Practices

Here, cut-and-get-out logging operations, inadequate fire protection, and other short-sighted actions have led to watershed soil erosion, downstream flooding, and loss of habitat for wildlife. Recreation opportunities are destroyed.

3. Poor Farming Methods

Overuse of land and repeated planting of the same crops, have exhausted the soil's fertility. The absence of contour farming leads to rapid runoff and results in erosion by wind and water.

4. Uncontrolled Growth of Suburbs

Lack of effective zoning and building regulations speeds decay. Open green space is chopped up into inadequate patches. "Bedroom" suburbs like this produce monotony, blight, and high crime rates.

5. Upstream Industrial Pollution

Industries that disregard downstream and downwind pollution degrade the entire watershed. Rural areas often encourage industrial parks without requiring adequate pollution controls.

6. Pollution from Mines

Mining companies abandon underground working without a thought that eventually they will cave in and create surface pockets or feed deadly acid water into streams. Others strip off valuable topsoil and leave ugly scars which add to stream pollution and deterioration of the area.

7. & 9. Faulty Industrial Zoning

Unregulated placing of industry pollutes city's air and water and downgrades value of adjacent property.

8. Improper Waste Disposal

Sewage treatment and waste disposal facilities lag behind population growth, hastening the poisonous suicide of the city.

10. The Polluted River

Pollution the full length of the river has made it an open sewer. Fish cannot live in it, people dislike drinking it even after costly purification. Swimming is impossible, and boating unpleasant.

11. Poorly Managed Traffic

A source of air pollution, frustration, and sudden death, poorly planned traffic facilities—added to substandard mass transportation—strangle the Central City.

12. Trapped by Towers

As the population grows and open space is lost to monstrous high-rise apartments, city dwellers become imprisoned by their own "progress." They live an elbow-to-elbow existence. The more fortunate breathe filtered air at home and at work. Others sneeze and snuffle through smog-filled days and nights.

Prepared by the U.S. Department of the Interior

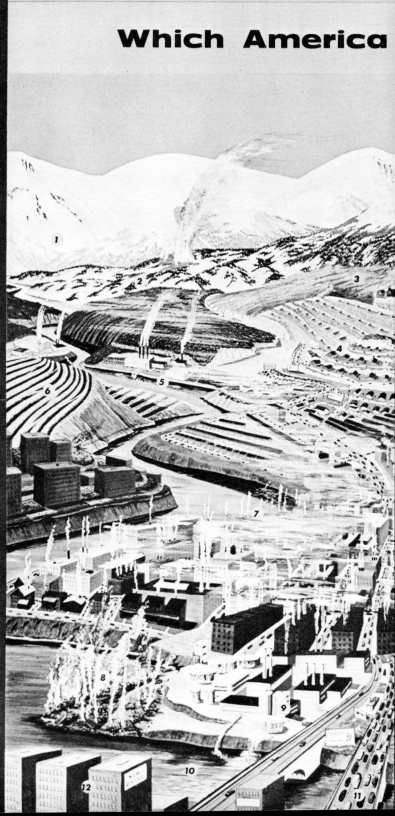

C H A R T

Do You Choose?

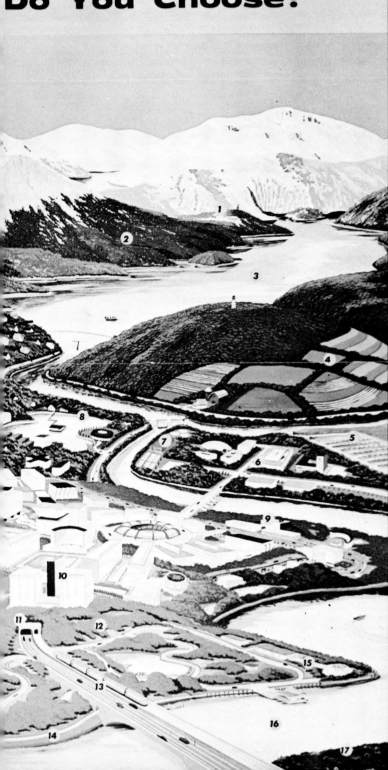

A GOOD PLACE TO LIVE

The balance of Nature and the quality of man's environment can be maintained in an increasingly populous watershed if sound conservation practices are followed. Some of the benefits are listed below and are keyed to the right half of the illustration.

1. Proper Forestry and Mining
Good forest management means selective cutting, fire protection, and planting new trees. Such practices promote continuing yields of forest products. Strip-mined areas have been re-covered with topsoil. Planting holds the soil in place and keeps streams silt-free.

2. Space to Roam
Wilderness areas are protected, providing assured wildlife habitat, a healthy forest base for the watershed, and outdoor recreation for all.

3. Multipurpose Reservoir
Flood control, power generation, municipal and industrial water supply source, and outdoor recreation facilities are some of the benefits of this reservoir.

4. Farm Land Management
Rotation of crops and grasslands, contour strip planting, wildlife hedgerows, all make this farm flourish while protecting the health and quality of the land.

5. Irrigation
Water provided by a diversion dam and a high-line canal turns normally non-productive land into fertile farms.

6. Industrial Parks
Planning and zoning provide attractive and efficient clustering of industry, to the benefit of both industry and city. Sources of industrial water and air pollution are controlled within the regulated industrial park complex.

7. Fish Hatchery
Hatcheries provide fish to supplement stocks in reservoirs, streams, and lakes.

8. Satellite Communities
Self-contained communities like this offer the services and advantages of close-in suburban living. The beauty of the natural terrain and setting is carefully preserved.

9. Waste Disposal
Efficient sewage plants treat effluents from city systems, keeping the river clean. Refuse is burned to generate power in plants equipped with air pollution abatement devices.

10. The Beautiful City
Careful planning and development provide a beautiful, livable Central City environment. Area-wide master plans control the city's growth, provide a smooth traffic flow, and promote work and living patterns oriented not to technology but to people.

11. & 13. Highways and Rapid Transit
Recessed and underground superhighways, combined with a rapid transit system that extends to the suburban satellite communities, provide efficient movement of people and goods to and from the Central City. With home-to-work rapid transit, private car use is reduced. Combining highway and rapid transit operations uses less open space and requires fewer river crossings.

12. City Park and Recreation Areas
Planned parks like this provide the Central City with large wedges of open space and afford many forms of recreation and cultural facilities for the city dweller.

14. Footpaths and Bicycle Trails
Trails follow the natural terrain of the river banks from city to headwaters.

15. Green Spaces
Through proper planning and zoning, abundant open space in and around the city is preserved. This green space provides a natural source of beauty and recreation opportunities.

16. The Clean River
Pollution control and good watershed management keep the river clean, making it a recreational delight.

17. Scenic Easements
Scenic easements along river banks protect the natural beauty of the river. Pollution control is made easier and bank erosion prevented. Outdoor recreation opportunities abound in the natural areas preserved

such as terrain, temperature, and precipitation will influence the occurrence of certain diseases such as malaria and encephalitis. In addition, the biological and social environments within which the agent and host interact will determine the occurrence and distribution of disease among population groups. For example, social and cultural conditions may strongly influence one's exposure and susceptibility to disease. Furthermore, some social factors may act as direct causes of disease or may increase or decrease the probability that disease will occur in a given population.

In order to understand disease and the disease process, epidemiologists must investigate all the factors leading to the disease. Because of the shift in mortality from infectious disease to chronic disease in our population today, social and psychological processes as causes of disease are replacing specific infectious agents. Hence, the prevention of illness is becoming more a matter of changing the habits, customs, and life-styles of individuals. To this end, epidemiology will aid us in our attempts to identify the specific factors associated with disease and the interrelationships that affect the occurrence and the course of health and disease in our modern technological society. Any change in the agent, host, or environment may upset the ecological equilibrium that had previously evolved and may enhance the occurrence and distribution of disease in population groups. For example, changes in the agent (a new strain of virus), the host (prolonged exposure to stress), or the environment (irrigating former arid lands for agricultural purposes thereby providing breeding places for mosquitoes) may destroy the ecological equilibrium previously attained.

Human ecology and epidemiology are not considered to be radical new approaches to the study of health and disease. The emerging epidemiological multiple causation approach within the broad context of ecology promises an exciting breakthrough in the attempt to more fully understand the complexities of medical and public health problems in the world today. Basic progress toward the solution of many of our present health concerns will depend upon the application of sound ecological and epidemiological principles. Table 1–1 illustrates some of the current health problems having ecological implications.

Table 1–1 Selected Current Public Health Problems with Ecological Implications

Population explosion	Alcoholism and drug abuse
Malnutrition and obesity	Suicide
Air pollution	Mental illness
Water pollution	Accidents
Sewage and waste disposal	Problems of the aged
Medical and health quackery	Urbanization

Suchman, a prominent medical sociologist, very aptly alludes to some of the emerging trends in public health that further underscore the need to seek ecological solutions.[24]

1. Changes in the nature of disease. Social and psychological processes as causes of disease are replacing specific infectious agents. Changes in one's life-style have become a crucial factor in the treatment of disease. Changes

24. Edward Suchman, *Sociology and the Field of Public Health* (New York: Russell Sage Foundation, 1963), p. 182.

in the age patterns of disease have caused public health to be concerned with the intrauterine child, the neonate, and middle-aged and elderly persons. Also, early detection and rehabilitation have become the symbols of public health today. The increased numbers of elderly people have created new demands for long-term care and special facilities (e.g., nursing homes, home care).

2. Changes in social and environmental conditions. Modern technology has created new public health problems such as air pollution, radiation, accidents, quackery, and the like. The breakdown of social and family supports has increased the importance of mental illness, alcoholism, and drug abuse.

3. Changes in medical care practices and organization. The rapidity of new medical discoveries has led to the expansion of medical specialists, with a corresponding decrease in the number of general practitioners. This in turn has created problems with respect to the integration of medical services and in the continuity of patient care. The high cost of medical care has led to rapid expansion of health insurance plans and has increased social and political pressure for national health insurance. Serious shortages in medical and nursing personnel have led to the development of quasi-medical personnel such as nurse's aids, physicians assistants, and so forth.

4. Changes in public health practice. The prevention of illness is becoming more a matter of changing the habits, customs, and life-styles of individuals than of immunizing populations. New methods of health education are needed to produce behavior change. Cultural differences among population subgroups require special emphasis and attention for the public health worker. Utilization of medical services rather than establishment of services is the concern today. Public health educators must learn how to motivate people to utilize services.

5. Changes in public opinion and behavior. Health is now perceived as a right rather than as a privilege. Medical care has become a necessity of life and an essential part of any social welfare program.

SUMMARY

In summary, the public has become aware of ecology as a science vitally important for the survival of future generations. It is up to us as teachers to help students realize that if man continues to devastate the earth, plunder his natural resources, and decimate his fellow man he may be headed for his own ultimate destruction. Students need to become aware of the fact that the successful survival of the human race depends upon the condition of all other environmental factors, both living and nonliving. In short, modern man's health depends upon how well he can adapt to and manipulate his environment without creating additional upsets in the ecosystem. To this end, epidemiology may indeed be a valuable tool for ecologists in understanding the complex forces and their interrelationships that influence the occurrence and distribution of health and disease in population groups.

Discussion Questions

1. Distinguish between the following paired terms: ecology and ecosystem, population and community, human ecology and epidemiology.
2. Describe the basic informal "laws of ecology."
3. Of what importance is the food web in ecology?
4. How does the process of eutrophication occur?

5. What is the difference between descriptive and analytical epidemiology? between prospective and retrospective study?
6. Briefly describe some of the early concepts of disease and their contribution to our culture or understanding of the disease process.
7. Why is the germ theory considered to be inadequate for explaining the occurrence of many of the disease problems today?
8. Describe the multiple causation and stress theories of disease.
9. Describe the importance of the agent-host environment relationship in epidemiology.
10. What are the most important trends in public health today?

References

Ackerman, Lloyd. *Health and Hygiene*. New York: Ronald Press Co., 1943.

American Public Health Association Program Area Committee on Environmental Health. "Description of Environmental Health." *American Journal of Public Health,* June 1965, pp. 928–930.

Bettmann, Otto. *A Pictorial History of Medicine*. Springfield, Ill.: Charles C Thomas, 1956.

Cassel, John. "Potentialities and Limitations of Epidemiology." In *Health and the Community,* eds. A. Katz and J. Felton. New York: Free Press, 1965.

Commoner, Barry. *The Closing Circle*. New York: Bantam Books, Inc., 1971.

Dubos, René. *Man, Medicine, and Environment*. New York: New American Library, 1968.

Dubos, René. *Mirage of Health*. New York: Doubleday & Co., 1961.

Ehrlich, P., Ehrlich, A., and Holdren, J. *Human Ecology: Problems and Solutions*. San Francisco: W. H. Freeman & Co., 1973.

Fox, John, Hall, Carrie, and Elveback, Lila. *Epidemiology—Man and Disease*. New York: Macmillan Co., 1970.

Guerrin, R. F., and Borgatta, E. "Socio-Economic and Demographic Correlates of Tuberculosis Incidence." *Milbank Memorial Fund Quarterly* 43, no. 3 (1965): 281–288.

Handler, Philip. "In Defense of Science: The End of the Beginning," *Vital Speeches of the Day*. 15 September 1971, p. 715.

Holmes, Thomas. "Multidisciline Studies of Tuberculosis." In *Personality, Stress and Tuberculosis,* ed. P. Sparer. New York: International Universities Press, 1956.

Mechanic, David. *Medical Sociology—A Selective View*. New York: Free Press, 1968.

Murdoch, W. W., ed. *Environment, Resources, Pollution and Society*. Stanford, Conn.: Sinauer Associates, Inc., 1971.

Selye, Hans. "Recent Progress in Stress Research with Reference to Tuberculosis." In *Personality, Stress and Tuberculosis,* ed. by P. Sparer. New York: International Universities Press, 1956.

Selye, Hans. *The Stress of Life*. New York: McGraw-Hill Book Co., 1956.

Stans, Maurice. "Wait a Minute: The Good Old Days That Never Were." *Vital Speeches of the Day*. 1 September 1971, p. 690.

Suchman, Edward. *Sociology and the Field of Public Health*. New York: Russell Sage Foundation, 1963.

Chapter 2
SOCIOCULTURAL
INFLUENCES
ON
HEALTH

How do social and cultural factors influence one's perceptions of health and illness?

What conditions appear to be responsible for the low-income orientation toward preventive medicine?

To what extent is the quality of medical care that Americans receive related to social and economic variables?

How can schools help meet the health needs of children who would otherwise be deprived of this attention?

Implicit in any discussion of health is some conception of the nature of health and illness. That is, whenever health is considered or mentioned in a conversation, we conjure up some meaning to the term. This is not to suggest, however, that interpretations or conceptions of health and illness are similar among all people. Regardless of one's personal concept of health, certain states of ill health would undoubtedly be viewed as illnesses. For example, when one is on a hospital's critical list and has been administered the last rites of the Church, most would agree that the person is indeed very ill. Under less extreme circumstances, people may disagree over what constitutes healthy and unhealthy states. Moreover, how individuals respond to their individual perceptions of illness and positive health further demonstrates the variant health orientations in our society. Even among persons faced with what appear to be similar health problems or choices coping behaviors differ, especially when health is assigned different positions of importance in their individual value systems.

Among the multiple ecological forces that influence health attitudes, behaviors, and values, social and cultural variables are extremely important. In a school setting successful health instruction hinges upon the teacher's willingness and capacity to recognize the relationships between children's sociocultural experiences and their orientations toward health. Before attempting to modify health attitudes and behaviors, one must identify existing behaviors, understand how these were developed, and discover their meanings to children. Educators have learned that when teaching children to read readiness activities should be related to the child's life experiences.

Fig. 2–1. Typical home in middle-income neighborhood. . . . educational programs must take in to account the diverse socioeconomic experiences of children.

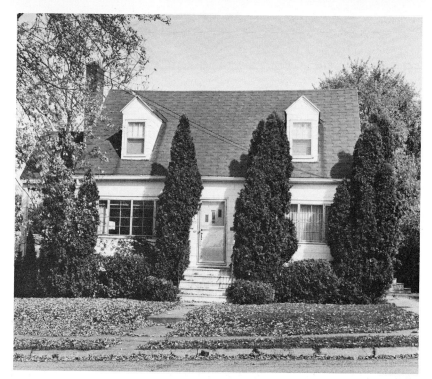

Fig. 2–2. Home in low-income neighborhood.

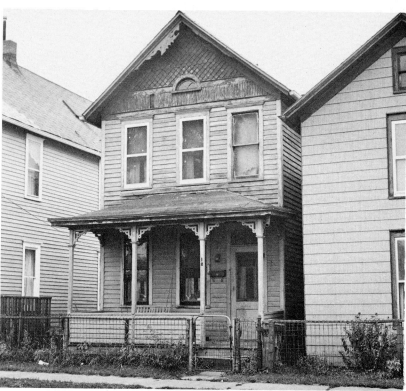

For example, when learning to recognize the letter r, youngsters from socio-economically deprived families might respond to a picture of a rat but not to an illustration of a rotisserie. Even though the application of this educational principle enhances the relevance of learning, it is frequently overlooked in health teaching. Efforts to develop and implement a health education program that fails to capitalize on the social and cultural experiences of children are educationally unsound and socially irresponsible. The purpose of this present chapter is to acquaint teachers with social and cultural factors that influence health status and shape the health attitudes of children.

Health is an abstraction employed when one considers his or others' relative levels of physical and mental well-being. To most people health is a subjective assessment that typically reflects how one feels and to what extent he is able to perform his functions. The popularity of this concept notwithstanding, health may also be conceived as a social value, the importance of which is weighed against other values held by the individual. For example, when family income is severely limited and securing food and shelter are dominant life goals, concepts of health and illness will differ from those of families who are not preoccupied with basic survival needs. Ordinarily when middle-class Americans experience physical discomforts such as headache or fever, they consider themselves ill. Their response to such distress might include staying home from school or work. Some would no doubt seek the counsel of their family physician. Would the same behavior be manifest in a family living under less favorable socioeconomic circumstances? Consider, if you will, a man struggling to raise eight children on an annual income of $3,000. This income figure is not unrealistic, for one-fifth of nonwhite United States families had an annual income of less than this during 1971.[1] Actual incapacitation, rather than moderate discomfort, would be a more likely criterion of sickness among people living under such unfortunate circumstances. Economically deprived individuals often consider themselves ill only when a condition is so severe and disabling as to prevent them from providing for their urgent physical necessities. Anything short of this may not be interpreted as illness. In other words, the life-style of some people is such that as long as they are able to "keep going," they are neither sick nor in need of medical attention. The essential point is that socially influenced attitudes toward health may allow some complaints or disorders to be so tolerated, commonplace and seemingly natural, as to become compatible with the individual's definition of sound health.

Behavioral scientists recognize that family attitudes toward health are internalized by the child during the socialization process. By the time the child reaches school age many of these attitudes have become functional components in his total health behavior. Hochbaum points out that "These health attitudes are passed on by parents to their children, partly intentionally, partly through their examples, and partly in various subtle and imperceptible ways of which neither they nor the children are aware."[2]

SOCIAL DEFINITIONS OF HEALTH AND ILLNESS

1. U.S., Department of Commerce, Bureau of Census, *Statistical Abstract of the United States: 1973*, 94th ed. (Washington, D.C.: Government Printing Office, 1973).
2. G. M. Hochbaum, *Health Behavior* (Belmont, Calif.: Wadsworth Publishing Co., 1970), p. 48.

Naturally, when the teacher and her pupils differ in their understandings of what constitutes positive health and illness, neither party can communicate effectively with the other. This is apparent in the following excerpt from an interview with a member of a low-income family:

> "I wish I really knew what you mean about being sick. Sometimes I've felt so bad I could curl up and die, but had to go on because the kids had to be taken care of, and besides, we didn't have the money to spend for the doctor—how could I be sick? . . . How do you know when you're sick, anyway? Some people can go to bed almost any time with anything, but most of us can't be sick—even when we need to be."[3]

How would an elementary school age child react to his teacher's health lesson if each was operating from a different frame of reference? If the lesson was totally foreign to the child's experience, he might conveniently tune out the teacher's message. Perhaps he would consider the teacher's point of view unrealistic and even silly since his own views of health emanated from a background vastly different from his teacher's experience. Naturally, attitudinal and perceptual differences always exist between teachers and younger, less-experienced learners. The essential point is that these differences should not be intensified by other dissimilarities in the social world from which each has emerged.

HEALTH NEEDS OF POVERTY GROUPS

The United States is often regarded as a nation of unprecedented wealth and abundant opportunity where individuals, regardless of socioeconomic, ethnic, or other circumstances, can substantially improve their lives. Few would argue the point that exciting opportunities do indeed exist. However, the notion that all citizens have equal access to these opportunities is dangerously naive. Inequities pervade many aspects of life, but are particularly apparent when health care is concerned. In spite of the fact that our gross national product—the internationally recognized measure of a nation's affluence—exceeds that of any other country, millions of Americans do not share this wealth. Physician's services, for instance, are not readily available to many people. Modern diagnostic and therapeutic facilities are virtually nonexistent in some areas. Knowledge of the basic principles of preventive medicine is lacking, particularly in the lower socioeconomic groups where low levels of education tend to compound the problem. Health scientists are in general agreement that our health care delivery system has been relatively unsuccessful in responding to the health needs and expectations of minority groups and the poor. In essence, unequal access to optimal health exists in this country. This situation is responsible for needless illness, disability, and death. Moreover, its far-reaching effects seriously jeopardize the extent to which deprived individuals are able to capitalize on other opportunities including education that could improve their lives. Conditions of poor health and poverty form a vicious cycle that has entrapped an estimated forty million Americans.

3. E. L. Koos, *The Health of Regionville* (New York: Columbia University Press, 1954), p. 30.

The poor usually live in conditions which undermine physical and mental health—malnutrition, crowded and unclean housing, inadequate heating and sanitary facilities, substandard working conditions, poor provisions for personal hygiene. Illness generated or exacerbated by these conditions prevents or handicaps many of the poor from making use of the education, training, and employment opportunities which could lift them out of poverty. These limitations are compounded for the children of the poor.[4]

One of the purposes of this chapter is to examine health conditions among the poor and discuss how these are related to the child's school experience. For purposes of discussion, poverty is broadly conceived as a state of extreme deprivation, the causes of which involve complex economic, psychological, social, racial, educational, and geographic factors. Poverty involves more than a lack of money. Low level of education, lack of job security, discrimination, isolation from the mainstream of society, and other factors interact to create a way of life that is intolerable by present-day standards. Though an estimated two-thirds of America's poor are white, a larger proportion of blacks than whites is poor. According to the United States Census Bureau, black Americans are three times as likely as whites to be living in poverty.[5] This discussion of poverty and health focuses on low-income groups, nonwhite Americans (of whom approximately 92 percent are black), and others whose life-styles deprive them of the level of preventive and therapeutic health care enjoyed by the majority of citizens.

Meager incomes, scant or nonexistent savings, and little hope for improving their situation give rise to the feeling of powerlessness that characterizes people in poverty. Among poor children this orientation is most tragically apparent in their fatalistic attitude toward health and their resignation to illness. Time orientation is widely recognized as another significant attitudinal difference between the poor and the nonpoor. Affluent Americans are generally able to contemplate the future, establish goals based upon their perceptions, and direct themselves toward the goals they have established. Poor people, on the other hand, are more frequently oriented to the present and show reluctance to think or plan in terms of the future. Perhaps this orientation is related to the feeling of powerlessness that has convinced them that in spite of their best efforts their influence on the future is negligible. Any single explanation of this phenomenon would be a gross oversimplification. In any case, the tendency to live and think in terms of the present is clearly part of the low-income life-style. More important, this attitudinal posture has broad health implications, especially in the field of preventive medicine. Widely accepted health practices including regular medical and dental checkups, prenatal care, and immunization for preventable diseases, all of which require some concern for the future, may be of

4. U.S., Office of Economic Opportunity, *The Comprehensive Neighborhood Health Service Program*, OEO Guidance no. 6128–1 (Washington, D.C.: Government Printing Office, 1968), p. 3.
5. U.S., Department of Commerce, Bureau of Census, *Consumer Income*, Series P-60, no. 77 (Washington, D.C.: Government Printing Office, 7 May 1971).

little consequence to those who live primarily in the present. This is not to suggest that poor people are not concerned with their health. The truth of the matter is that poor people are unable to enjoy the luxury of preventive health care. Consequently, their way of life imposes a distinct health disadvantage when compared to nonpoverty groups.

> In almost every phase of health care and behavior, the poor behave differently from the middle class and the more affluent sectors of American society. They have higher prevalence rates for many diseases, including schizophrenia. They have less accurate health information. Illness is defined differently. They are less inclined to take preventive measures, delay longer in seeking health care, and participate less in community health programs. When they do approach health practitioners, they are more likely to select subprofessionals. And, under the care of professionals, they are apt to be treated differently from better-off patients.[6]

INEQUALITIES IN HEALTH STATUS

By many standards, health conditions in the United States have shown dramatic improvement in recent decades. The average life expectancy has increased from 59.7 years in 1930 to 71.2 years in 1972. Deaths of infants during the first year of life declined from 99.1 per 1,000 live births in 1915 to 16.7 per 1,000 live births reported in 1974. While these statistics reflect encouraging trends in the health status of the American people, they do not reveal the vast health inequities that exist within this population.

The health disadvantage of poor people begins at conception and usually lasts throughout life. Health authorities agree that adequate prenatal care is one of the best measures to promote the health of both unborn infants and expectant mothers. Benefits of this care are realized during gestation, at delivery, and in the postnatal period. Women from low-income groups less frequently receive adequate prenatal care than do their counterparts living under more affluent conditions. Public health authorities consider the infant mortality rate (deaths of children under one year of age per 1,000 live births) to be a sensitive index of health conditions within a population. Each year, significant differences in infant mortality rates are noted when comparisons are made of groups differing along income, racial, and educational lines. Unquestionably, the higher rates among deprived people are, in part, the result of a lack of medical supervision during pregnancy. Nonwhite infants born to low-income and poorly educated parents consistently show the highest mortality rates (fig. 2–3). There is considerable evidence that medical care during pregnancy and childbirth is especially urgent for low-income expectant mothers, for they often face greater hazards than pregnant women from more affluent families. In support of this view, the National Center for Health Statistics has indicated that low birth weight (5 pounds, 8 ounces or less) is more common in low-income nonwhite families. The risk of mortality is about thirty times greater in the first

6. U.S., Department of Health, Education, and Welfare, *Low-Income Life-Styles*, edited by L. M. Irelan, Welfare Administration Publication no. 14 (Washington, D.C.: Government Printing Office, 1968), p. 51.

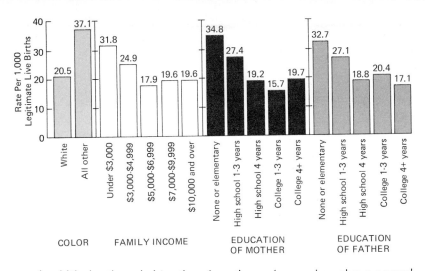

Fig. 2–3. Infant mortality rates by color, family income, and education of the parents in the United States, 1964–1966. (From U.S. Public Health Service, *Health of Children:* 1970, PHSP no. 2121.)

month of life for those babies than for others of normal or above normal birth weight.

Many of those who manage to survive the rigors of birth and infancy continue to face greater health hazards than their more affluent age-mates. Data from 42,000 household interviews were compiled by the federal government in 1968. About two-thirds of the children from this cross section of American families had visited a physician during the year of the survey. However, only one-half of the children from low-income, low-educated, and nonwhite families included in the survey had seen a doctor during the year. For the most part, these doctor visits were for medical emergencies, rather than for preventive care. This tendency for poor people to seek medical care only when a crisis develops is not only a result of limited income, but also a manifestation of their limited future-orientation. Many times treatment is delayed sufficiently long that the condition requires extensive and long-term treatment. When hospital care is required, nonwhite children and those from poor families are hospitalized for periods averaging twice as long as those for other children. Not only does this protracted hospitalization impose severe economic hardships on families, but it also places heavy demands on our overburdened health care delivery system.

Dental health The National Center for Health Statistics reported that in 1968 the average number of dental visits by children (under age 15 years) from families with less than $3,000 annual income was 0.4. In contrast, children from families with income more than $15,000 made an average of 2.3 visits to a dentist.[7] The less frequent dental visits by low-income children represents their failure to receive needed dental care, rather than a superior level of dental health. In general, children from low-income families have more untreated decayed teeth than do children whose parents are able to afford dental care. The relationship between income and the number of decayed and filled teeth is shown in figure 2–4. The data demonstrate that

7. U.S., Department of Health, Education, and Welfare, Public Health Service, *The Health of Children: 1970,* PHSP no. 2121 (Rockville, Md.: National Center for Health Statistics, 1970).

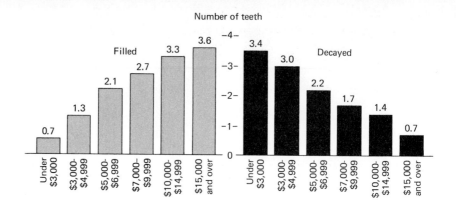

Fig. 2–4. Average numbers of decayed and filled primary and permanent teeth per child age six to eleven years by family income in the United States, 1963–1965. (From U.S. Public Health Service, *Health of Children: 1970*, PHSP no. 2121.)

dental caries (decay) is no respecter of family income. Children from families with annual income of at least $15,000 showed an average of 4.3 treated and untreated decayed teeth. Those from the lowest income families had, on the average, 4.1 decayed teeth. As family income increased, however, so did the likelihood of having carious teeth attended to by a dentist.

Nutrition Hunger and malnutrition are not restricted to the peasants of underdeveloped and overpopulated countries. Millions of American boys and girls go to bed hungry each night and arrive at school the next day even hungrier. There are conflicting estimates of the number of malnourished in the country, but most authorities place the number at about ten million, and some as high as twenty million. This tragic situation persists despite the fact that since 1950 total farm production has increased by 40 percent. Grain storage bins bulge at the seams, and surplus food commodities are destroyed in order to maintain favorable market prices. How can one justify the fact that in this nation, the most abundant the world has ever known, millions of families subsist on diets that by any standards are submarginal?

Contrary to popular opinion, malnutrition does not arise solely from lack of money to buy food. Surveys of school children have shown that surprising proportions of these youngsters do not eat breakfast. Others are victims of overnutrition (overeating). However, when poor people are considered, lack of money must be cited as one of several major causes of their nutritional deficiencies. "They have learned from years of experience to assuage their hunger with such inexpensive foods as black-eyed peas, grits, beans, sometimes potatoes, and maybe a little fatback—foods that fill the stomach but do not by themselves adequately nourish.[8]

To assume that lack of money for food is the sole cause of hunger and poor nutritional practices is to appreciate only part of the problem. Nutritionists have long recognized that ignorance of fundamental nutritional principles is a primary cause of malnourishment. People either lack knowledge of what constitutes an adequate diet, or they use poor judgment in spending their food dollar. Effective nutrition education can provide the information and motivation to cope with these dimensions of the nutrition problem. In fact, nutrition education must be an integral part of any

8. M. S. Stewart, *Hunger in America*, Public Affairs Pamphlet no. 455 (Washington, D.C.: Public Affairs Press, 1970), p. 2.

program to improve the nutritional status of economically deprived or poorly informed families. The classroom teacher faces a major challenge when involved in nutrition education, for it often involves the modification of food-buying practices, methods of food preparation, and culturally influenced eating patterns. Behavior change depends upon the extent to which long-standing beliefs, attitudes, and habits, stemming from diverse sociocultural experiences, can be modified.

Teachers who work with low-income children will rarely, if ever, encounter clinical cases of rickets, scurvy, or other classical dietary deficiency diseases. Poor nutrition, particularly that associated with a lack of food, is usually manifest in more subtle ways. Perhaps this explains why some conditions resulting from poor dietary habits may be mistakenly attributed to other causes. There is convincing evidence, for example, that malnutrition during infancy and early childhood can lead to retarded physical and mental development.[9] Children who suffer nutritionally may have a shorter attention span than their well-nourished classmates. They may appear disinterested in classroom activities. Consequently, achievement and success in school are affected. Disease transmission is favored by the highly contaminated environments and crowded living conditions characteristic of some low-income homes. When children living under these circumstances subsist on poor diets, which lowers their resistance to acute infections, the situation is compounded. They tend to be ill more frequently and for longer duration than those who are well nourished and who live under more favorable conditions.

Empty or poorly filled stomachs have broader though less obvious implications for school personnel. A hungry child can be a disruptive influence, particularly if he is unable to attend to the learning task with which his class is involved. Some teachers and school administrators have reported that poorly fed pupils sometimes coerce their classmates into sharing lunch or lunch money with them. On occasion they may resort to stealing in order to obtain food money. While most people consider these behaviors to be antisocial, it must be borne in mind that they may represent the only way the child knows to satisfy his need for food.

Since malnourishment affects one's physical, emotional, and intellectual performance, schools have shown increased interest in improving the nutrition behavior of school children and their families. Comprehensive nutrition education programs require the involvement of both instructional and noninstructional school personnel. They also involve deliberate efforts to reach the parents of children. Classroom teachers provide the major thrust in these efforts, and success or failure is often dependent upon their interest and concern. Their educational background and daily contact with pupils facilitate the development of nutrition education experiences that can best meet pupils needs.

CULTURAL INFLUENCES ON HEALTH

Culture is broadly defined as a set of beliefs and behaviors that are shared by most members of a society and which distinguishes them from members of other societies. Hochbaum has referred to the term *health culture,* which he defined as follows:

9. M. S. Read, "Malnutrition and Mental Retardation," *Journal of Nutrition Education* 2, no. 1 (1970): 23–25.

. . . the total structure of beliefs and practices concerning health and illness that are shared by all or most members of a society or of any large specific population segments of a society—that is, a structure that sets them apart from members of other societies or other population segments of the same society.[10]

In general terms, Hochbaum identified health cultures as primitive, pseudoscientific, and scientific. Primitive groups believe in witchcraft, voodoo, and the supernatural as causes of disease. They often place great faith in tribal healers, believed to possess magical healing powers. Folk medicine is an example of the application of pseudoscientific health practices that have been passed down through the generations. Although some folk medicine beliefs have a scientific rationale, their acceptance is primarily based on pseudoscience and tradition.

Our modern society has largely rejected primitive notions concerning disease causation. Belief in natural causes of illness, rather than in supernatural causes, distinguishes the health orientation of most Americans from that of primitive cultures. This sophistication notwithstanding, residual influences of diverse cultural heritages still exist. Health cultures brought to our shores by immigrants are modified, become altered in succeeding generations, and eventually disappear. To varying degrees they are manifest in health superstitions, folk remedies, and other practices not in keeping with scientific knowledge. First generation Italians, for example, frequently believed that when food was being prepared in their homes a visiting pregnant woman should taste the food. Failure to do so would, they believed, result in some defect in her unborn child. By the third generation, folklore such as this is often rejected and replaced by beliefs having a scientific basis. The phenomenon of cultural integration in America makes it difficult to isolate health styles that set apart a particular ethnic or cultural group. Likewise, the interaction of social and economic variables with one's cultural beliefs precludes attempts to isolate pure cultural factors that influence health. The so-called culture of poverty is a good example of this. Many of our poor are members of minority groups. They are, in addition, socially, educationally, and economically disadvantaged. Naturally, their health orientation is a composite of ecological variables, rather than of cultural variables, or of any other single consideration. Nevertheless, the task at hand is to show how culture can influence health. Perhaps the best opportunity to accomplish this is to examine American Indian culture. Even then, qualification is necessary, for Indian customs and traditions have been dramatically influenced by the white man's culture.

The Navajo are most numerous of all American Indian tribes, constituting approximately 20 percent of the estimated 800,000 Indians in this country. In some ways Navajo health beliefs more closely approach those of their ancestors than those of the general United States population. According to Crockett, "The Navajo traditionally has believed that illness occurs when by some means the patient falls out of harmony with the forces of nature."[11] Restoration of this balance is the essential purpose of Navajo

10. Hochbaum, *Health Behavior,* p. 44.
11. D. C. Crockett, "Medicine Among the American Indians," *HSMHA Health Reports* 86, no. 5 (1971): 403–404.

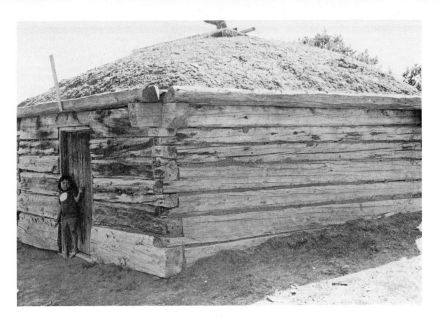

Fig. 2–5. A young Navajo girl stands in front of her hogan. (U.S. Department of Agriculture photo.)

health rituals. A distinctive hierarchy of tribal practitioners rely upon ancient tribal beliefs to heal the sick. Men identified as singers or chanters, diagnosticians, and herbalists each assume different roles in ministering to the health needs of tribal members. These rituals do not necessarily preclude treatment by qualified medical doctors. If a professional physician happens to be present, he may be consulted and permitted to provide treatment. Not infrequently, patients' families will insist that the sick person also be treated by Navajo practitioners. This reliance upon traditional health practices indicates how important cultural beliefs are among present-day Navajos and their health orientation.

HEALTH STATUS OF AMERICAN INDIANS

Health conditions among American Indians tend to parallel those of other low-income ethnic groups. Deaths from disease associated with poor sanitation and substandard housing (e.g., tuberculosis, gastritis) have declined sharply in recent years but are still more common than in the general population. Otitis media (inflammation of the middle ear) has the highest incidence of all acute conditions that pose significant danger to health. This condition is particularly common among Indian children less than five years of age. If not treated properly, otitis media may involve serious scarring of the eardrum and subsequent hearing loss. Further evidence of the improvement in health conditions among Indians is shown by the fact that infant death rates have declined more than 50 percent since 1955. Encouraging though this may appear, infant Indian death rates in 1973 were about one and one-half times higher than those recorded for other Americans.

HEALTH SERVICES AMONG AMERICAN INDIANS

Health services are presently available to about 400,000 Indians through the Indian Health Service (IHS) of the United States Public Health Service. Physicians and other IHS personnel have overcome many of the cultural barriers

Fig. 2–6. Navajo nutrition aides prepare a Navajo breakfast using foods supplied by the U.S. Department of Agriculture. (U.S. Department of Agriculture photo.)

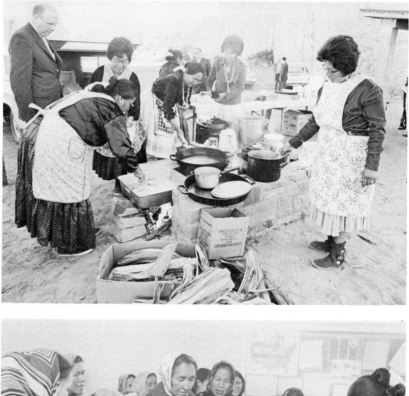

Fig. 2–7. Navajo women are shown involved in a cooking demonstration. Here, foods supplied by the U.S. Department of Agriculture are used to prepare a meat roll, mush, and a peanut butter cake. (U.S. Department of Agriculture photo.)

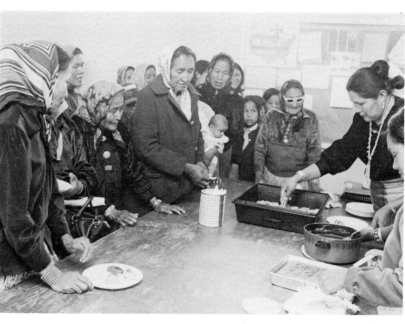

that once denied Indians access to modern medical care. Today, over fifty hospitals staffed by the IHS are operated almost exclusively for Indians. Additional inpatient and outpatient services are available in clinics maintained principally for this population. Increased access to these facilities has brought about remarkable improvements in health status. Most notable of these is the declining rate of neonatal deaths (deaths of those under twenty-eight days old). In 1970, this rate had been reduced to 14.2 deaths per 1,000 live births, a rate slightly less than that for the general population. Improved prenatal care and an increase in the proportion of medically attended, in-hospital deliveries were largely responsible for this progress. Unfortunately, during the postneonatal period (twenty-eight days up to one year) death rates for Indian children remain significantly higher than for non-Indians. Authorities suggest that this is due mainly to the poor living conditions, lack of sanitation, and absence of medical supervision that the Indian infant experiences when he leaves the hospital and is exposed to the deprivation and health culture of tribal life. Improvement in the health status of American Indians has been realized, but much remains to be accomplished. The ultimate objective is to help these people achieve an overall level of health that is comparable to that of the majority of citizens. How quickly and successfully this goal is reached will depend on two principal conditions: success in creating an increased awareness and acceptance of modern health technology and ability to provide improved health resources to our Indian population.

Apart from those who teach on Indian reservations or work with Alaskan natives, relatively few teachers face a situation as anachronous as that posed by Navajo culture. Yet no classroom is entirely devoid of health beliefs and attitudes that are, to some extent, influenced by the cultural backgrounds of pupils. Though these influences are commonly expressed as superstitions, misconceptions, and old wives' tales, their existence can undermine effective instruction. Some, such as the belief that warts will appear on the skin if one handles a toad, are quite harmless. The mistaken notion that you should "feed a cold and starve a fever" is a rather common idea that is moderately harmful. Other beliefs and practices such as taking a laxative to relieve abdominal cramps are extremely dangerous since appendicitis may exist and could be aggravated by a laxative. Health beliefs and folk practices that present the greatest harm potential deserve top priority in the instructional program. Overcoming these beliefs is a difficult undertaking, for children have prolonged and intimate contact with family members who undoubtedly share and support their mistaken notions concerning health.

Health conditions in rural America can be appreciated by recognizing two different, yet interdependent, conditions: geographic location and economic status. It is especially important for those who work with rural children to understand how these two factors affect the availability and quality of health care and, ultimately, the health status of rural youth.

In one sense, most of our fifty-four million rural residents are deprived in terms of health. Regardless of family income, they are more or less isolated from specialized medical personnel and adequate health facilities. Counties showing the lowest population densities have disproportionately smaller numbers of health care facilities, physicians, and other health care providers. For purposes of analyzing the demographic dimensions of health care problems, the United States Public Health Service has classified counties according to the following groups:

Group 1: *Greater metropolitan*—counties with 1 million or more inhabitants
Group 2: *Lesser metropolitan*—counties with 50,000 to 1 million inhabitants

HEALTH IN RURAL AREAS

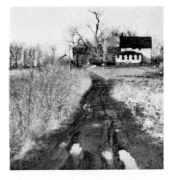

Fig. 2–8. Geographic isolation deprives many rural residents of access to health care.

Group 3: *Adjacent*—counties contiguous to metropolitan areas; population range from 500 to 508,500 inhabitants

Group 4: *Isolated semirural*—counties containing at least one township with 2,500 or more residents

Group 5: *Isolated rural*—counties not included in the above four groups

This classification system is used in Table 2–1 to illustrate the relationship

Table 2–1 Medical Doctors and Hospital Facilities Per 100,000 Population, United States and County Groups, 1966

Personnel and Facilities	United States	County Group 1/				
		1	2	3	4	5
		Number				
Physicians in patient care	125	171	123	73	81	43
General practice	33	34	28	35	36	33
Specialists plus hospital-based physicians	92	137	95	38	46	8
Hospitals	2.9	1.8	1.9	4.0	5.3	6.3
Hospital beds	381	401	381	323	412	209
		Percent				
Percentage of population	100	35.8	30.6	15.7	14.7	3.2

Source: Taken from U.S., Department of Agriculture, *Rurality, Poverty and Health*, Agricultural Economics Report no. 172, 1970.

between county groups and the availability of medical facilities and physicians. Of particular note is the shortage of specialists and hospital-based physicians in isolated rural areas. As a consequence, residents of these remote areas do not have access to the quality of care that is available in urban settings. Geographic remoteness from physicians and health facilities further places rural dwellers at a disadvantage. The location problem is aggravated by difficulties related to the provision of emergency care services. While some rural regions boast competent rescue teams and emergency care personnel, many lack vital ambulance or mobile treatment services. Treatment (and even discovery) of emergency cases is often delayed, with tragic results. In view of this and other factors, it is not surprising that rural accident fatality rates are higher than those of urban areas.

Environmental conditions in rural sections increase the risks of illness. Disposal of household wastes, for instance, is handled on an individual home basis, rather than by elaborate sewage systems such as one finds in cities. Inadequate septic tanks and other sewage disposal facilities will almost inevitably lead to outbreaks of communicable diseases in rural areas. Another increasing concern is the provision of ample, safe, and desirable water supplies. Private wells usually provide water for farm families. Use of fertilizers and other chemicals may lead to the contamination of wells. Increasing concentrations of animal wastes, the results of feeding larger numbers of livestock in confined areas, adds to the problem of maintaining safe farm water supplies. Clearly, the geographic character of nonurban areas creates health hardships that are distinctly rural. As was mentioned previously, the general lack of health personnel deprives many rural families of vital health care. One approach to alleviating this health crisis in rural regions is through the establishment of comprehensive public health programs in county or

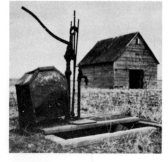

Fig. 2–9. Private water supplies that are poorly maintained pose serious health hazards to rural residents.

multicounty health departments. These programs stress preventive medicine and provide professional counsel and services in areas otherwise remote from health personnel and facilities. Some essentially rural states lack the local health agencies required to provide such programs.

Economic status is the other major consideration having a profound influence on the health of rural residents. Approximately 25 percent of our total population lives in rural areas. Within this group live an estimated 40 percent of the nation's poor. Poverty not only exists in rural America; it is also rampant. According to Wershow, deprivation may actually be a greater problem in a rural setting than in a city ghetto:

> . . . . It is perhaps even worse to grow up and live in a rural slum because there are almost no services available to rural poor. They are just as poor, just as miserable, only more invisible—up the dirt roads and unmarked paths of our backwoods. About the only choices the rural poor have are to starve quietly in the country or to leave for the city, and the uncertain "benefits" of urban poverty.[12]

Irrespective of income, race, or level of education, rural residents face a serious health care disadvantage.

MIGRANT AND SEASONAL WORKERS

Problems of the rural poor are compounded in two subgroups of this population. The first of these groups is comprised of an estimated three million seasonal workers who move within and between states to harvest crops. At the peak of crop seasons, virtually every state employs migrant workers. Florida, New York, Michigan, Texas, and California are reported to hire them in the greatest numbers. Most of these workers and their families are poorly educated and many do not speak English. They lack basic health information and are unfamiliar with doctors and hospitals in their areas of temporary employment. To make matters worse, their occupational mobility often results in loss of residency status and a consequent loss of eligibility for some health and welfare benefits. At least 75 percent of our seasonal and migratory work force fail to qualify for any welfare programs. A large percentage of these people work in counties where there is neither a commodity distribution program nor a food stamp program. School administrators have reported that migrant children are delayed as much as three weeks in some instances before they can qualify for free school lunches. Living conditions for agricultural migrants range from adequate to deplorable, the former being the exception rather than the rule. Even in those migrant camps where facilities appear adequate, the number of workers and their families actually occupying a building may far exceed the number of residents for which the building was certified. As a consequence, gastrointestinal illnesses (e.g., diarrhea) and other conditions associated with crowded and unsanitary living are common. The incidence of skin disease and respiratory infection is unusually high.

Since passage of the Migrant Health Act of 1962, migrant living conditions have improved somewhat. Designed to help communities provide

12. H. J. Wershow, "Pathogenesis of Urban Slums," *Journal of American Medical Association* 215, no. 12 (1971) 1959–1962.

basic health services for migrant workers and their families, this legislation has been responsible for family clinics and programs in public health nursing, health education, sanitation, and nutrition in regions employing seasonal labor. Continued efforts are desperately needed to provide the health programs and resources required to meet the needs of this group. To date, projects funded under the Migrant Health Act have not been developed in many geographic areas where the need is most urgent.

Another rural subgroup that faces severe health disadvantagement consists of several million poor Negroes who have moved to metropolitan areas from the rural countryside of southern states. These people have settled mainly in Detroit, Chicago, Los Angeles, Boston, New York, and other large northern and western cities. For many, the move represents a futile effort to escape the pathetic social and economic conditions of the rural South. Unfortunately, their migration frequently adds to their misery, for they are poorly equipped physically, educationally, vocationally, and emotionally to make the transition to inner-city life. Cities have been relatively inept in many instances in responding to the health, social, and economic needs of this group. Disillusioned with northern urban life, many of these migrants have returned to their former homes in the South.

ATTITUDES TOWARD HEALTH CARE

From the previous discussion, it is painfully clear that those in greatest need of health care are the ones most frequently denied this care. Earlier in the present chapter this disparity was explained in terms of limited income, low level of education, and geographic remoteness from health personnel and facilities. In other words, the health consumer with little money, limited education, and an unfavorable geographic situation was singled out as the cause of his own health disadvantagement. Should the deprived consumer bear the entire blame for the situation in which he finds himself? New insight may be gained by considering the organization and operation of the health care system to which these people have limited access. If the health care system as it is conceived in this country fails to accommodate the social, economic, educational, and cultural differences that are represented by our citizens, the existing health care system itself is a barrier to adequate health care.

In general, medical authorities recommend the private physician approach to utilization of medical care. In all probability most people subscribe to this notion and find it quite satisfactory. Many consider this the ideal arrangement, for it encourages a stable physician-patient relationship that offers personal, systematic, and total care. Those who utilize this private practice health care model recognize the need for effective communication between practitioner and patient. This relationship, like other beneficial social relationships, involves an interaction, the success of which depends upon some degree of mutual trust, respect, understanding, and acceptance.

Rosenstock's view of private practice health care suggests that this approach may not be equally appealing to all social and economic groups:

> It would be well to recognize that the professional referral and care systems are middle-class institutions conceived by middle-class planners, oriented toward rationality in health matters, gen-

erally staffed by representatives of the middle class, and in the United States, at least, involving a system of financial arrangements that are more feasible for the middle class to manage than for the lower class. It does not seem surprising that members of the non-middle class may be reluctant to enter this foreign world.[13]

Virtually all families with incomes in excess of $10,000 have their own physicians. Lower-class families, by contrast, are much less likely to do so. One study of public aid recipients revealed that only 16 percent of families interviewed had private physicians. This finding reflects not only economic, but also social, psychological, and cultural reasons for their failure to use the private physician approach to medical care.

Race is another variable that appears to influence willingness to engage private physicians. When income and occupational levels remain constant, blacks less frequently have private doctors than do their white counterparts. Some medical sociologists explain that culturally influenced patterns of consumption and spending account for this trend. Others believe that the elusive factor of psychological distance between black patients and white physicians may be responsible. The claim is made that blacks of any income level prefer to avoid the psychological threat (or actual indignities) that results from contact with highly educated, affluent, upper-class physicians. In any case, it has been observed that blacks show a marked preference for health care in public clinics, rather than with private physicians. While an evaluation of the health care provided in these public facilities is beyond the scope of this discussion, it is widely acknowledged that public clinic care tends to be more impersonal, episodic, and fragmented than the care one would expect from a close relationship with a single family doctor. That the impersonal public clinic may actually protect clients from the threat of rejection by a doctor is a very real possibility. Generally speaking, one may receive adequate health care from either privately practicing physicians or those employed in public clinics. What is important is that those who need medical care receive it. Unfortunately, this is not always the case, even when the opportunity exists. Consultation with and advice from friends, relatives, and other nonmedical people are preferred by many socioeconomically deprived families. This practice reflects more than a nonaccepting attitude toward traditional medical care. It carries with it the hazards inherent in inaccurate diagnosis, delayed treatment, and protracted use of folk remedies and patent medicines.

Limitations of time and space have precluded a comprehensive discussion of the attitudes that people hold toward health care. An effort has been made to convince the reader that one's attitudinal posture concerning health care has an influence on his health status. It should be clear though that greater efforts are needed in order to fully appreciate the sociocultural genesis of health care attitudes. For until this is understood, especially among poor people and minority groups, attempts to change behavior will be futile.

13. I. M. Rosenstock, "Prevention of Illness and Maintenance of Health," in *Poverty and Health: A Sociological Analysis*, eds., Kosa, Antonovsky, and Zola (Cambridge: Harvard University Press, 1969), p. 188.

IMPLICATIONS FOR THE SCHOOL HEALTH PROGRAM

Regardless of whether one teaches children from the inner city, the rural countryside, or the affluent suburb, the discussion in this chapter will be useful. Concern has focused primarily on the health needs of deprived people. Of necessity we have generalized about the health characteristics of this segment of society. It is vitally important to recognize that, regardless of other obvious similarities, wide variations may exist in health attitudes, values, and behaviors within a group. Some children judged poor by other standards receive adequate medical care and reflect health concerns and values that are essentially middle class. On the other hand, one should not be too surprised when she encounters youngsters from affluent families whose "health style" is somewhat deprived. The essential point is that the health orientation of children or their families should not be stereotyped or prejudged by their reference group affiliation or their personal background.

Teachers, administrators, and other school personnel have a vested interest in child health. For even the most inexperienced classroom teacher recognizes that the malnourished pupil is handicapped since his ability to concentrate and sustain physical and mental activity is hampered. Frequent illnesses lead to erratic school achievement. Furthermore, those who receive limited health supervision in the home and come to school ill may pose a health hazard to themselves and others in their class. In short, a child whose health suffers is a liability to himself, to others, and to the educational system facilitating his development. Because of this fact, schools have traditionally assumed responsibility for child health, particularly when health needs impede the learning process and are unmet by other social institutions.

HEALTH SERVICES IN SCHOOLS

School health services are defined as those techniques employed by physicians, dentists, nurses, dental hygienists, teachers, and the like, to appraise, protect, and promote the health of pupils and school personnel. Needless to say, these services comprise a vital component of the comprehensive school health program. A rather detailed discussion of this subject is found in chapter 8. Nevertheless, at this point it is useful to comment on common socially and culturally related health needs and their implications for the school health services program.

Most schools make an effort to appraise the health status of pupils. Admittedly, the efforts are sometimes inadequate, and as is true of other school programs, the quality of health services is a reflection of school board, administrative, and teacher awareness of and concern with the needs of children. Health services include but are not limited to health observation, screening of vision, hearing and dental health, and health examinations. These procedures assume added importance in schools where children do not have family physicians to provide the services. In the absence of both family physician and school health services a child with a hearing loss may experience severe speech and learning difficulties. The child with organic heart damage may be permitted to engage in school activities that are too strenuous for him. Youngsters whose vision problems go undetected may continue to be classified as slow learners by their unsuspecting teachers.

Well-staffed school health service departments require the services of a physician, usually on a part-time basis, to administer medical examinations. School nurse-teachers or, in some localities, public health nurses, as well as dental hygienists, dietitians, psychological services personnel, and health educators, are members of the health service team. The school's role does not end when health defects or abnormalities are detected, even though schools are not permitted to provide medical treatment. Often it becomes necessary for health service workers to convince families of the need for medical follow-up to correct remediable conditions. When families are unable or unwilling to purchase needed eyeglasses for their child or to pay for the treatment of other health problems, adequate follow-up measures pose a special challenge to school personnel. To facilitate the follow-up, school nurses or other representatives of the school must be able to work with families, sometimes with an incredible amount of patience. Moreover, it is necessary that they be familiar with public aid programs, service organizations, and other community health resources that can help deprived families receive the medical care they need.

SCHOOL HEALTH INSTRUCTION

Classroom teaching would be greatly simplified, but much less exciting and challenging, if all children shared such a broad range of life experiences that individual differences were virtually nonexistent. If this absurd situation prevailed, instructional personnel could easily be replaced by mechanized procedures that would program every child in the same manner. Clearly, this approach represents the antithesis of current educational thought with its emphasis on individualized instruction, nongraded schools, and open classrooms. Several factors, not the least of which is the impact of one's sociocultural experience, have led educators to consider each child as an individual, a product of his unique ecological circumstances. Strangely enough, of all the basic understandings of human behavior, none is violated more frequently and unknowingly than the phenomenon of individual uniqueness. Insensitivity to pupil differences is most paradoxical among some younger teachers, for as a group this new breed is keenly aware of other sociocultural inequities. Being aware of social needs is one thing; however, understanding the classroom implications of these needs is quite a different matter. If the findings and trends reported throughout this chapter are to be of pragmatic value to teachers, their educational implications must be explored further.

Identifying health needs   The effectiveness of a teacher is, in part, a product of how well she knows her pupils, how well she relates to them, and how cognizant she is of their diverse health orientations, attitudes, and behaviors. Obviously no teacher has ever or will ever come to know her clients as thoroughly as she might wish to. Teacher insights do not happen spontaneously, but require considerable time, effort, and skill. An open, accepting, and flexible classroom atmosphere is essential if the children are to behave naturally and express themselves. Opportunities to reveal health attitudes and other behavioral clues in structured and unstructured settings will enable teachers to pinpoint specific child health needs. Simple though classroom observation of health behavior may appear, it requires an astuteness that some adults have not developed. Perceptions and interpretations of classroom behavior can be easily distorted by two major elements of the communication process. The first of these is stereotyping, the tendency to view members of a social or cultural group as being similar in all respects to every other affiliate of their group. Stereotypers are unable to judge persons as individuals possessing characteristics that set them apart from other members of their social, economic, cultural, religious, ethnic, or other group. Thus, one must exercise extreme caution when considering the health needs of the diverse groups represented in the school. Human understanding and interpersonal relationships are further undermined by ethnocentrism. This phenomenon causes one to view his own reference group with uncritical favor and use the values of his own group to judge others. Individuals so inclined consider the ways of their group to be superior to those of others. Prejudgment of others is the insidious by-product of both stereotyping and ethnocentrism. Since educators possess no immunity to either of these processes, they must cultivate the objectivity necessary to avoid these and other barriers to effective communication.

Children express themselves Primary graders are ordinarily quite open and frank in the classroom once they overcome initial anxieties, feel comfortable in school, and develop a sense of confidence in themselves and trust in their teacher. Where this sense of security abounds, classes buzz with conversation, each child anxious to be heard. While educational traditionalists are inclined to view classes of this type with slight disfavor, the free and open climate has distinct advantages. Admittedly it is sometimes necessary to impose a structure that provides opportunities for all children to express themselves. Kindergarten teachers, for instance, have long used "show and tell" as a way to encourage self-expression. Over the years this simple technique has yielded an incredible amount of child and family health information. Magazine pictures can also be used to encourage children to express their knowledge and beliefs about health matters. This approach is a simple application of the projective technique and is most useful with individuals and small groups. By explaining what is happening in a picture, or why someone is doing something, children interpret the picture in terms of their own experience. Outcomes of this and similar activities provide a basis for "instant teaching" and subsequent learning experiences. Discussions of children's crayon drawings and the use of experience charts are enjoyable activities that can satisfy this same end.

Older children also respond positively in an open, nonthreatening classroom environment. Unlike most younger children, they ordinarily possess the skills and maturation required to prepare impromptu stories, role play, become involved in small group projects, and engage in similar activities that will provide pertinent health information for the teacher. With these observations serving as a starting point, the stage is set for the type of instruction that is relevant to pupils' past experiences and future health needs.

It was noted earlier in this discussion that social factors exert a powerful influence on the relative importance of health matters to individuals. No single ecological ingredient is more critical to health teaching, pupil motivation, and instructional relevance. Conceived properly, health instruction can be one of the most popular and exciting of all areas of study, for the pupils themselves are the subjects of the instruction. Therein lies the key to successful health teaching.

Often pupil interest and enthusiasm reach a low point when health is taught as an end in itself, rather than as a means to an end. For example, it is generally recognized that instruction about personal cleanliness should be stressed with young children, particularly those from low-income families. When taught that one should bathe simply because it makes one clean, some children are not motivated. Being clean makes little sense to them. However, when personal cleanliness is treated as a means of helping one to attain something of value to him, the success potential of instruction increases. I am reminded of a practice teacher who had been badly frustrated in her efforts to encourage children to brush their teeth. When asked why she believed this dental health instruction was important, she replied, "So the kids will avoid cavities and unnecessary tooth loss." As reasonable as this outcome appears, it neither justified toothbrushing as far as the children were concerned, nor answered other questions they were pondering. Why should anyone brush his teeth, use dental floss, and visit his dentist regularly? So what if you lose all your teeth? Aren't you better off when you have false teeth? If instruction is based on the premise that positive dental health is a virtue, or an end in itself, it is clearly doomed. Unless the instructional emphasis is on the relationship between sound dental health and that which has value to pupils, the teacher's efforts may be in vain. The desire for pleasing personal appearance, need for peer acceptance, and the ability to eat and enjoy different foods often convince younger children that healthy natural teeth do serve a purpose. Junior high school students often appreciate this fact when they understand that success in careers (e.g., instrumental music, professional modeling) and relationships with members of the opposite sex are influenced by one's dental health status. In short, successful health teaching, regardless of the topic, depends largely upon the pupil's ability to relate this experience to himself and to whatever is important in his life.

Nutrition education   Food and nutrition habits have been identified as areas of health need among those who are socially and economically deprived. Awareness of children's existing dietary patterns, food preferences, and nutrition knowledge is a useful prerequisite to classroom nutrition education. Because these behaviors are firmly rooted in one's social and cultural heritage, they are highly resistant to change. Improving dietary habits and nutritional status is a painfully slow process that demands skill, patience, understanding, and ingenuity. Many efforts fall short of their goal because educators mistakenly believe that middle-class food and nutrition habits should or could be imposed upon children from nonmiddle-class families. Actually, many foods common to low-income diets are nutritious and should be retained because of their economic necessity and cultural importance. Often these diets need only to be supplemented with additional protein or other nutrients. Expectations of success in nutrition education are greater when one works within the nutritional practices of a group and builds upon this framework. For example, the common practice of eating three meals a day has no special merit from a nutritional standpoint. The usual times at which these meals are eaten have evolved as a scheduling convenience and not as a health necessity. It follows, therefore, that the child who prepares most of the food he eats when he becomes hungry should not be taught that three meals a day are essential to sound health. Obviously, in this situation the instructional emphasis should be on food selection based upon the Basic Four Food Groups. Using these groups as a guide it is surprising how much latitude one has in food selection while meeting basic nutritional requirements. A breakfast consisting of a bowl of soup, a grilled cheese sandwich, and a raw potato can be nutritious if additional nutrients are included in one's total dietary pattern. Breakfasts do not have to include cereal, juice, eggs, toast, and milk or other typical breakfast foods in order to make a contribution to one's nutritional status.

Tasting parties are fun for children and often succeed in introducing them to new foods. Kosher food, soul food, oriental food, and special low-cost dishes may be introduced in the classroom in conjunction with health or social studies units of instruction. Identifying, preparing, serving, and tasting vegetables, fruits, and other foods will introduce youngsters to foods they enjoy but were previously unaware of. Ideas for new foods may arise from a field trip to a local supermarket as part of a unit on community helpers (e.g., the local grocer) or health (e.g., keeping food safe). An important aspect of these and other nutrition education experiences is the involvement of parents as frequently as possible, for changes in child nutrition are facilitated when family eating practices are modified.

Hot breakfast and school lunch programs provide additional opportunities to change health behavior. Schools whose clients are from minority and low-income groups often place high priority on school feeding programs. Increasing recognition is being given to these efforts as laboratory experiences where children can practice the nutrition principles emphasized in the classroom. In addition, this living laboratory provides an excellent opportunity for teachers to observe children and thereby evaluate the effectiveness of their teaching and identify further nutritional needs. One common criticism of school feeding programs as they relate to socioeconomically deprived children is that they are administered poorly. Children who are able to pay for their lunches do so, but those who qualify for free meals are frequently singled out as welfare recipients because of the mechanics of the program. Forcing children to stand in a special free lunch line or providing them with easily identifiable free lunch tickets strips them of dignity and self-esteem. While these procedures are inadvertently instituted, they tend to point up how insensitive educators can be to the feelings and needs of children. The most serious outcome of activities of this type is that it creates negativistic attitudes toward hot breakfast and lunch programs which obviously could militate against nutrition instruction in the classroom.

Health providers and their services   Since many children do not receive adequate medical care and, in fact, never see a physician or dentist until a crisis exists, the school can help in acquainting children with roles of members of the health care team. Beginning in the school itself, children can come to know the school physician, nurse, dental hygienist, guidance personnel, and others who comprise the health service staff. Involvement of these professionals in the instructional program adds a new dimension to learning and acquaints children with those who look after their well-being. Timely scheduling of their classroom visits has an additional advantage when arranged prior to routine health-screening procedures. Otherwise anxious children will understand what to expect during vision or hearing screening and be more likely to accept and understand these procedures. Health personnel in the greater community should not be overlooked as instructional people. Representatives of health agencies can describe the services they provide to all members of the community. If field trips are planned, the services of parent helpers should be enlisted with preference given to those who might benefit from knowing about the programs of particular health agencies. Local health departments, since their programs are often comprehensive and freely available to all, deserve special consideration as sources of instructional support and field trip sites.

Personal cleanliness and hygiene   Health instruction should respond to the personal hygiene needs of children. While these needs are often most evident among children from socially, educationally, and economically deprived families, they are not restricted to these families. In general, children from all income levels need instruction in this area. Personal hygiene habits are least resistant to change among the very young and consequently deserve priority in the primary grades. Continued emphasis is desirable throughout the intermediate and junior high school years. Those classroom behaviors that reduce the spread of infectious diseases should be stressed and reinforced, especially when they are not emphasized in the home. Covering the mouth while sneezing and coughing, using handkerchiefs (and, more appropriately, disposable tissues), keeping hands away from the face, and washing hands before eating and after using the rest room are basic health habits deserving attention. Because children share instructional materials (e.g., crayons, books) and work in close proximity with others, the spread of infectious diseases is enhanced in the classroom. By observing sound personal hygiene habits, children help to protect themselves as well as their classmates. Helping young people to become aware and considerate of others is, after all, a fundamental goal of primary education, and can be approached quite easily through health teaching.

SUMMARY

Social, cultural, and economic factors are ecological influences having important health implications for children in the elementary and middle grades. The general purpose of this chapter is to convince the reader that one's perceptions of illness and health, the extent to which health care is accessible to him, and the manner in which the individual utilizes health services and facilities are all affected by these ecological entities.

Children who have been denied access to quality health care often operate at a distinct disadvantage in school. Moreover, their chances of living long and productive lives, free of disability, may be significantly less than those of their more affluent classmates.

Obviously, a school is not in a position to rectify all of the health inequities manifest in its students. However, health needs of those children whose life-style deprives them of optimal health can be partially met in the elementary and middle grades. Success in this regard is largely dependent upon teachers' knowledge of individual differences and how skillfully they can relate the instructional program to the diverse social, cultural, and economic backgrounds of their pupils.

Discussion Questions

1. What evidence exists to support the view that all Americans do not have equal access to adequate health care?

2. Describe general characteristics of the low-income life style that may be incompatible with health maintenance programs.
3. Support or refute the belief that poor people place lower value on their health than do middle-class Americans.
4. How can one justify current school concern with the total health needs of children?
5. To what extent do you believe that "equal health care for all people" is a realistic or unrealistic national goal?
6. Describe specific techniques teachers can use to better understand the health orientations of their pupils.
7. What factors have contributed to the health care crisis in rural America?
8. In your judgment, which elements of the middle-class orientation toward health should not be imposed upon less affluent groups?
9. React to the authors' contention that the school lunch program provides rich educational opportunities.
10. Describe a unique teaching technique or learning experience that you believe would help children learn the importance of one or more personal hygiene practices.

References

Crockett, D. C. "Medicine Among the American Indians." *HSMHA Heath Reports* 86, no. 5 (1971): 403–404.

Hochbaum, G. M. *Health Behavior.* Belmont, Calif.: Wadsworth Publishing Co., 1970.

Koos, E. L. *The Health of Regionville.* New York: Columbia University Press, 1954.

Read, M. S. "Malnutrition and Mental Retardation." *Journal of Nutrition Education* 2, no. 1 (1970): 23–25.

Rosenstock, I. M. "Prevention of Illness and Maintenance of Health." In *Poverty and Health: A Sociological Analysis,* eds. Kosa, Antonovsky, and Zola. Cambridge: Harvard University Press, 1969.

Stewart, M. S. *Hunger in America* (Public Affairs Pamphlet no. 455). Washington, D.C.: Public Affairs Press, 1970.

U.S., Department of Commerce. Bureau of Census. *Consumer Income,* Series P-60, no. 77. Washington, D.C.: Government Printing Office, 7 May 1971.

U.S., Department of Commerce. Bureau of Census. *Statistical Abstract of the United States: 1973.* 94th ed. Washington, D.C.: Government Printing Office, 1973.

U.S., Department of Health, Education and Welfare. *Low-Income Life-Styles.* Edited by L. M. Irelan. Welfare Administration Publication no. 14. Washington, D.C.: Government Printing Office, 1968.

U.S., Office of Economic Opportunity, Health Services Office, Community Action Program. *The Comprehensive Neighborhood Health Service Program,* OEO Guidance no. 6128-1. Washington, D.C.: Government Printing Office, 1968.

Chapter 3
THE
GENETIC
ASPECTS
OF
HEALTH

What are the moral, legal, sociological, and scientific issues that might arise due to the application of knowledge of the genetic code?

What is meant by the genetic-environmental spectrum of human disease?

What ecologic variables influence length of life?

The role of heredity in determining the health status of the human organism is extremely complex and dependent in part upon its interaction with numerous environmental variables. One's physical and mental well-being are products of the interplay between his genetic endowment and the physical and sociocultural environment which one constantly interacts with in his daily living. Neither the genetic nor the environmental factors are held constant throughout an individual's total life span, but are continually changing and exerting their dynamic influence on health. Against the genetic background various environmental influences such as climate, nutrition, drugs, chemicals, toxins, socioeconomic status, utilization of health services, and general living conditions and life-style contribute greatly to the health status of the individual.

It is generally accepted that certain forms of diabetes mellitus are genetically determined, although the precise genetic mechanism is still unknown. Pathologically, the disease is usually due to failure of certain specialized cells in the pancreas to produce enough of the hormone insulin which is needed for the normal utilization of blood sugars by the body. Upon the diagnosis of the disease, dietary reduction of sugars and starches may be prescribed along with injection of insulin to maintain health and remove the symptoms. Thus, diabetes may be controlled by manipulating the environment; however the treatment process will not alter the diabetic genes possessed by the patient. Obviously, an environment that supplies insulin is favorable to individuals who carry the genes for diabetes.

The ingenuity of the human race in developing modern technological innovations is continually altering the environment. We are now employing chemical compounds previously unknown to combat anxiety and illness, spraying others upon our agricultural plants to destroy pests, and using others to pollute our streams and atmosphere. Certain modern drugs such as thalidomide previously used successfully as a tranquilizer in nonpregnant women when taken in the early stages of pregnancy led to the birth of deformed infants without arms and legs and other gross abnormalities. Some of the most potent drugs used in medicine have been identified as being mutagenic or capable of inducing change in the genetic structure of body cells. Recent developments in genetics are helping to make clearer the complex interactions between heredity and environment and the implications for the health of present and future generations.

THE GENETIC CODE

Major scientific advances in understanding the mechanisms of the transmission of genetic traits have resulted from studies involving the chemical composition of chromosomes. It was discovered that the chromosomes of all organisms ranging from the lowly bacteria to higher forms of plant and animal life including man are similar in respect to chemical composition. Different genes of the same organism as well as genes of different organisms are composed of the same class of chemical substances called nucleoproteins. The nucleic acid fraction of the nucleoproteins of all chromosomes consists almost entirely of deoxyribonucleic acids (DNA).

The chromosomes include many DNA molecules that convey the genetic information in coded form to direct the development of the organism. Each gene as a section of a chromosome is either a whole DNA molecule or just part of one. DNA is a highly complex molecule which is structurally similar to that of a twisted rope ladder. The two spiral strands of the helix are held together by hydrogen bonds between the bases. The bases—adenine, guanine, cytosine, and thymine (A,G,C,T)—are arranged in a specified order; that is, the adenine base is always linked to thymine and guanine is always bonded to cytosine.[1] Thus, the two spiral chains are exact complements of each other, so that if the double spiral chain separates into two single strands, each can re-form an exact copy of the original double structure by bringing together the four bases (A,C,T,G).

Structurally, the spiral strands are elongated, and along the length of each are situated the four bases which are arranged in a specified order in which the bases code for one or other of the twenty amino acids whose place and nature determine the genetic instructions that are transmitted to the body's cells.

The DNA molecules are situated in the cell nucleus, whereas the cytoplasm contains a related protein known as ribonucleic acid (RNA) which accepts and interprets the genetic instructions as to pattern and form transmitted by the DNA. The genetic instructions are transferred from the DNA to the RNA via a special messenger form referred to as transfer RNA. Once the gene's DNA has transferred its genetic information to the RNA messenger, the latter directs the formation of particular protein substances from the amino acids that are available. Many of the proteins are enzymes which enable vital chemical reactions to take place within the cell. DNA may be referred to as the "chemical master which lays down the genetic law, while RNA is its creature which enforces it."[2] Thus, every cell possesses an or-

1. Philip Handler, ed., *Biology and the Future of Man* (London: Oxford University Press, 1970), p. 31.
2. Amram Scheinfeld, *Your Heredity and Environment* (New York: J. B. Lippincott Co., 1965), p. 175.

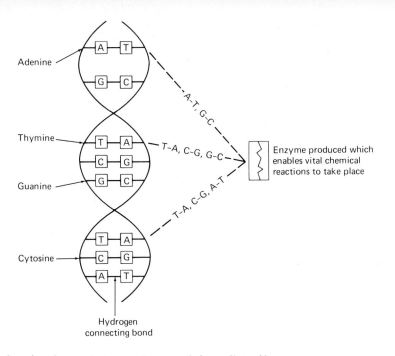

Adenine

Thymine

Guanine

Cytosine

A-T, G-C

T-A, C-G, G-C

T-A, C-G, A-T

Enzyme produced which enables vital chemical reactions to take place

Hydrogen connecting bond

Fig. 3–1. This drawing represents a cross section of DNA, which is the basis of a gene. Shown are the spiral strands and the four bases: A, T, G, C. (Adapted from Scheinfeld, *Your Heredity and Environment,* Lippincott, 1965.)

ganized code of genetic instructions, and the cell itself acts as a computer in terms of interpreting the coded information.

With an understanding of the genetic code has now come the distinct possibility of our complete mastery of evolution and control of human heredity. It is staggering to think of the sociological, religious, and moral consequences of producing superhuman beings, geniuses, and Greek Adonises in the laboratory. However, a more direct benefit to future mankind may be in the alleviation and control of genetic defects and diseases. The potentialities for the twenty-first century in the prevention of chronic disabilities, illness, and lifesaving from genetic diseases and disorders appear most impressive and promising for future generations.

HEREDITY AND DISEASE

Some scientists feel that all diseases of mankind possess a genetic component and result from basic hereditary flaws in protein, fat, or carbohydrate metabolism. It is generally thought that genes tend to produce their effects through metabolic pathways that are controlled by various chemical enzymes. Biochemical processes under genetic control help to determine individual metabolic variations related to the functioning of vital body organs and systems, reaction to stress, the onset and severity of communicable and chronic disease, and health, aging, and longevity.

It is extremely difficult to determine which specific diseases are of true genetic origin and which may be categorized as congenital. In addition, scientists often refer to certain diseases as being familial or tending to appear in generations of families. It is therefore not uncommon to see educated individuals using these terms interchangeably to denote or imply the same connotation.

A disease, defect, or abnormality is considered to be hereditary if such condition is caused by one or more defective genes. *Congenital* refers to the fact that the abnormality was present at birth. It may be acquired in the uterus by virtue of various metabolic, hormonal, infectious, toxic, nutritional, genetic, environmental, or other influence acting on the embryo or fetus to distort its development. Congenital abnormalities may therefore be either acquired during the developmental process of the child during the prenatal period or may be of true genetic origin. For instance, a child with a congenital heart defect may have acquired the abnormality during embryonic development by virtue of the damaging effects of the virus of German measles on the developing heart structure. On the other hand, it is possible that the congenital heart defect was caused by a defective gene or genes transmitted from the parent or parents to the offspring. However, since neither of these operating conditions can be scientifically verified in many cases, we thus label the condition a congenital heart defect since it was present in the child at birth.

Syphilis at times has been referred to erroneously as being a hereditary disease. Congenital syphilis may be acquired *in utero* by the developing infant through infection by the mother. Obviously, the father could not transmit the spirochete through his genes; however, the organism *Treponema pallida* could be transported in the man's seminal fluid along with the spermatoza. Once the initial infection of the mother occurred, the disease could be transmitted to the developing child during the prenatal stage or even during the process of birth itself when the child became infected as he passed through the birth canal. Generally, the spirochete passes through the placenta to infect the child during the prenatal stage of development. Fortunately, with the modern scientific methods availabe, syphilis can be controlled both in the mother and in the developing fetus through antibiotic therapy since antibiotics also pass through the placenta structure.

The mere fact that a condition is congenital (present at birth) or familial (appears in the family) does not necessarily mean that it is hereditary. Certain behavioral traits and styles of living peculiar to certain families may increase the risk of their members contracting certain diseases. For instance, the relationship between the behavioral trait of cigarette smoking and lung cancer is well established and well documented by scientific evidence. It has also been observed that mothers who breast-feed their infants for long periods of time (seventeen months or more) have a lower risk of developing breast cancer than those who employ more modern technological methods available. Thus, the child-rearing practices of the mother may exert a significant influence insofar as the development of breast cancer is concerned. Some authorities feel that this preventive relationship may be accounted for in part by the presence of certain hormonal factors which operate within the female who breast-feeds her child. Other familial practices such as dietary habits of consuming foods rich in saturated fats and sugars may account in part for the appearance of coronary heart disease in certain families for generations.

Many diseases and disorders affecting human beings follow the simple Mendelian laws of hereditary transmission, while others are quite complex in genetic function. Some diseases are labeled genetic since they involve the chromosomes but display little tendency to appear or run in families. Other disorders are not yet fully understood in terms of adequate assessment of their true genetic operation. Not all character traits are inherited in a simple manner. When the transmission of a trait within a family does not follow one of the more recognized patterns, that is, it depends upon a number of genes acting in concert, it is referred to as multifactorial or polygenic inheritance. Intelligence and stature, for example, are dependent upon the control and effect of many pairs of genes, as is the inheritance of clubfoot and cleft lip. There is growing evidence that polygenic inheritance patterns may also account for many of the more common medical problems such as hypertension, high levels of serum cholesterol, and diabetes mellitus.

What one inherits is to a limited extent counterbalanced by one's ability to react to various environmental conditions. Equipped with superior genes for physical and mental growth and development, an individual's health status may be retarded by poor dietary practices, lack of adequate health and medical services, or improper health protective attitudes and behavior. (These realities were elaborated upon in chapter 2.) In addition our intellectual capabilities may be hindered by the lack of sufficient motivation and/or the failure of the environment to provide the necessary stimuli.

HEREDITY AND ENVIRONMENTAL INTERACTION

Figure 3–2 illustrates the concept of human diseases as being represented on a spectrum ranging from those diseases which are largely environmental in causation to those which are more directly influenced by heredity. At the extreme end of the genetic-environmental spectrum one may observe specific diseases such as muscular dystrophy, cystic fibrosis, Huntington's chorea, and some metabolic and chromosomal disorders that are largely genetic in origin.

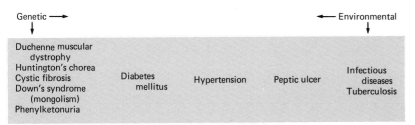

Fig. 3–2. This diagram illustrates the genetic environmental spectrum of human disease. (Adapted from Emery, *Heredity, Disease and Man*, University of California Press, 1968.)

Muscular dystrophy is a chronic disease characterized by the weakening and wasting away of the body's voluntary muscles. The disease is progressive, and there is no known treatment for halting the progress of the loss of muscular strength. More than two-thirds of the estimated 200,000 victims in the United States are children between the ages of three and thirteen years. The most common form of muscular dystrophy (Duchenne) is inherited and in some cases is due to a sex-linked recessive gene that afflicts males about three times as often as females.[3] Respiratory diseases such as the common cold may present serious problems to afflicted children if the muscles of breathing are involved.

Cystic fibrosis is a hereditary disorder that is transmitted by a recessive gene. It is a generalized disorder of the exocrine or duct glands that secrete mucus, saliva, tears, and sweat. Abnormally thick discharges of mucus produce blocking of the respiratory passages in the lungs. In addition, the ducts of the pancreas become clogged, and therefore the digestive enzymes are unable to function properly. Colds and other respiratory diseases also present serious hazards to the victims of cystic fibrosis. This particular disease affects

3. *Muscular Dystrophy—The Facts* (New York: Muscular Dystrophy Association of America, 1970).

approximately one out of 1,000 newborn infants and is frequently referred to as the "greatest killer" of white children. Cystic fibrosis appears to be nonexistent in Oriental children and rare in blacks.[4]

The genetically determined inability to convert phenylalanine, an essential amino acid, into tyrosine which is metabolized by other enzyme systems results in a disorder called phenylketonuria (PKU). The high concentration of phenylalanine in the blood causes mental retardation because it is an inhibitor of enzyme systems of the brain.[5] PKU can be detected within the first few days of life, and placing the infant on a special low-phenylalanine diet can prevent further retardation. This disorder is inherited as a recessive trait and occurs in approximately one out of 10,000 births.

Huntington's chorea is a degenerative disease of the central nervous system characterized by emotional and physiological deterioration of the victim. It is inherited as a pure Mendelian characteristic that behaves as a dominant gene, with the result that one-fourth to one-half of the offspring of the patient develop the disease (usually in their late thirties or early forties). At the present time there is no known cure for this disorder.

Down's syndrome (mongolism) results from an error in the total number of chromosomes that find their way into the cells. As a result of this autosomal (determines characteristics other than sex) aberration the child has forty-seven chromosomes instead of the usual forty-six. Children afflicted with this disorder are both physically and mentally retarded. This disorder appears to show some relationship to the age of the mother. There is one chance in fifty of a woman in her forties giving birth to a mongoloid child, while the corresponding risk for a woman in her twenties is one in 2,000.[6]

At the environmental end of the spectrum, science has determined that susceptibility to pulmonary tuberculosis is inherited. However, only a relatively small number of genetically predisposed individuals ever develop the disease because stress, nutritional status, general health, and exposure are of greater importance in the causation of tuberculosis than is genetic susceptibility. In between the two ends of the spectrum, both genetic and environmental factors appear to share influence in disease causation. For example, peptic ulcer is twice as common in the siblings of ulcer patients than is found in the general population, but it is also well documented that stress is a major contributing factor in the causation of this disorder. Peptic ulcer is now being diagnosed with increasing frequency in children. Some pediatricians feel that the increased stress placed on children by parents and school may be a factor in the rising incidence of this disorder. The sharp increase noticed in children, particularly among boys, the apparent higher risk in the upper socioeconomic strata, the greater number of mixed marriages among the parents of peptic ulcer patients, the high proportion of parents of peptic ulcer cases who themselves had the same condition, and the evidence of marital discord in the family distinguish childhood peptic ulcer from many other long-term childhood disorders.[7]

4. Benjamin Kogan, *Health: Man in a Changing Environment* (New York: Harcourt, Brace & World, 1970), p. 239.
5. C. L. Anderson, *Health Principles and Practice*, 5th ed. (St. Louis: C. V. Mosby Co., 1972), p. 141.
6. Dorothy Davis, "Predicting Tomorrow's Children," *Today's Health* 46 (January 1968): 32–37.
7. Harry Sultz et al., "The Epidemiology of Peptic Ulcer in Childhood," *American Journal of Public Health* 60, no. 3 (1970): 498.

Thus, from the foregoing discussion it might be surmised that in some diseases such as cystic fibrosis the environment plays only a small part in causation. While in others such as tuberculosis the environment becomes omnipotent as a contributing factor in causation. But, whatever the disease or the role played by heredity, one should be aware that some individuals are inherently more vulnerable than others. As will be explained later in this chapter, one's sex will determine whether or not certain hereditary diseases and defects will manifest themselves in the host.

How long is the human organism capable of living? What is the relationship between longevity and various ecological factors such as heredity, race, sex, biological influences, body build, physical condition, occupation, and environment? Discussion of these questions has been of keen interest to the human race since Eve tempted Adam with an apple, and probably no question is fundamentally more important to any of us than How long will I live?

Human life is indeed a very personal affair. The complete life cycle begins with conception, continues with infancy, and passes through childhood, adolescence, maturity, and old age, and finally terminates in death. Many lives are cut short before individuals complete their expected life cycle: an accident, a disease, or a war may interrupt the process at any stage for certain individuals. However, it is certain that all of us must eventually reach that final stage in our life cycle, for there is a natural span of life, a limit that is imposed upon life itself.

LIFE SPAN AND LIFE EXPECTANCY

Life span and *life expectancy,* while often used interchangeably in the literature, are entirely different concepts. *Life span* refers to the maximum biological time limit that is imposed upon life itself. While *life expectancy* refers to the average length of life that a person born during a certain period of time can be expected to live under the conditions that exist during that time period. Table 3–1 shows the life expectancy or average length of life during certain periods of history.

Table 3–1 Life Expectancy During Selected Eras

Time Period	Life Expectancy (yrs.)
Roman	22
Middle Ages	33
1789 (U.S.)	36
1854 (U.S.)	41
1900 (U.S.)	50
1972 (U.S.)	71

Life span   Probably the most extreme record of longevity cited in the literature is that of Thomas Parr, an English farmer who died in 1635 at the reputed age of 152 years.[8] A Dane, Christen Drakenbery, is said to have attained 146 years of age, while the Soviet Union at times has publicized cases of individuals reputedly 150 years or older. The United States also has laid

8. Alex Comfort, *Aging: The Biology of Senescence* (New York: Holt, Rinehart & Winston, 1964), p. 91.

claim to the longevity record by recording several individuals who lived to be 120 years of age and over. The Bible cites extraordinary instances of longevity and sets the age of Adam as 930 years and of Seth of 912 years; however, the figures presented in the Bible were most likely based on methods of calculating years that were entirely different from those employed today. In general, the extraordinary ages that have been cited were credited to persons for whom no reliable and authentic records were available. There has been no apparent change in the life span of human beings since historical records have been kept. Life span is set at between 110 to 115 years—the age to which authentic records indicate that the oldest person lived. An exact figure cannot be presented for the human life span as there is always the possibility that another individual will surpass the previous maximum that had been established.

The maximum ages attained by various animal groups cover a broad range for which there is no simple explanation. Life span tends to be correlated with large size, but there are numerous exceptions, even within families. Species life span appears to be fairly fixed and predetermined by genetic factors. The longest lived animals probably are the tortoises, with fish, birds, and human beings not far behind. Table 3–2 presents the life span reported for various members of the animal kingdom.

Table 3–2 Life Span of Selected Animals

Animal	Life Span (yrs.)
Tortoise	150
Elephant	77
Chimpanzee	39
Horse	40
Crocodile	60
Carp	50
Toad	36
Sturgeon	100
Golden eagle	80
Vulture	117
Dog	25
Cat	25

Life expectancy The dramatic increase in life expectancy at birth during the twentieth century has had profound social consequences for Americans. On the one hand, it has resulted in a record proportion in the number of aged persons in the community—a group that represents special problems of health, income, and adjustment. On the other hand, it has made possible the prolongation of family life and has increased the length of one's occupational life.

The greatest gain in life expectancy between 1900 and 1972 occurred at birth. In 1900, the life expectancy at birth was 49.2 years, while the corresponding figure for a child born in 1972 is 71.2 years. The shortest overall gain in life expectancy occurred at the opposite end of the human life cycle. At age 85 years, the net gain in life expectancy between 1900 and the present was approximately one year.

The major reason for the tremendous gain in life expectancy at birth between these time periods can be attributed largely to the lowering of the infant mortality rate. Thus, we have not changed the limits of life, but we have simply changed the concentration of cases into the older population groups. The application of medical and scientific knowledge has made it possible for individuals to live longer by controlling the infectious diseases which in the past exerted a heavy toll on the earlier age groups.

Life expectancy is a hypothetical measure that is often employed to measure the health status of a population. Expressed as a number derived from a life table, it indicates for a given period of time the average lifetime to be expected by a population group if at each successive age the group experiences the mortality rates that were prevalent during that period of time. Life tables appear to be somewhat conservative estimates since a child born in a particular era will undoubtedly face continually improving conditions during his estimated seventy-one years of life.

GENETIC AND ENVIRONMENTAL INFLUENCES ON LIFE EXPECTANCY

One of the most striking genetic factors that influence life expectancy is sex. The average length of life in 1971 was 75.6 years for white females and 68.3 for white males. Thus, the life expectancy among white females exceeds that for white males by 7.3 years. In 1956, the females outlived the males by 6.4 years and in 1900 by only 2.9 years.

Death rates for males are higher than for females at every age and the superiority of the female sex is evidenced even before birth when her chances of being born dead are much smaller than those of the male.[9] Moreover, the mortality advantage that the female possesses is not uniform along the entire age span as it is greater for some age periods than for others. (fig. 3–3). In infancy, the mortality rate for boys is approximately 34 percent higher than that for female infants. The overall mortality disadvantage that the male faces increases with age and reaches its highest peak between the ages of fifteen and twenty-four years during which young men are exposed

9. Jacob Yerushalmy, "Factors in Human Longevity," *American Journal of Public Health* 53, no. 2 (February 1963): 150.

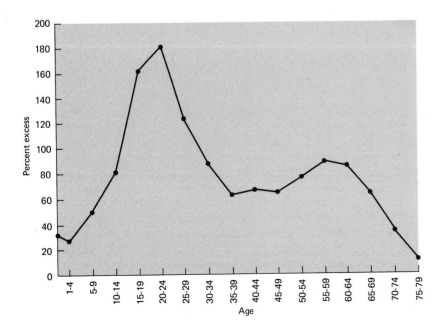

Fig. 3–3. Diagram illustrating the percent excess of male mortality over female mortality by age in the United States in 1971. (From U.S., National Center for Health Statistics, *Facts of Life and Death*, 1974, p. 8.)

to mortality risks that are over two and one-half times greater than those for the female sex. This is due in part to the higher accidental death rate found among males during this particular age period. However, accidents as a cause of death do not account for the entire mortality difference found between the sexes. It may also be noticed that a second mortality peak occurs in the late fifties when the death rate for men is almost double that for the female sex. The excess death rate for the male during this age period is largely due to the higher mortality experienced by men with respect to cardiovascular diseases. Again, however, this particular cause of death does not account for the entire mortality difference. Throughout his entire life span, the male experiences a higher mortality rate from most all of the diseases known to medical science with but few exceptions. Notably among these exceptions is diabetes mellitus, which claims over 30 percent more female deaths.

Table 3–3 Sex Differences in Causes of Death During Infancy Among Babies Born in United States, 1970

Cause of Death	Male Infants Rate per 100,000	Female Infants Rate per 100,000	Excess of Boy Over Girl Deaths (%)
Congenital abnormalities	341.2	308.9	16
Septicemia	22.6	17.9	32
Accidents	57.1	50.7	18
Meningitis	14.8	10.7	45
Bronchitis	11.8	08.4	47
Influenza and pneumonia	154.8	114.8	41
All other diseases of respiratory system	19.9	12.8	63
Certain causes of mortality in early infancy	1,262.7	923.1	44
Asphyxia of newborn (unspecified)	267.1	201.4	39
Immaturity (unqualified)	224.4	180.9	30
All causes	2,113.2	1,614.6	37

Source: Data from U.S., Department of Health, Education, and Welfare, Health Resources Administration, National Center for Health Statistics, *Vital Statistics of the United States*, vol. 11, 1973.

Table 3–4 Average Remaining Lifetime in Years at Specified Ages by Sex, 1971

Age	Male	Female
0	68.3	75.6
1	68.6	75.8
5	64.8	72.0
10	60.0	67.1
15	55.1	62.2
20	50.5	57.3
25	46.0	52.5
30	41.3	47.7
35	36.7	42.9
40	32.1	38.2
45	27.7	33.6
50	23.6	29.2
55	19.7	24.9
60	16.2	20.8
65	13.2	17.0
70	10.5	13.4
75	8.3	10.2
80	6.5	7.5
85	4.9	5.2

Source: U.S., Department of Health, Education, and Welfare, Health Resources Administration, National Center for Health Statistics, *Facts of Life and Death*, 1974, p. 8.

Note: Figures are for the white population only.

Table 3–3 shows the sex differences as to the causes of death among infants born in the United States during 1970. In practically all classifications as to cause of death, male infants show an excess of deaths over female infants. Also, when we contrast the average remaining lifetime at specified ages by sex, it is quite noticeable that the female enjoys a distinct advantage (Table 3–4). Scientific evidence clearly indicates that biologically speaking the female is the vastly superior sex.

The relative roles of endogenous (biological) and exogenous (environmental) factors which may account for the sexual differences found in life expectancy have not been clearly delineated by scientific research. However, Scheinfeld suggests three basic reasons for the relative superiority of the female with respect to longevity that appear to have scientific merit.[10]

First, the general sexual differences with respect to bodily makeup and chemical functioning may endow the female with certain advantages in resisting and fighting disease. The clearest evidence appears in the role of

10. Scheinfeld, *Your Heredity*, p. 217.

the sex hormones in that the female produces proportionately more of the estrogens and the male more of the androgens. Several studies have shown that the death rate from heart disease among men treated with female hormones (estrogens) was about half that of control groups which did not receive the female hormones. Also, it has been observed that the female is biochemically more variable than the male in many respects which may be due in part to changes that occur in body chemistry during menstruation and pregnancy. It is possible that this variability helps the female to adjust to stress, disease, and other adverse conditions better than her male counterpart.

Second, the male is more likely to inherit certain specific diseases and defects which may place him in an unfavorable position with respect to mortality and morbidity. Scientific investigations have shown that sex-linked conditions such as color blindness and hemophilia are more common among males than among females. Sex-linked conditions result from defective genes which are carried on the X chromosome. At conception the female receives two X chromosomes (one from each parent), while the male receives only one X chromosome from his mother and the Y chromosome from his father. Thus, the male is apparently more vulnerable to these defects since there is no corresponding gene on the opposite Y chromosome to neutralize the effects of the gene which causes the defect. In order to produce a sex-linked defect in the male, only one defective gene is needed. In contrast, the female needs two defective genes to produce a defect since the chances are greater that there will be a normal gene on the other X chromosome to offset the effects. (Figure 3–4 shows the genetic transmission of color blindness.) Other conditions that are considered to be sex linked include some forms of nearsightedness, enlarged cornea, defective iris, optic atrophy, nystagmus, and muscular dystrophy (Duchenne type).

In addition, there are other genetic conditions that discriminate predominately against the male sex, as in the case of baldness. The genetic explanation for the presence of the sexual differences that are observed with respect to baldness is that the tendency for baldness results from a special

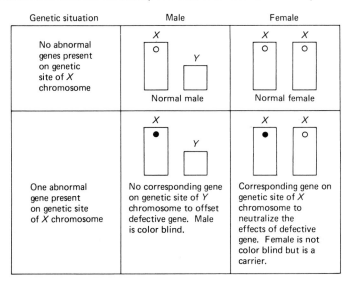

Fig. 3–4. Scheme to demonstrate patterns of sex-linked inheritance. Illustrated here is the genetic transmission of color blindness. Note: Males can transmit color blindness only to their daughters because the defective gene is carried on the X chromosome and not on the Y chromosome.

THE GENETIC ASPECTS OF HEALTH

type of gene that is referred to as "sex limited" or "sex influenced" because it is usually only within the male biochemical environment that the effects are able to assert themselves. The sex-limited gene is not carried on the X chromosome, but is found in one of the other twenty-two chromosomes. Thus, the genes can be inherited equally by both sexes; however, the sex-limited gene tends to behave as a dominant among males and as a limited recessive in females. One theory that is frequently advanced to explain this genetic phenomenon is that the biochemical makeup of the sexes influences the manner in which the gene expresses itself. For instance, in the female the lack of an excess of male androgens and the absence of their effects prohibits the hair from falling out, even when the gene is present. Conversely, in males the excess of male hormones makes the hair follicles more vulnerable to the effects of the sex-limited gene.

Interestingly, gout is also suspected of being a sex-limited disease. There is some evidence to suggest that the predisposition to this ailment is caused by a metabolic defect associated with the presence of a dominant gene which tends to raise the level of uric acid in the blood. Gout afflicts approximately twenty times more men than women, although the gene for the predisposition is equally received by both sexes. It is suggested that the biochemical environment of the female tends to suppress the effects of the inherent genetic predisposition to the disease. However, gout becomes much more prevalent in the female after menopause, which appears to indicate that the biochemical differences that had existed between the sexes begins to narrow and becomes more similar with the termination of the childbearing period in the female.

Third, the sociocultural environment has played a role in producing the excess male mortality. This appears to be especially significant with respect to accidents where the male experiences a higher mortality rate. Approximately 70 percent of the deaths due to accidents occur in the male sex. Also, the higher mortality rates experienced by the males in large urban cities and in the upper socioeconomic groups suggest that certain modes or styles of living may place an unequal stress on males. It is possible that the male is subjected to more internal stress than the female, with a consequent higher incidence of coronary heart disease and ulcers. Other suggested related factors include the male's inattention to preventive health behavior: exercise, diet, and general neglect in securing an annual physical examination.

Furthermore, it has been observed that the excess male mortality is not peculiar to only the United States, but is common throughout the world. The differences in the death rate between the sexes are greatest where life expectancy is highest and tends to widen as each country's mortality rate declines. Evidence that the greater female longevity is conditioned in part by the environment is seen in underdeveloped countries. The poorer the living and health conditions are in a country (as reflected by higher death rates and lower life expectancy), the smaller is the excess of male over female life expectancy. In Bolivia, the life expectancy of both sexes is 49.7 years. In India, the life expectancy for the male is 45.2 years and for the female 46.6 years. Hence, the innate advantage of the female cannot assert itself because of the unfavorable environmental conditions that affected both sexes. Also, where the infant mortality rate is highest (reflecting the worst environmental conditions), the excess of male over female mortality is lowest, as seen in Peru where the excess is only 7 percent. By contrast, in the United

States, the excess of male deaths over female deaths is almost 34 percent higher during the first year of life.

It appears that the more medical science and technology improve the environment, the greater the life expectancy becomes for both sexes, but the excess of female over male life expectancy increases. That is, the better the environment, the more likely the female becomes capable of asserting her inherent biological advantage with respect to longevity as evidenced by the 7.3 year advantage that the American female possesses over the male. The poorer the general environment, the less likely the female is able to express her biological or genetic advantage.[11] The continued and increasingly greater advantage of the female with respect to longevity over the past several decades is most remarkable and surprising in view of the diminishing differences between the sexes in many behavioral and social-cultural patterns with respect to employment, occupation, smoking, drinking, and recreational practices. This suggests that the genetic and biochemical differences between the sexes must exert a potent influence which tends to favor the female more than the male.

RACE AND LIFE EXPECTANCY

In 1900, the life expectancy at birth for the Negro population was 32.5 years for the male and 35 years for the female, which represents a total of approximately 16 years less than that expected for the white population. By 1971, the differences in life expectancy at birth for the nonwhite population as compared to the white population had diminished to approximately six and a half years. Table 3–5 shows that the excess of white over nonwhite life

Table 3–5   Average Remaining Lifetime in Years at Specified Ages by Sex and Race, 1971

Age	Male*	Excess of White Over Nonwhite Life Expectancy	Female†	Excess of White Over Nonwhite Life Expectancy
0	61.2	7.1	69.3	6.3
1	62.3	6.3	70.2	5.6
5	58.6	6.2	66.5	5.5
10	53.7	6.3	61.6	5.5
15	48.9	6.2	56.7	5.5
20	44.4	6.1	52.0	5.3
25	40.3	5.7	47.3	5.2
30	36.2	5.1	42.7	5.0
35	32.2	4.5	38.3	4.6
40	28.3	3.8	34.0	4.2
45	24.6	3.1	30.0	3.6
50	21.2	2.4	26.1	3.1
55	18.1	1.6	22.5	2.4
60	15.2	1.0	19.0	1.8
65	12.9	0.3	16.1	0.9
70	10.9	—0.4	13.7	—0.3
75	10.6	—2.3	12.6	—2.4
80	10.2	—3.7	10.8	—3.3
85	9.5	—4.6	9.0	—3.8

Source: Adapted from U.S., Department of Health, Education, and Welfare, Health Resources Administration, National Center for Health Statistics, *Facts of Life and Death,* 1974, p. 8.

  * Figures for nonwhite groups are for Negroes only. However, Negroes comprised 95% of the nonwhite population.

  † Figures represent the difference in total number of years in the average remaining lifetime between white and nonwhite populations.

11. Scheinfeld, *Your Heredity,* p. 341.

expectancy at birth is 7.1 years for the male and 6.3 years for the female. The narrowing in the life expectancy between the white and nonwhite populations over the past several decades has been largely due to the decline in the communicable disease death rate and its resultant impact on lowering the infant mortality rate.

Similar to their white counterparts, black females have a higher life expectancy at birth than black males, and the differences between the life expectancy of the sexes have also increased during the past seven decades. At age 70 years and over the life expectancy for the black population is greater than that expected for the white population. Possible explanations for this phenomenon suggest that there may be a considerable understatement of mortality experiences by the black population due to inaccurate reporting of deaths or that blacks who reach the age of 70 years and above may be of hardier constitution.

It is anticipated that as the nonwhite population makes continued economic and social advances and as the benefits of modern medical care and public health programs are made increasingly available to nonwhites, the differences that exist in life expectancy between the races should diminish greatly. Nevertheless, differences in longevity do exist today and reflect the numerous economic, cultural, and attitudinal factors that play a significant role in the reduced life expectancy of the nonwhite population.

OCCUPATION AND LIFE EXPECTANCY

The effects of various occupations on one's health and longevity may be both direct and indirect. The morbidity and mortality rates of workers engaged in occupations involving mining and construction may be influenced directly by the higher probability of accidents and exposure to dusts which contain a large percentage of silica. On the other hand, the environment that individuals create for themselves based upon the wages that they receive determines the circumstances of their life. When salaries are deficient, a relatively low standard of living may be imposed upon workers and their family, the consequences of which may be expressed in terms of inadequate food and clothing, crowded and unsanitary living quarters, the need for the wage earner to stay on the job when ill, the lack of utilization of medical facilities, and numerous other handicaps that impinge on health and longevity. Mortality studies indicate that the death rate for workers and their spouses increases as the economic scale is descended.

Industrial accidents claim approximately 14,200 lives annually and result in 2.5 million disabling injuries.[12] The highest death rates are reported in the mining, quarrying, construction, and agricultural groups. Coal miners, granite cutters, sandblasters, and metal miners who are exposed to large quantities of silica dust experience higher death rates from tuberculosis and silicosis.[13] Mortality from pneumonia is high among welders, metal and coal miners, mill workers, and bartenders and below average in clerical, agricultural, and skilled occupations. Besides the social and economic influences which affect death rates, workers appear to be more susceptible to disease where specific occupational hazards exist such as fatigue from strenuous

12. *Accident Facts* (Chicago: National Safety Council, 1974).
13. Louis I. Dublin, *Factbook on Man from Birth to Death* (New York: Macmillan Co., 1965), p. 284.

labor, presence of irritating gases and dust, decreased atmospheric pressure, dampness, heat, long-continued repetitive motion, and exposure to inclement weather.

Scientists, teachers, social workers, engineers, clergymen, farmers, and clerical workers tend to have the highest longevity rates of all of the occupational groups. Miners, musicians, tailors, policemen, taxi drivers, laborers, painters, firemen, and bartenders have a lower life expectancy than that found in the general population. In a study conducted in England and Wales it was observed that clergymen at the age of twenty-five years had an expectation of life that was five years greater than that of the general male population for the same age group. Physicians appear to have little advantage in longevity as based on records which indicate that their life expectancy is the same for the general population at age twenty-five years.[14] Apparently, the advantages of medical knowledge are not sufficient to counteract the strenuous hours required by their profession.

In summary, the differences in longevity between various occupational groups may be due not only to the nature of the work involved, but also to the attitudes, habits, personality, temperament, and living conditions of the personnel engaged in their work activity. Recent studies have suggested that life expectancy may be affected more by the living conditions that are associated with occupation than by the occupation itself. Several studies conducted in England have found that the wives of men in various occupational classifications have mortality rates proportionate to their hsubands' rates. The wives of laborers had the highest death rates as contrasted to the wives of professional men who had the lowest mortality rates. Also, several health studies have shown that lower socioeconomic groups tend to perceive health differently than higher socioeconomic groups. Lower socioeconomic groups tend to delay in seeking medical care and are generally less oriented toward preventive medicine. Thus, the wage earner that is found in the low-income group will seek out medical services only as a last resort, that is, when it interferes with job performance. In general, lower socioeconomic groups tend to experience higher mortality rates and lower life expectancy. Conversely, high socioeconomic groups experience low death rates and longer life expectancy.

OTHER INFLUENCES AFFECTING LIFE EXPECTANCY

Individuals who are moderately or markedly overweight have a higher death rate than those who are of average weight.[15] However, obesity sometimes accompanies other diseases such as coronary heart disease, atherosclerosis, diabetes, and gallbladder, liver, and kidney disorders. Each of these diseases by itself could shorten life expectancy. On the other hand, persons who are extremely underweight also tend to have a higher than average mortality rate. It is likely that extreme underweight may cause an individual to be more susceptible to infection or may accompany a particular disease such as tuberculosis, pneumonia, or nutritional defect which produces a shorter life expectancy.

14. Dublin, *Man From Birth to Death,* p. 405.
15. U.S., Department of Health, Education, and Welfare, *Obesity and Health* (Washington, D.C.: Government Printing Office, 1966), p. 26.

Various studies concerned with body stature indicate that short men tend to have above average mortality rates, whereas their taller counterparts possess death rates somewhat below average.[16] Stature by itself does not appear to directly affect longevity: the environment that contributes to accelerating or retarding the growth process appears to be the key factor. Better standards of nutrition, medical care, and level of living may influence not only growth and development, but also longevity.

Heavy drinking of alcoholic beverages is related to a shorter life expectancy due to accidents and diseases that are associated with the misuse and abuse of alcohol. Also, the general physical debilitation that often accompanies the deleterious effects of large amounts of alcohol over long periods of time exerts a tremendous impact on the life expectancy of the heavy drinker. However, there is no scientific evidence to indicate that drinking alcoholic beverages in moderation affects man's longevity.

Alcoholism predominantly affects males by a six-to-one ratio and is particularly common in certain occupations such as those involving nonroutine, pressure, and decision-making responsibilities. It is also more frequently found in certain nationalities—Scandinavian, Nordic, and Polish—in contrast to its relative infrequency among Greeks, Italians, and Jews.[17]

Cigarette smoking is a major cause of lung cancer and is an important factor in the development of emphysema, chronic bronchitis, and heart disease. Cigarette smokers experience substantially higher rates of death and disability than their nonsmoking counterparts in the population. Thus, cigarette smokers tend to die at an earlier age and experience more days of disability than comparable nonsmokers. Studies indicate that heavy cigarette smokers have a life expectancy eight years less than that of nonsmokers.[18]

Marital status appears to be related to longevity in that the overall mortality rate for all age groups is lower for the married population than for the single population. However, the mortality rate may reflect the better care and the more favorable environment generally experienced by married individuals. Also, it should be observed that many individuals do not marry because of poor physical or mental health.

OUTLOOK FOR FUTURE GAINS IN LONGEVITY

It appears that existing knowledge in medicine and public health will continue to be applied more intensively and widely to specific population groups in the United States and other countries. The greatest future gains in longevity undoubtedly will occur in those countries where infant mortality is at its highest and the environmental conditions the worse. In the developed countries, including the United States, future gains in life expectancy will be moderate at best. The mortality rates in infancy and childhood are already so low that future decreases in death rates at these ages would add little to the average length of life.

The greatest potential source for increasing longevity is in the reduction of deaths from cardiovascular and renal disorders. Reducing deaths from

16. Scheinfeld, *Your Heredity*, p. 349.

17. John Hanlon, *Principles of Public Health Administration* 6th ed. (St. Louis: C. V. Mosby Co., 1974), p. 462.

18. U.S., Department of Health, Education, and Welfare, *A Physician Talks About Smoking* (Washington, D.C.: Government Printing Office, 1971), p. 7.

accidents and pneumonia would only have a minor effect on longevity at ages sixty years and over, while deaths from other causes would have a greater potential impact on longevity. Future progress in longevity will depend largely on the magnitude of the reductions in mortality from the chronic and degenerative diseases.

SUMMARY

The study of the genetic factor in health and disease is especially difficult since the genetic composition of each individual differs, the generation time is fairly long, the number of offspring are small, and controlled mating is not feasible. In addition, it is very difficult to separate the environmental variables from the genetic influences as to possible initiating and contributing factors in disease causation. In some diseases such as Huntington's chorea the genetic component is quite explicit. In others such as the communicable diseases, the environmental factors appear to predominate. Between these two extremes, the environmental and genetic factors operate with varying degrees of importance. Finally, it should be understood that genes interact with their environment, and all genetic processes must be considered within the context of their ecosystems.

In the final analysis it appears that heredity tends to establish the pattern of genetic potential for longevity, but reaching or realizing the potential depends to a great extent upon the environmental influences one encounters. Positive values, attitudes, beliefs, and practices toward health and medical care enable us to reach our maximum potential. Our health status is greatly influenced by the sociocultural environment that surrounds us as we seek to adjust to the demands of living. One's culture helps him to formulate and shape his values and attitudes toward health and medical care. Other ecological factors such as socioeconomic status, education, sex, race, occupation, habits, and level of living aid in determining overall health status and longevity potential.

Discussion Questions

1. Briefly explain the genetic code.
2. What is the basic difference between a congenital condition and a familial condition?
3. Explain the genetic environmental spectrum of disease.
4. What is the difference between life expectancy and life span?
5. Why do women appear to be biologically superior to men? What factors may account for their greater life expectancy?
6. How is race related to life expectancy?
7. What is the relationship between occupation and longevity?
8. What is the outlook for future gains in longevity?

References

Accident Facts. Chicago: National Safety Council, 1974.

Anderson, C. L. *Health Principles and Practice*. 5th ed. St. Louis: C. V. Mosby Co., 1972.

Comfort, A. *Aging: The Biology of Senescence*. New York: Holt, Rinehart & Winston, 1964.

Davis, D. "Predicting Tomorrow's Children." *Today's Health* 46 (January 1968): 32–37.

Dublin, Louis I. *Factbook on Man From Birth to Death.* New York: Macmillan Co., 1965.

Handler, P., ed. *Biology and the Future of Man.* London: Oxford University Press, 1970.

Hanlon, John. *Principles of Public Health Administration.* 6th ed. St. Louis: C. V. Mosby Co., 1974.

Kogan, Benjamin. *Health: Man in a Changing Environment.* New York: Harcourt, Brace & World, 1970.

Muscular Dystrophy—The Facts. New York: Muscular Dystrophy Association of America, 1970.

Scheinfeld, Amram. *Your Heredity and Environment.* New York: J. B. Lippincott Co., 1965.

Sultz, Harry, et al. "The Epidemiology of Peptic Ulcer in Childhood." *American Journal of Public Health* 60, no. 3. (1970): 498

U.S., Department of Health, Education, and Welfare. *Obesity and Health.* Washington, D.C.: Government Printing Office, 1966.

U.S., Department of Health, Education, and Welfare. *A Physician Talks About Smoking.* Washington, D.C.: Government Printing Office, 1971.

Yerushalmy, Jacob. "Factors in Human Longevity." *American Journal of Public Health* 53, no. 2 (February 1963): 150.

Chapter 4
GROWTH
AND
DEVELOPMENT

What are some predictable patterns of growth and development?

How may the growth process affect a child's attitudes and behavior?

What are the educational and social implications of the secular trend with respect to adolescent development?

Growth is usually defined as an actual increase in the size of a body part or of the whole organism in terms of cell division. Development refers to the increasing maturity of the structure and function of a body part. While growth of the organism may be evaluated on the basis of weight and length, the evaluation of development is somewhat hindered by the absence of well-established criteria. Today, it is common practice for most educators to combine the terms *growth* and *development* in order to permit a broader connotation to be made.

Growth and development comprise a dynamic process which may be divided into four distinct areas: physical, intellectual, emotional, and social. All of these areas are interrelated as the individual functions as a whole organism within the environment. If one of the parts becomes disturbed, the entire organism may be affected in some manner. For example, a child's height or lack of it, obesity or scrawniness, energy levels, and various physical handicaps may have a decided impact upon the child's attitudes and behavior both within and outside the classroom.

This chapter will concentrate mainly on the physical dimension of growth and development. Subsequent chapters will incorporate information relating to the other areas.

The mean or average birth weight of a newborn child is approximately 7½ pounds. During the first three months the average infant gains about 2 pounds a month and doubles his birth weight by five months of age. The child generally triples his birth weight by the end of the first year, and his weight is quadrupled by the end of the second year. From age two years until the ninth or tenth birthday the annual increment in weight averages about 5 pounds. During adolescence a rapid gain in weight occurs that corresponds in both sexes with gains in height. The adolescent acceleration occurs

**PATTERNS
OF
PHYSICAL GROWTH
AND
DEVELOPMENT**

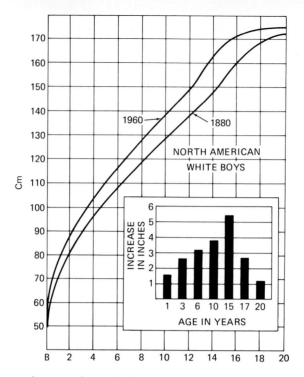

Fig. 4–1. Schematic curves of mean stature for 1880 and 1960. Inset shows differences between the curves at selected ages. (From H. V. Meredith, "Change in the Stature and Body Weight of North American Boys during the last 80 years," in *Advances in Child Development and Behavior*, Academic Press, 1963, p. 90.)

NORTH AMERICAN
WHITE BOYS

earlier in girls, with the most rapid spurt beginning at ten to twelve years of age, while for boys the accelerated weight gain occurs two years later.

The average infant measures about 20 inches in length at birth. By the end of the first year the infant will have increased his birth length by 50 percent. At age four years, he will have doubled it. From age six years to adolescence the mean annual increase in height is approximately 2 inches. As in weight, the adolescent acceleration of height generally occurs in girls at ages ten to twelve years and for boys at from twelve to fourteen years of age. From thirteen years in girls and fifteen years in boys the rate of growth in height rapidly decelerates. Growth generally ceases in girls around seventeen to nineteen years of age but may continue in boys at a slow rate beyond age twenty years.[1]

Over the past century, investigators have been accumulating evidence to support the fact that today' children grow faster, experience the adolescent growth spurt earlier, reach puberty sooner, and attain their final adult height earlier. Data that support these secular trends are not confined only to American children but involve a diversity of national and ethnic groups as well.

Meredith in his comprehensive review and analysis of growth data over a period of eighty years found that the average fifteen-year-old white male was 5¼ inches taller and 33 pounds heavier than his counterpart from the earlier decades (fig. 4–1).[2] Reviews of physical growth studies of Negro

1. E. Watson, and G. Lowrey, *Growth and Development of Children* (Chicago: Year Book Medical Publishers, 1967), p. 86.
2. H. V. Meredith, "Change in the Stature and Body Weight of North American Boys During the Last 80 Years," in *Advances in Child Development and Behavior*, eds. L. Lipsett and C. Spiker (New York: Academic Press, 1963), p. 90.

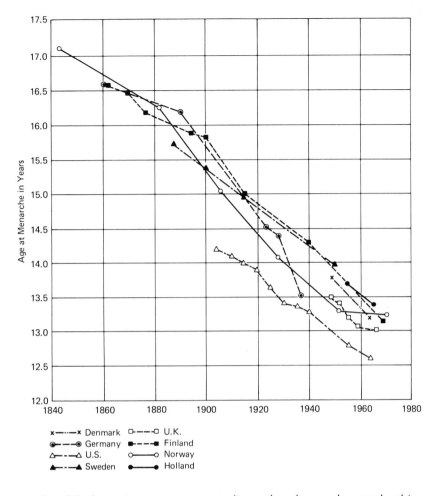

youths while limited to some extent indicate that the secular trends of increasing size and earlier maturation are also true for blacks. [3, 4]

The secular trend with respect to the earlier occurrence of the first menstrual period (menarche) may be observed by examining the data presented in figure 4–2. Females in the United States have been experiencing the menarche approximately three to four months earlier each decade of life. In 1900, the average American girl had her first menstrual period (menarche) after her fourteenth birthday; today it occurs around 12.5 years of age. Males have also shown a similar pattern of earlier sexual maturation, with puberty occurring two years later than for females. Tanner reported the median menarcheal ages of Western European females ranged from 12.8 to 13.2 years of age.[5] By contrast, females residing in underdeveloped areas of

3. W. M. Moore, "The Secular Trend in Physical Growth of Urban North American Negro Schoolchildren," *Monographs of Society for Research in Child Development* 35, no. 7 (1970): 70.

4. J. M. Tanner, "Sequence, Tempo, and Individual Variation in the Growth and Development of Boys and Girls Ages Twelve to Sixteen," *Daedalus* 100, no. 4, (1971): 929.

5. Tanner, "Sequence, Tempo, and Individual Variation," p. 928.

the world such as that found in the Highlands of New Guinea and in Central Africa had a median menarcheal age of 17 and 18 years, respectively.

While most of the differences between population groups with respect to these secular trends have been generally attributed to better nutritional practices, other ecological factors are also probably involved. The lowering incidence of certain diseases such as poliomyelitis and the development of vaccines to prevent several of the communicable diseases that formerly afflicted many children during their critical growth periods have probably all contributed in part to these secular trends.

The trend toward earlier age of sexual maturity has also had a significant impact on the social behavior of children with respect to boy-girl relationships. In 1963 Havighurst made the following observation:

> Within the past generation, the ages at which boys and girls begin dating, going to boy-girl parties, learning to dance, and other precursors of courtship and marriage have all decreased, so that junior high school is now a theater of rather active social life of a sort which formerly was thought more appropriate for the senior high school.[6]

Recently the heterosexual interests of children have become dramatically more pronounced in the elementary school as evidenced by the earlier initiation of dating behavior and formulation of boy-girl friendship patterns within this group. Parents of elementary school girls are expressing considerable concern regarding their daughters early interest in boys and their desire to use lipstick, training bras, eye makeup, and other manifestations of sex appeal. Correspondingly, the behavioral practices for boys are now being expressed in earlier patterns of dating, smoking, drinking, and use of drugs.[7] Other reports have also indicated that the total percentage of students engaged in drug-taking behavior such as cigarette smoking, drinking, and using drugs has increased significantly during the past several years.[8, 9]

As a consequence of these and other trends in the society, the more progressive elementary schools have attempted to cope with these problems by incorporating units of sex education, mental health, and mood-modifying substances into their curriculum. Furthermore, some administrators have become cognizant of the need to restructure the school system because of the accelerated growth patterns of adolescents. Accordingly, it has been suggested that the sixth grade be taken out of the present elementary system and in combination with the seventh and eighth grades form a new structure, that is, that a middle school be formed.[10] This should

6. R. J. Havighurst, "Do Junior High School Youth Grow Up Too Fast?" *Bulletin of National Association of Secondary School Principals* 22 (1963): 160.
7. R. E. Muuss, "Adolescent Development and the Secular Trend," *Adolescence* 5, no. 19 (1970): 278.
8. U.S., Department of Health, Education, and Welfare, Health Services and Mental Health Administration, *Teenage Smoking—National Patterns of Cigarette Smoking Ages Twelve Through Eighteen in 1968 and 1970*, HSM Publication no. 72–7508 (Rockville, Md., 1972), p. 6.
9. Illinois Interagency Drug Education Development Committee, Office of Superintendent of Public Instruction, *Teaching About Drug Abuse* (Springfield, Ill., 1971), p. 10.
10. Muuss, *Adolescent Development,* p. 281.

enable the educational system to more adequately cope with the concomitant problems associated with pubescence and the adolescent period of growth and development.

The various body systems and their organs have their own unique rates of growth and development. At birth the head is relatively more mature than the rest of the body and therefore larger in size. The average child at birth is approximately 20 inches long, with the head comprising at least 5 of these inches. If all parts of the body were to develop at the same rate, the average six-foot adult would have a head 18 inches long. However, after the first year of life the chest circumference becomes increasingly larger in proportion than the head as the growth of the latter gradually slows down. The extremities of the body are shorter than the trunk at birth but grow more rapidly later in life. During adolescence the major gain in height can be attributed to the growth of the lower segment of the body with most of the growth in height being due to the acceleration of trunk length rather than to length of legs.[11] Generally, the body structures that reach their adult status earliest are the head, hands, and feet.

The change in body proportions during childhood and adolescence underscores a general principle of growth. That is, the organism follows a cephalocaudal (head to tail) pattern of development.[12]

Since the proportions of head, trunk, and extremities vary with the growth of the body, a shifting of the center of gravity of the body occurs that influences both body posture and balance. The center of gravity in the newborn is near the lower point of the breastbone (xiphoid), and throughout early childhood it remains above the umbilicus. It is just below the umbilicus at five or six years of age and is below the ilium or the lowest division of the small intestine by thirteen years of age.[13] Posture is strongly influenced by the growth of skeletal, muscular, and neuromuscular mechanisms that mature with advancing age. Health educators are in general agreement that so-called poor posture is very seldom detrimental to the physical health of the child unless it is the result of some pathological condition. Good posture, however, is certainly desirable from an aesthetic point of view, but the old idea of criticising children to stand or sit straight in the classroom because it is detrimental to their health is outmoded.

The direction of motor development and control also follow the cephalocaudal principle. Thus, the infant can lift his head before his trunk, control his arms before his legs, and sit upright before he stands. Motor skills are dependent upon a number of factors such as the physique the child inherits, maturation level, and the amount of practice that the child has had with respect to a given activity. Children who are behind in the development of motor skills required for certain play activities such as ball throwing may be ridiculed by their peers. Some elementary teachers react as if developmental age were synonymous with chronological age in that they insist on forcing certain motor skills on all children before they may be ready both physically and mentally. In addition, they often plan the same set of ex-

11. Muuss, *Adolescent Development*, p. 911.
12. L. E. Robinson, *Human Growth and Development* (Columbus, Ohio: Charles E. Merrill Publishing Co., 1968). p. 50.
13. Watson and Lowrey, *Growth and Development*, p. 121.

periences for all children instead of attempting to individualize their educational efforts to match the competencies of the child.

Sexual differences among children of the same age are sometimes ignored in the planning and evaluation of educational experiences. Garn and Clark concluded from their study of sex differences in oxygen consumption that boys have a special need for more activity than girls at both elementary and junior high levels.[14] Often boys are forced to conform to activity programs which do not provide a natural outlet for their different energies and activity needs. Furthermore, it is a common observation that preschool, kindergarten, and first grade girls have less difficulty than boys in pleasing their teacher and achieving better grades on their written work. The coordination of motor control in boys is not equal to that of females at these earlier grade levels.[15] However, schools often place the same demands on all children and evaluate their progress upon how well they perform certain designated tasks, without giving due consideration to the unique differences that exist between the sexes.

GROWTH CURVES OF BODY ORGANS

Certain organ systems of the human body display fairly definite patterns of growth. Scammon has identified four major types of postnatal tissue growth.[16] These are illustrated diagrammatically in figure 4–3 where each type is shown as the percentage increment from birth to age twenty years. The first may be labeled the general type which includes the body as a whole and most of its external dimensions, with the exception of the head and neck as the growth of the head is more closely related to the growth of the brain. The kidneys, spleen, respiratory and digestive organs, aorta and pulmonary trunk, blood volume, musculature as a whole, and skeleton as a whole all follow the general type. This type of growth shows a rapid increment during early infancy, a slowing down during late infancy, and a slow,

14. S. Garn, and L. Clark, "The Sex Differences in Basal Metabolism Rates," *Child Development* 24 (1952): 215–224.

15. B. Wright et al., *Elementary School Curriculum: Better Teaching Now* (New York: Macmillan Co., 1971), p. 59.

16. R. E. Scammon, "The Measurement of the Body in Childhood," in *The Measurement of Man* by J. Harris, C. Jackson, D. Patterson, and R. E. Scammon (Minneapolis: University of Minnesota Press, 1930).

Fig. 4–3. Growth of the various parts and organs of the body drawn to a common scale by computing their value at successive ages in terms of their total postnatal increments from birth to age 20 years. (From J. Harris et al., *The Measurement of Man*, University of Minnesota Press, 1930.)

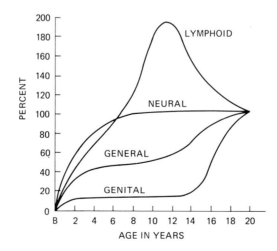

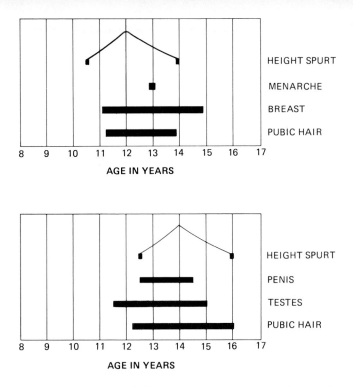

AGE IN YEARS

AGE IN YEARS

steady increment during childhood followed by a rapid spurt of growth during the onset of puberty.

The growth of the neural type which includes the brain and its parts—dura, spinal cord, optic apparatus—and many head dimensions reaches 60 percent of the total growth by two years and 90 percent at six years of age. Genital growth, which includes the reproductive system and its parts, is quite unlike the pattern of neural growth in that there is a minimal increment in infancy followed by virtually no growth until the onset of puberty after which a 90 percent increment occurs. Figures 4–4 and 4–5 display the sequence of events of puberty in girls and boys.

The lymphoid type including the thymus, lymph nodes, tonsils, and adenoids reaches a maximum increment at eleven years of age followed by diminution during the next nine years. Failure in the past to recognize the physiological increase in lymphoid tissue of the tonsils and adenoids at this age period may have been responsible for many unnecessary tonsillectomies and adenoidectomies.

By examining figure 4–3 we can observe that an eight-year-old child has attained only 10 percent of mature development with respect to genital tissue growth, 50 percent of skeletal growth, 95 percent of neural growth, and 120 percent of lymphoid growth.

The differences between the sexes in their rates of growth are readily observable to upper elementary and junior high school teachers. Teachers of this age group are most likely to have in the same class a majority of girls who have reached the menarche and many boys who have not yet entered the period of pubescence (see figs. 4–6 and 4–7). Also, girls between the ages of eleven and thirteen years are generally taller on the average than boys of

SELF-CONCEPT AND BODY IMAGE

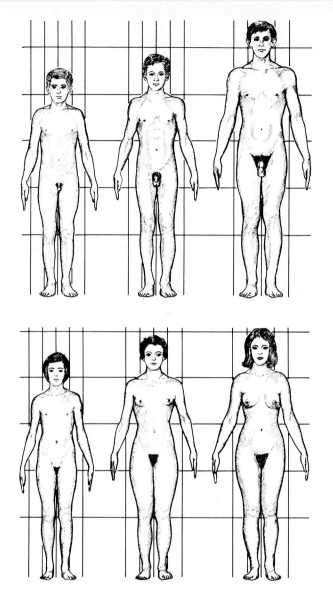

Fig. 4–6. Three boys, all of the chronological age of 14.75 years, showed a similar variation in the range of their development. Evidently some boys have entirely finished their growth and sexual maturation before others even begin theirs. This drawing is based on photographs made by Tanner and colleagues at the Institute of Child Health, University of London. (From "Growing Up," in *Life and Death and Medicine,* by J. M. Tanner. Copyright © 1973 by Scientific American, Inc. All rights reserved.)

Fig. 4–7. Three girls, all with the chronological age of 12.75 years, differed dramatically in development according to whether the particular girl had not yet reached puberty (*left*), was part of the way through it (*middle*) or had finished her development (*right*). This range of variation is completely normal. This drawing is based on photographs made by Tanner and colleagues at Institute of Child Health, University of London. (From "Growing Up," in *Life and Death and Medicine,* by J. M. Tanner. Copyright © 1973 by Scientific American, Inc. All rights reserved.)

the same age. Not only are the girls more physically mature duing this period, but they are also more likely to display a greater degree of social and emotional maturity. Such a situation is often observed at school functions where boys may feel awkward and ill at ease because of their developmental immaturity in comparison to that of the girls. These differences in physical, emotional, and social maturity gradually diminish as the boys reach pubescence, but nevertheless persist to create problems throughout the school years.

Children are intensely interested in their own rate of growth and development. Being too short or too tall, too thin or too fat, or just being different is what creates concern for the child. Peer conformity or the desire to be alike is a strong motivating factor in influencing the attitudes and behavior of children. The school child whose growth and development deviates from that of his classmates is likely to be concerned, especially if he perceives the deviation within his own sex and age group to be quite excessive. His growth and development may be normal for his particular, unique growth pattern but abnormal as judged by his standards when he compares himself with his peer age group. Table 4–1 shows the physical

Table 4–1. Physical Growth Standards for Children from Age 5 to 15 at 5th, 50th, and 95th Percentiles

	Boys					
	Height in Inches			Weight in Pounds		
Age	5th P	50th P	95th P	5th P	50th P	95th P
5	40.3	43.4	46.4	33.0	40.3	47.6
6	42.8	45.9	49.0	36.0	44.7	53.4
7	44.8	48.1	51.4	40.3	50.9	61.5
8	46.9	50.5	54.1	44.4	57.4	70.4
9	48.8	52.8	56.8	48.0	64.4	80.4
10	50.6	54.9	59.2	51.4	71.4	91.4
11	51.9	56.4	60.9	53.3	78.9	102.5
12	53.5	58.6	63.7	60.0	86.0	113.5
13	55.2	61.3	67.4	65.3	98.6	131.9
14	57.5	64.1	70.7	75.5	111.8	148.1
15	61.0	66.9	72.8	88.0	124.3	160.6
	Girls					
5	40.6	43.4	46.2	32.2	40.9	49.6
6	42.8	45.9	49.0	35.5	45.7	55.9
7	44.5	47.8	51.1	38.3	51.0	63.7
8	46.4	50.0	53.6	42.0	57.2	72.4
9	48.2	52.2	56.2	45.1	63.6	82.1
10	49.9	54.5	59.1	48.2	71.0	95.0
11	51.9	57.0	62.1	55.4	82.0	108.6
12	54.1	59.5	64.9	63.9	94.4	124.9
13	57.1	62.2	66.8	72.8	105.5	138.2
14	58.5	63.1	67.7	83.0	113.0	144.0
15	59.5	63.8	68.1	89.5	120.0	150.5

Source: Adapted from F. Falkner, "Some Physical Growth Standards for White North American Children," *Pediatrics* 29: 467–474.

growth standards for white North American children from 5 to 15 years of age at the 5th, 50th, and 95th percentiles. It may be observed that at age 12 years boys may vary between the 5th and 95th percentiles by as much as 10.2 inches in height and 53.5 pounds in weight. Correspondingly, girls at the same age may vary as much as 10.8 inches in height and 61 pounds in weight. This table simply presents a general picture for children, and when one uses it as a standard, the individual variation in children's growth must not be overlooked.

The rate of maturity may pose some special problems with respect to self-acceptance. Boys who are early maturers may find certain advantages in that their peer culture idolizes strength, tallness, and athletic prowess. Slow-maturing males are at a definite disadvantage with respect to activities involving athletics at the junior high level. The absence of secondary sex characteristics may also serve to remind the slow maturer of his perceived inferiority. The boys' locker room or shower room may be a place of embarrassment for him as he is subjected to ridicule by the early maturers.

Early-maturing girls may also have rather unique problems associated with accelerated development. The early maturer may well find that her new drives and interests are not shared by her nonpubescent girl friends. She may feel conspicuous and out of place in playground and school activities because she is the biggest girl in her class and literally towers over the boys. The accompanying weight gain associated with her increase in height may also influence her to diet at a time when sound nutrition is essential. Menstruation may present a problem if the girl has not been prepared for her new feminine role. We recall the familiar story repeated many times by elementary teachers:

> . . . Jane came to me in tears. She returned from the girls' bathroom and told me that she was bleeding and was afraid. . . What do I tell Jane? That the educational system failed? . . . That her parents failed in their responsibility? . . .

Height, weight, appropriate masculine or feminine physique, all influence the child's self-perception. However, we as teachers must also understand that self-concept does not suddenly develop at adolescence. A child's concept of his unique self has been emerging and forming throughout preadolescent life as he reacts and interacts with his family, peers, and other individuals within the total environmental structure. The child who enters adolescence with an adequate self-concept is probably better equipped to handle the challenges of his changing body and the problems of adjustment that are associated with growth and development. It must be stressed that each child's growth and developmental pattern is unique and that a wide range of individual differences do exist. Children should grow and develop properly according to their age, sex, body type, and genetic endowment and within certain standards that are generally accepted by the medical profession.

ECOLOGICAL FACTORS AFFECTING GROWTH AND DEVELOPMENT

The ecological factors that influence growth and development are multiple in nature and extremely complex in their interrelationships. From the time of fertilization of the ovum until death, each phase of development is influenced by the interplay of inherited genes and the many external factors whose roles began at conception. In the assessment of growth and development of a child all variables should be considered: genetic, congenital, racial, socioeconomic status, nutritional, illness, hormonal, physical activity, and other possible influences.

HEREDITY

It is general knowledge that height, weight, and body build are all influenced to some degree by heredity, some more strongly than others. Fairly high correlations exist with respect to stature and weight of siblings. It has also been observed that the rate of growth is more alike among siblings than among nonrelated individuals.[17] In some families patterns of accelerated growth and early maturation are the rule, while in others growth and maturation are somewhat slow and delayed. Parents, teachers, and youth

17. Watson and Lowrey, *Growth and Development*, p. 39.

workers should not be too hasty to conclude that just because the child's parents are short the child also will be short. As Scheinfeld relates:

> Short parents may be of several genetic types: (1) Where both are of consistently short ancestral stock and probably carry predominantly "short stature" genes, in which case all their children will probably be short; (2) where both parents are of ancestry with "mixed stature" genes, in which case they may have children of various heights, grading up to quite tall; (3) where parents are short not because of their genes, but because their growth was suppressed by adverse environments, in which case all their children will tend to be taller than they.[18]

Furthermore, stature is not dependent alone upon the action of a single gene but is the result of the action of many genes (multifactorial or polygenic inheritance), all of which influence growth and development in some manner. Additionally, whatever genes for shortness or tallness a child inherits, their effect can be greatly accelerated or retarded by the many ecological factors that exert their influence on the developing child.

ENDOCRINE GLANDS

The pituitary, thyroid, parathyroid, adrenal, pancreas, and gonads all secrete powerful hormones that influence growth and development. The function of these glands is influenced by some degree by heredity as well as by other factors such as disease, psychological deprivation, emotional crises, dietary intake, and other acquired disorders. Many important studies are now being conducted by the National Institute of Child Health and Human Development (NICHD) to determine the specific effects of the various hormones on growth and organ function, the mechanism underlying these effects, and the changes in the production of various hormones that occur during different growth periods. Recent findings[19] of several studies supported by NICHD indicate that: (1) The hypothalamus (a portion of the brain that controls several biological drives such as thirst, hunger, fear, and sex) may be important in the control of the functioning of the pituitary gland. When experimenters electrically stimulated the hypothalamus, they observed that the growth hormone was secreted from the pituitary gland. This finding suggests several new avenues for clinical studies that may be aimed at alleviating retarded growth in children. Presently, the availability of the growth hormone which is obtained entirely from the pituitary gland of human beings is severely limited. Current efforts are underway to develop a synthetic hormone that can be made more readily available to children with growth problems. (2) A relationship between severely emotionally deprived children and retarded physical growth was also observed. This suggests that psychological deprivation may suppress pituitary function and thus inhibit the release of the growth hormone.

18. Amram Scheinfeld, *Your Heredity and Environment* (New York: J. B. Lippincott Co., 1965), p. 115.
19. Report of National Institute of Child Health and Human Development, "Child Health and Human Development: Progress 1963–1970" (Washington, D.C.: Government Printing Office, 1970), p. 23.

CONGENITAL DEFECTS

It is often difficult to determine whether a particular congenital abnormality was caused by factors inherent in the genetic structure or whether infectious, toxic, endocrine, nutritional, traumatic, and other prenatal pathogenic factors operating on the germ cell or within the pregnant woman were responsible for producing a particular defect. Abnormal development of the lower limbs and lower spine may occur in infants born of diabetic mothers or of pregnant women who have taken certain drugs such as thalidomide during early pregnancy. Various surveys have shown that if a pregnant woman contracts German measles (rubella) during the first several weeks of pregnancy there is a 60 percent chance that her child will be abnormal in some manner.[20] Congenital abnormalities associated with German measles are deafness, eye defects such as cataracts, heart disease, mental retardation, and microcephaly (abnormal smallness of head). These abnormalities may seriously arrest the growth and development of afflicted children physically as well as psychologically and socially.

SOCIOECONOMIC STATUS

Considerable evidence has been accumulated to indicate that at maturity the average difference in height between high and low socioeconomic groups of adolescents ranges from 8 to 20 centimeters, or an average of approximately 5 percent of their full mature height.[21] These differences more than likely reflect the presence of certain factors operating within the environment that tend to impede growth in the disadvantaged population. As was noted in chapter 2, such factors as higher disease rates, low levels of nutrition, lack of health information, inability to afford medical care, substandard housing, inadequate sanitary control, and other environmental and cultural influences all tend to leave their impact on the developing child. However, whatever the importance of these environmental and cultural factors might be, it should be understood that they also operate within the genetic sphere. For as anthropologists point out, some of the tallest statures are found in areas where the poorest nutritional and environmental living conditions exist.[22]

NUTRITION

Sound nutritional practices are of fundamental importance to the growing and developing child. The nutrients contained in food provide the building blocks for bones, muscle, and fat and aid in determining whether the body achieves its genetic potential with respect to size and shape. More important, the nutrients in food influence the development of organs and cells, thereby controlling their functional capacity throughout life.

Several major reports have amply documented the problem of hunger

20. A. Emery, *Heredity, Disease, and Man* (Berkeley: University of California Press, 1968), p. 206.

21. B. S. Bloom, *Stability and Change in Human Characteristics* (New York: John Wiley & Sons, 1964): 37.

22. Scheinfeld, *Your Heredity*, p. 111.

and malnutrition in the United States.[23, 24] In certain depressed areas such as in the southeastern states and Appalachia malnutrition is similar to that found in the underdeveloped nations of the world. Low levels of nutrition can produce adverse effects on physical growth and intellectual development. In a statement presented before the Senate Select Committee on Nutrition and Related Human Needs, Lowe summarized the effects of malnutrition in childhood by stating the following:

> 1. When a fetus receives inadequate nutrition *in utero,* the infant is born small, the placenta of his mother contains fewer cells than normal to nourish him, and his growth will be compromised;
>
> 2. When an infant undergoes nutritional deprivation during the first months of life, his brain fails to synthesize protein and cells at normal rates and consequently suffers a decrease as great as twenty percent in the cell number;
>
> 3. During the last trimester of pregnancy, protein synthesis by the brain is proceeding at a very rapid rate. Immediately upon delivery, this rapid rate decreases, although it still continues at a greater pace than at later times of life. In animals, this sharp decrease in protein synthesis immediately after birth occurs in both full-term and premature animals. The decrease in protein synthesis occurring in premature animals in all probability also occurs in premature human infants. If we can extend animal observations to the human situation, we have a logical explanation for one of the most distressing concomitants of prematurity; as many as fifty percent of prematurely born infants grow to maturity with an intellectual competence significantly below that which would be expected when compared with siblings and even with age peers.
>
> 4. Severe malnutrition suffered during childhood affects learning ability, body growth, rate of maturation, ultimate size, and if prolonged, productivity.[25]

Several studies have indicated that there are critical periods in the development of the growing child when malnutrition will adversely affect growth, some of which may be irreversible.[26, 27, 28] Apparently the earlier

23. Report by Citizens' Board of Inquiry Into Hunger and Nutrition in the United States, "Hunger U.S.A." (Washington, D.C.: New Community Press, 1968).

24. Report by American Public Health Association in Cooperation With Citizens' Board of Inquiry Into Health Services for Americans, "Health Crisis in America" (Washington, D.C.: American Public Health Association, 1970).

25. C. U. Lowe, Statement Before Senate Select Committee on Nutrition and Related Human Needs, 28 January 1969.

26. A. Schaefer, "Observations From Exploring Needs in National Nutritional Programs," *American Journal of Public Health* 56, no. 7 (1966): 1092.

27. H. W. Reese, ed., *Advances in Child Development and Behavior* (New York: Academic Press, 1971), p. 159.

28. J. Richmond and H. Weinberger, "Program Implications of New Knowledge Regarding the Physical, Intellectual and Emotional Growth and Development and the Unmet Needs of Children and Youth," *Supplement to American Journal of Public Health* 60, no. 4 (1970): 33.

malnutrition exists, the more devastatingly it will affect growth and development. Physical size, organ function, and mental development may be impaired under adverse environmental conditions that influence the quality and quantity of food that is available for consumption. Also, the effect of deprivation appears to be greatest during the periods of most rapid growth and least during periods of least rapid growth. At infancy and puberty the caloric requirements per unit of body weight are at their highest, and during the first six months of postnatal life, the infant requires more than twice the calories per pound of body weight that are needed by active adults. Inadequate nutrition during these critical periods of life may adversely influence normal growth and development.

DISEASE

Nutritional status also bears a relationship to immunity and resistance to disease. Since many of the substances associated with immunological phenomena are proteins, inadequate protein intake may lead to inferior production of antibodies.[29] The extent to which specific infectious diseases contribute to growth failure is difficult to assess due to the catabolism (destructive metabolism) resulting from all infections. Additionally, in disease there is often an accompanying reduction in dietary intake and an increased loss of nutrients in the feces and urine. In general, any severe prolonged illness is liable to produce some effect on growth and organ development. Diarrheal diseases may predispose infants and small children to much of the malnutrition observed in poverty areas of the United States and of the world.[30] Iron deficiency anemia, which affects between 30 to 70 percent of children in poverty areas, if severe can also result in growth retardation. A chronic disorder such as congenital heart disease may impair the growth and development of the entire body.

Teachers may observe that children who had been absent from school due to an illness such as regular measles (rubeola) may exhibit some weight loss upon their return to the classroom. Such children may also fail to show any clear evidence of a height gain over a short span of time. These conditions are most likely to be temporary, and often these children will resume their normal growth pattern.

PHYSICAL FITNESS AND ACTIVITY

An individual's level of physical fitness can be influenced by both genetic and environmental factors; however, substantial evidence indicates that regular suitable exercise is one of the essential variables in maintaining favorable health status throughout life. Exercise and activity have several recognized positive effects on the health of the individual. First, there is the benefit of maintaining general muscular tone throughout the body including the heart itself. Generally, the body muscles grow stronger with proper use and weaker with disuse. A second benefit from exercise is that involving its psychological effect. Proper exercise of the right degree and intensity produces relaxation and relief of nervous tension. Also, exercise and activity

29. Watson and Lowrey, *Growth and Development*, p. 368.

30. K. V. Bailey, "A Study of Human Growth in the Framework of Applied Nutrition Programs in the Western Pacific Region," *Monographs of Society for Research in Child Development* 35, no. 7 (1970): 47.

help in controlling overweight and obesity. Even though overweight and obesity may be due to a combination of genetic and environmental factors, the increased metabolic requirement resulting from exercise does help to control body weight if the caloric intake is not increased. Finally, the deepening of respiration caused by exercise tends to favor the function of the lungs in gaseous exchange and in the general condition of lung tissue. Exercise of almost any kind, suitable in degree and duration for a particular individual, plays a useful role in the physical and psychological health status of the child. Teachers and youth workers need to understand that exercise should be based on the age, sex, and physical and motor condition of the child, as well as upon individual interests. Children differ in these attributes and should not be graded in their physical education classes according to how many pushups, sit-ups, and cartwheels that they can perform to the delight of their instructor.

Some parents and teachers tend to compare the growth patterns of their children by employing the standard age, height, and weight tables that are found so abundantly in the literature. Several limitations should be stated in utilization of tables of this type to appraise the physical status of children. (1) Published charts that are available may be out of date because of the recent gains in the rate of development of children. Some of the age, height, and weight tables that are still being reproduced in printed matter were developed from data collected in the middle 1940s and 1950s. (2) Differences of opinion exist among authorities regarding the amount a child may deviate from the mean before he should be considered for referral. (3) The use of the mean as a standard index fails to consider the fact that each individual has his own unique and proper growth pattern. (4) The means for many of the standard tables are based upon a rather large population that includes many different subgroups that reflect the interaction of social class, race, health and nutritional status, and the influence of environmental conditions upon subsequent growth and development. (5) Tables of height and weight for given ages are often not representative of actual growth patterns since sexual maturation and growth spurts do not occur at the same chronological age in all children. (6) The problem of evaluating weight status in children from these tables is most complex. An accumulation of fat in children during the prepubertal period is a frequent occurrence and probably does not have the same significance as overweight or obesity that occurs sometimes in the early school years or after pubescence. Regardless of their limitations, charts of this type do provide an index for studying orderly development in children.

Several prepared types of growth profile charts have been developed to evaluate the physical growth of children. The Meredith physical growth record employs both weight and height measurements and provides a graphic indication of the child's growth status.[31] Separate forms are used for boys and girls as well as for children in the age groups four to eleven and eleven to eighteen years. Five normative zones ranging from tall to short

EVALUATION OF GROWTH AND DEVELOPMENT

31. Forms for both boys and girls may be obtained through the order departments of the American Medical Association, 535 N. Dearborn St., Chicago, Illinois, 60610, or through the National Education Association, 1201 Sixteenth St., N.W. Washington, D.C. 20036.

and from heavy to light are outlined on each form for plotting height and weight data. The particular zone into which a child's height and weight data are recorded indicates his position with respect to other children of the same sex and age. When a child's height and weight points do not lie in corresponding channels (e.g., light for weight and average zone for height), this fact may denote normal slenderness or an undesirable state of health. Further medical examination by a physician may indicate that the child has an infection or a nutritional problem or is medically normal and of slender build.

The Wetzel grid is based on the principle that normal growth proceeds along a channel characteristic of the individual's body build.[32] Physical status, level of physical development, and nutritional status may be objectively evaluated by proper interpretation of the recorded data.

Teachers may also use the height and weight data commonly found on the child's school health record to evaluate physical growth or may wish to develop their own growth charts.

Height and weight measurements should be undertaken at least three times during the school year. For example, height and weight measurements may be made early in September, in January, and in May. Height should be recorded to the nearest one-fourth inch and weight to the nearest half-pound. Children who fail to show a gain in weight for three or more successive months should be referred for appropriate action. This is also true for children who are grossly overweight or underweight and those who show fluctuating weight changes. Height is more difficult to assess since for any given year a child's gain in height may be very small, yet still be normal for him even though his age peers are becoming taller. However, failure to gain in height is most significant during the stages when growth should be accelerated.

Children are interested in observing their own rate of development, and his own growth record is something that a child can see and understand. Educationally, they can be used to reveal the relationship between growth and nutrition, sleep, rest, and exercise. Furthermore, growth charts may have the advantage of motivating children to change their health attitudes and behavior. Finally, it should be stressed that charts by themselves are not a substitute for physical examination and should never be used to compare children against each other. Growth and development are unique for a given individual, and charts only show the average child growing at an average rate.

SUMMARY
The rate of growth and development of children reflects the interface of genetic and environmental factors. Children inherit possible patterns of growth from their parents, while the environment dictates which of the patterns will be attained. Generally, children who inherit "tallness" genes and are reared in a positive environment tend to achieve their genetic potential. Conversely, children who are severely malnourished particularly during the growth period may not reach their optimal level of growth and development.

Interrelationships exist between many of the ecological factors affecting growth and development. Heredity, endocrine glands, congenital de-

32. Copies may be obtained through National Education Association Service, Inc., 1200 W. Third Street, Cleveland, Ohio.

fects, socioeconomic status, nutrition, disease, physical fitness, activity, and medical care all play a role in the growth process of the child. Teachers should understand the variability of growth patterns in children and be able to reassure students that each child develops at his or her own unique rate of growth.

Discussion Questions

1. What secular trends have been observed with respect to the growth and development of children?
2. Briefly discuss the various factors that may account for the emergence of these secular trends.
3. How have these secular trends influenced the social behavior of children?
4. What impact have these secular trends had on our educational institutions?
5. What are some of the basic principles of growth and development?
6. Discuss the relationship between physical growth and self-concept.
7. How are the various ecological factors related to growth and development?
8. What are the limitations of standard age, height, and weight tables in assessing the physical growth of children?
9. What standards can a teacher use in evaluating physical growth?

References

Bailey, K. V. "A Study of Human Growth in the Framework of Applied Nutrition Programs in the Western Pacific Region." *Monographs of Society for Research in Child Development* 35, no. 7 (1970): 47.

Bloom, B. S. *Stability and Change in Human Characteristics.* New York: John Wiley & Sons, 1964.

Emery, A. *Heredity, Disease, and Man.* Berkeley: University of California Press, 1968.

Garn, S., and Clark, L. "The Sex Differences in Basal Metabolism Rates." *Child Development* 24 (1952): 215–224.

Havighurst, R. J. "Do Junior High School Youth Grow Up Too Fast?" *Bulletin of National Association of Secondary School Principals* 22 (1963): 160.

Illinois Interagency Drug Education Development Committee. *Teaching About Drug Abuse.* Springfield, Ill.: Office of Superintendent of Public Instruction, 1971.

Lowe, C. U. Statement before Senate Select Committee on Nutrition and Related Human Needs, 28 January 1969.

Meredith, H. V. "Change in the Stature and Body Weight of North American Boys During the Last 80 Years." In *Advances in Child Development and Behavior,* ed. L. Lipsett and C. Spiker. New York: Academic Press, 1963.

Moore, W. M. "The Secular Trend in Physical Growth of Urban North American Negro Schoolchildren." *Monographs of Society for Research in Child Development* 35, no. 7 (1970).

Muuss, R. E. "Adolescent Development and the Secular Trend." *Adolescence* 5, no. 19 (1970): 278.

Reese, H. W., ed. *Advances in Child Development and Behavior.* New York: Academic Press, 1971.

Report by American Public Health Association in Cooperation with Citizens' Board of Inquiry Into Health Services for Americans, "Health Crises in America." Washington, D.C.: American Public Health Association, 1970.

Report by Citizens' Board of Inquiry Into Hunger and Nutrition in the United States, "Hunger U.S.A." Washington, D.C.: New Community Press, 1968.

Report of National Institute of Child Health and Human Development, "Child Health and Human Development: Progress 1963–1970." Washington, D.C.: Government Printing Office, 1970.

Richmond, J., and Weinberger, H. "Program Implications of New Knowledge Regarding the Physical, Intellectual and Emotional Growth and Development and the Unmet Needs of Children and Youth." *Supplement to American Journal of Public Health* 60, no. 4 (1970): 33.

Robinson, L. E. *Human Growth and Development.* Columbus, Ohio: Charles E. Merrill Publishing Co., 1968.

Scammon, R. E. "The Measurement of the Body in Childhood." In *The Measurement of Man* by Harris, J., Jackson, C., Patterson, D., and Scammon, R. E. Minneapolis: University of Minnesota Press, 1930.

Schaefer, A. "Observations From Exploring Needs in National Nutritional Programs." *American Journal of Public Health* 56, no. 7 (1966): 1092.

Scheinfeld, A. *Your Heredity and Environment.* New York: J. B. Lippincott Co., 1965.

Tanner, J. M. "Sequence, Tempo, and Individual Variation in the Growth and Development of Boys and Girls Ages Twelve to Sixteen." *Daedalus,* 100, no. 4 (1971): 929.

U.S., Department of Health, Education, and Welfare, Health Services and Mental Health Administration. *Teenage Smoking—National Patterns of Cigarette Smoking Ages Twelve Through Eighteen in 1968 and 1970,* HSM Publication no. 72–7508. Rockville, Md.: 1972.

Watson, E., and Lowrey, G. *Growth and Development of Children.* Chicago: Year Book Medical Publishers, 1967.

Wright, B., et al. *Elementary School Curriculum: Better Teaching Now.* New York: Macmillan Co., 1971.

Chapter 5
PSYCHOLOGICAL
DIMENSIONS
OF
HEALTH

Why does one encounter difficulty in developing a concise, yet comprehensive definition of mental health?

To what extent should teachers be concerned with the mental health of children?

What measures can be taken to reduce the stress potential of the school experience?

What classroom behaviors are indicative of early emotional difficulties that may eventually lead to serious behavior problems?

In what ways are the goals of American education consistent with the principles of positive mental health?

Since the turn of the century, knowledge of human behavior has advanced to the point where there is absolutely no doubt that man is more than a physical creature. Increasing significance has been placed on mental and emotional qualities as fundamental components of total health. Evidence shows that the mental and physical dimensions of health are interrelated, with one never completely independent of the other. High levels of physical well-being augment the likelihood of sound mental health, and vice versa. Emotional difficulties may actually precipitate physical illness. Conversely, individuals who experience bodily ailments often encounter emotional involvement as a consequence of their physical disorder. Over the years, public awareness of the significance of mental health has had a marked effect upon social institutions, including schools. As a result, specialized personnel are involved in school programs to enhance the educational experience of emotionally handicapped, neurotic, and borderline psychotic children. Necessary though these efforts are, they do not constitute a comprehensive approach to mental health in our schools. Actually, most children are not in need of services provided by trained psychological services personnel. Yet, all children manifest mental health needs that to a greater or lesser degree influence their performance in school. In brief, schools should not limit their mental health efforts to the needs of disturbed children, but should incorporate mental health principles in the total educational experience of each child. In addressing itself to this point, the Joint Commission on Mental Health of Children has summarized what it believes are the essential mental health functions of schools as follows:

> For the school to be a mentally healthy environment for growing children there must be a change in the concept of how this institution shall serve society through the children it educates. Its goals must be not only achievement but personality development, not only competence but ego strength, not only intellectual power but self-understanding and feelings of self-worth, not only adaptability but individuality, not only accommodation but initiative. The changes to be enacted involve all aspects of the school milieu–curriculum, teaching methods, teacher-child relations, administrative practices, and architectural design.[1]

VIEWS OF MENTAL HEALTH

That positive mental health facilitates learning and all other human activities is a truism. Nonetheless, when people are asked to describe what they consider to be characteristic of mentally healthy behavior, the diverse views expressed reveal marked differences of opinion. Teachers are not immune to the confusion and ambiguity inherent in the terms *mental health* and *mental hygiene*. Many are convinced that if a child has "adjusted" to the school environment, he exemplifies sound mental and emotional health. Interestingly enough, others argue that total adjustment to the routine and requiredness of school life is intolerable to those showing a high level of mental health. A surprisingly high proportion of teachers believe that pupils who are not troublemakers in class rank high on the mental health scale. Still others contend that a certain amount of aggressive and disruptive behavior is normal and should be tolerated in the classroom. Surprisingly, these conflicting interpretations of what constitutes normal and abnormal behavior are frequently expressed by teachers who work with similar grade levels, in the same corridor of the same school. In spite of elements of truth in each of the views just expressed, all suffer shortcomings that suggest serious flaws in the teachers' concepts of mental health. Obviously, educators lay no special claim to the conceptual dilemma in defining or conceptualizing mental health. In noting this fact, Kaplan explains that "There have been many attempts to define mental hygiene, but this field is a hybrid which eludes precise definition. It consists not only of a body of knowledge, but also a way of life, a set of values, and a quality of interpersonal relationships."[2] The question of normal or abnormal, usual or unusual, and desirable or undesirable is substantially more definitive when physical health is concerned. When abnormal deviations in body temperature, blood pressure, or white blood cell count occur, a physician knows that disease is present. Since the body is a physical object, it lends itself to scientific measurement and scrutiny. The mind is really a concept, so that its activities defy the precise measurements that have been useful in distinguishing physical health from illness. Consequently, measurements of mental processes

1. Joint Commission on Mental Health of Children, *Crisis in Child Mental Health: Challenge for the 1970's* (New York: Harper & Row, 1969), p. 77.

2. L. Kaplan, *Foundations of Human Behavior* (New York: Harper & Row, 1965), p. 323.

and their behavioral implications have not yet attained this degree of clarity or sophistication. This fact is abundantly clear from the lack of agreement among authorities who have commented on the human qualities they believe to be indicative of positive mental health. Katz and Lewis state that "Mental health denotes the emotional stability, intellectual efficiency, and social effectiveness of people."[3] According to Menninger, mentally healthy people adjust to the world, maintain an even temper, and, among other qualities, possess a happy disposition.[4] With regard to "adjustment," some authorities depart from Menninger's view. Riesman explicitly recognizes that mentally sound individuals may indeed adjust to outside pressures and influences, but they also demonstrate an autonomous spirit that enables them to resist adjustment to some of these forces.[5] Menninger's belief that happiness is a criterion of sound mental health has also received some degree of criticism. Jahoda, for example, has emphasized that happiness or contentment in a situation calling for tension, emotional turmoil, and grief could be a manifestation of mental disturbance, rather than positive mental health.[6] Thus, in addition to assessing the nature of a behavior, Jahoda suggests that its relative normality or abnormality is dependent upon the setting in which the behavior takes place. Still another example of diverse views of mental health, one somewhat more philosophical than others discussed, is provided by Fromm, who speaks of mental health as ". . . the grasp of reality inside and outside ourselves, that is, by the development of objectivity and reason."[7] A somewhat different view has been expressed by Carroll, who believes that mental health is really a point of view possessed in varying degrees by different people.[8] In his opinion, this point of view includes self-respect and respect for others, understanding and tolerating the limitations of self and others, the belief that all behavior has an underlying cause, and an appreciation of the basic needs that are motives for behavior.

Irrespective of the obvious difficulties involved in defining and assessing mental health, there exists a pressing need to develop broad and operationally useful views of mental health that provide guidelines for a clearer understanding of human behavior and healthy personality. Only when operating from such a framework can educators hope to broaden their views of others and progress toward the goal of promoting the positive mental health of all children.

Partly as a result of the lack of agreement on a satisfactory definition of mental health, some mental hygienists have chosen to equate it with healthy personality development.[9] This posture enables one to approach the topic

3. B. Katz, and R. Lewis, *The Psychology of Abnormal Behavior,* 2nd ed. (New York: Ronald Press, 1961), p. 611.

4. K. Menninger, *The Human Mind,* 3rd ed. (New York: Alfred A. Knopf, 1937), p. 1.

5. D. Riesman, N. Glazer, and R. Denny, *The Lonely Crowd* (New Haven: Yale University Press, 1950).

6. M. Jahoda, *Current Concepts of Positive Mental Health* (New York: Basic Books, Inc., 1958).

7. E. Fromm, *The Sane Society* (New York: Holt, Rinehart & Winston, 1955), p. 69.

8. H. Carroll, *Mental Hygiene: The Dynamics of Adjustment,* 4th ed. (Englewood Cliffs, N.J.: Prentice-Hall, 1964).

9. S. Jourard, *Personal Adjustment: An Approach Through the Study of Healthy Personality,* 2nd ed. (New York: Macmillan Co., 1963).

of mental hygiene by way of a reasonably objective theory of personality development, while avoiding the semantic pitfalls inherent in the term *mental health*. Regardless of how carefully constructed any definition of mental hygiene or of healthy personality might be, it will suffer one or more inadequacies. Yet, this does not preclude the need for educators and others in the helping professions to have some conceptual basis for understanding healthy personality.

TOWARD A CONCEPT OF MENTAL HEALTH

Mental health may be conceived as a behavioral continuum extending from optimal mental health (optimal personality development) at one extreme to profound mental deterioration at the other. Severe mental and emotional disorders (psychoses) and many less incapacitating mental disturbances are quite obvious and can be diagnosed by trained personnel. However, the vast majority of people, including most school children, do not exhibit pathology of this magnitude. Neither do they enjoy that hypothetical quality known as optimal mental health. As it turns out, most individuals fluctuate nearer to the positive extreme of the mental health scale than to the mental illness end. Since most people show variations in behavior along this continuum, it is clear that different individuals can be expected to manifest behaviors that are indicative of sound mental health part of the time and actions that are less mentally healthy at other times. Conceptual difficulties arise from the fact that no precise position on the continuum distinguishes healthy from unhealthy behavior. No forced dichotomy can be imposed to separate actions that are reflective of mental health or of illness. To further confuse the issue, situational conditions often determine whether one's actions should be judged normal or pathological.

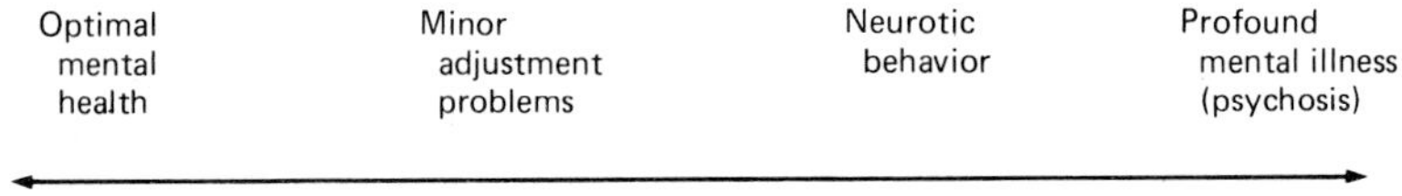

Fig. 5–1. Mental health continuum.

Optimal mental health	Minor adjustment problems	Neurotic behavior	Profound mental illness (psychosis)

To illustrate the importance of situational variables in assessing the quality of behavior, a few examples may be in order. Civilized cultures do not tolerate homicide. Those who commit brutal acts of this type are likely to be judged deranged or emotionally disturbed. Yet, in certain social settings, homicide has been regarded in an entirely different manner. Nazis embraced the belief that Jews were an inferior group and should be eliminated. To the supporters of this ideology, the tragic slaughter of millions of European Jews was not only nonpathological, but was also desirable and acceptable behavior. This illustration shows how group norms and expectations affect one's perception of what constitutes normal or abnormal, acceptable or unacceptable, and healthy or unhealthy behavior.

In addition to group norms and other social influences, there are other ecological elements that can determine whether a given behavior is mentally healthy or unhealthy. Hallucinations occur when one perceives something in the absence of sensory stimuli. Under usual circumstances, these phenomena are regarded as symptoms of mental deterioration. However, space researchers have observed that when in total sensory isolation for protracted periods of time man will usually hallucinate. In other words, by simply modifying the physical environment, behavior that would otherwise be undesirable is quite normal and expected. The essential point is that the mental health qualities of behavior have meaning only when one understands the ecological setting in which the behavior takes place. Social factors, cultural patterns, group norms, and environmental conditions are among the ecological elements that cause people to behave as they do. More important, these factors determine to what extent behavior should be interpreted as mentally constructive or corrosive. As the following illustration shows, this fundamental principle of mental health has direct application in the classroom:

> Ronald is a seventh grade pupil who makes repeated overt attempts to antagonize his English teacher. It appears that he almost welcomes the reprimands that invariably follow the class disruptions that he causes. His teacher is at her wits' end after having tried everything she can think of to discourage his frequent annoyances. In her view, his behavior is atypical and indicates an emotional problem that is beyond her control. She has decided that the next time Ronald upsets the class he will be referred to the school psychologist for an evaluation.

Without a doubt, Ronald's actions in class would be a source of concern to most teachers. Many would be inclined to remove him physically from class, using one of several options available to them. Perhaps others would place Ronald on detention, hoping that this punishment would change his behavior. Rather than take any immediate punitive action, the alert teacher would try to understand the reasons for his actions. Suppose that the boy's actions were designed to attract his teacher's attention. Perhaps this was the only way he knew of reaching out and gaining her favor. To Ronald, even a reprimand was more desirable than being ignored by the only teacher he really liked. In short, his behavior was designed to gain attention. In this context his classroom actions would be indicative of a normal personality motive. This is not to imply that his disruptions should have been tolerated. Imagine, on the other hand, that the boy's frightful conduct was his method of retaliating against a threatening parent, with the teacher serving as a symbol of parental authority. Under these circumstances his actions indicate the need for professional help. Similar behaviors may arise from entirely different motives, each reflecting different levels of mental health, and each requiring different responses by his teacher. The salient point in this example is that mental health is reflected more in the manner in which behavior is used than in the behavior itself. Annoying, unusual, or obnoxious conduct often takes on new significance when one gains insight into its underlying causes. While classroom teachers have neither the time nor the expertise to understand every motive of all their pupils, they should at least maintain an open mind when assessing the actions of children. This tendency not to prejudge and not to condemn solely on the basis of an overt act creates a climate that enhances the probability that reactions to behavior will promote, rather than undermine, healthy personality development.

CRITERIA FOR ASSESSING MENTAL HEALTH

The purpose of this discussion is to provide a measure of clarity to the vague notion of mental health. Up to this point our comments and examples may have only muddied the conceptual waters. However true this may seem, the intent has been to create an awareness of the need for a framework that will be useful in understanding people and promoting the healthy development of their personalities. As a final effort toward this end it is useful to consider the findings of Jahoda's synthesis of mental health criteria that have been suggested by different mental health authorities.[10] For our purposes, Jahoda's conclusions are particularly helpful because they reveal consistent themes or recurrent qualities that mental hygienists believe to be essential concomitants of positive mental health. Briefly summarized, the criteria enumerated by Jahoda include the following:

Attitudes of an individual toward his own self   The relevance of positive attitudes toward self is a recurrent theme in the literature. Important in this regard are feelings of self-confidence, self-esteem, and self-respect, all of which express a judgment that the self is essentially "good," capable, and strong. The need for a realistic assessment of self is extremely important, for it enables one to distinguish between what he actually is and what he hopes to be ideally. In recognizing self-limitations, the mentally sound individual believes these to be outweighed by positive characteristics he possesses.

Growth, development, and self-actualization   Many writers have expressed the belief that the essential quality of mentally healthy people is their tendency toward "becoming," understanding, and realizing their own potential. It is almost as if the individual were unfolding and moving forward in his effort to become the person he is capable of being. Serious questions may be raised concerning the likelihood that one ever realizes his full potential, understands himself thoroughly, or becomes self-actualized. Albert Schweitzer, Martin Luther King, Jr., and perhaps Eleanor Roosevelt have come as close to this ideal as have any other individuals in recent decades. While very few can expect to reach the heights of personal development attained by these rare persons, the fact remains that some degree of motivation or drive toward becoming or self-actualization is a positive sign of healthy personality.

Autonomy   As a characteristic of those who enjoy positive mental health, autonomy has been variously described as self-determination, independence, and self-containment. Decision making and the extent to which a person is influenced by other individuals or events are related to autonomy. Autonomous persons regulate their behavior from within, consistent with their own personal standards and inner organization of values, needs, and beliefs. This is the external dimension of autonomy. In addition, the autonomous personality has the ability to maintain a stable keel when confronted with adverse environmental conditions. Of course, tolerance of adversity is suggestive of mental and emotional soundness only when one perceives the threatening situation accurately. Even then, there are many instances (e.g., impending disaster) when even highly stable personalities would show a degree of instability. Characteristically, however, they would show less instability for shorter duration than would less autonomous persons.

10. Jahoda, *Current Concepts*, p. 23.

Perception of reality At first glance, accurate reality perception appears to be such an obvious characteristic of the healthy personality as to deserve little attention in this discussion. That is, people who are emotionally sound tend to see their surroundings accurately, while the mentally ill are more or less out of touch with reality at least part of the time. Unfortunately, perception of reality is not quite so simple a matter. There are, in fact, several ways one may perceive the same situation realistically. If one employee sees his job in terms of its limitations while another worker performing the same job perceives it according to its advantages, are not both perceptions correct? Jahoda stresses the following point:

> Mentally healthy perception means a process of viewing the world so that one is able to take matters one wishes were different without distorting them to fit these wishes—that is, without inventing cues not actually existing. To perceive with relative freedom from need-distortion does not mean, of course, that needs and motives are eliminated, nor that they have no function in perception. The requirement is of a different nature: the mentally healthy person will test reality for its degree of correspondence to his wishes or fears. One lacking in mental health will assume such correspondence without testing.[11]

Reality perception is also related to the ability to correctly interpret the feelings and actions of others, to arrive at distortion-free conclusions regarding the behaviors of others, and to consider the feelings of others worthy of concern. In a word, healthy personalities have the capacity to express empathy. The earlier example of the behavior problem presented by Ronald is illustrative of a teacher who no doubt could have benefitted from a greater measure of empathy.

Environmental mastery Success and adaptation are two themes commonly mentioned in conjunction with environmental mastery. These broad mental health qualities are said to include the ability to love and be loved, feelings of adequacy, efficiency in meeting situational requirements, the capacity for adaptation, and effectiveness in problem solving.

By no means does Jahoda's summary represent a precise definition of mental health. Neither does it comprise a totally adequate framework that is universally accepted by mental hygienists. Nonetheless, it does suggest subjective behavioral parameters within which one may operate to better understand their own behavior and that of others.

The concept of *personality* is nearly as elusive as the term *mental health*. This fact is borne out by Hall and Lindzey's review of the literature which identified at least fifty different definitions of personality.[12] This is not to say that fifty divergent points of view were found, for many were discovered to be similar. For instance, many of the definitions emphasized the impor-

THEORETICAL APPROACHES TO PERSONALITY

11. Jahoda, *Current Concepts,* pp. 51–52.
12. C. Hall and G. Lindzey, *Theories of Personality* (New York: John Wiley & Sons, 1957).

tance of the individual and his relationship to his environment. Other views stressed the theme of individual uniqueness and were, in that sense, compatible. With respect to the multiplicity of personality definitions, Thorpe emphasizes the following essential:

> The very breadth and scope of the various definitions of personality, extending back in time to man's earliest philosophical attempts to understand his own nature, forward to sober considerations of what man should or must be like to survive and build a constructive society, embracing both dimensions in terms of scientific, philosophical, or clinical observations on the problem, make it impossible to present a single final definition of the term. There seems no reason, however, to assume that this is either necessary or desirable. It is essential, nevertheless, that the student be aware of the many points of view regarding the nature of personality, their contributions to the science of man, and their value in understanding the problems of mental health.[13]

PSYCHOANALYTIC VIEWS

Sigmund Freud, a Viennese physician (1856–1939), is believed to have developed the first comprehensive framework for understanding personality. Recognized as the founder of classical psychoanalytic theory, Freud departed from the traditional study of consciousness and was the first to point out the importance of the unconsciousness. In his view, urges, drives, and repressed feelings, lodged in the mind's unconscious depths, control the conscious thoughts and actions of people. The concepts of id, ego, and superego were also suggested by Freud and have nearly as much validity today as when originally developed.

Id represents man's erotic drives and the organic needs for food, elimination, and physical contact. It is these primitive id demands that dictate infantile behavior. As the child grows and becomes aware of others and the world, new perceptions give rise to reasoning power (ego) that eventually permits one to control the primitive id. Once the child's social experience expands, group norms and social controls assume added importance as influences on his behavior. *Superego* is the Freudian term for conscience. It develops as a result of ethical and moral values established by the individual, and its function is to exercise conscious control over unacceptable or inappropriate id tendencies.

A group of contemporary psychoanalysts, represented by Erich Fromm and Karen Horney among others, have to some extent rejected or modified the original views of Freud. This group of psychoanalysts is commonly referred to as the neo-Freudian school. While recognizing the importance of innate biological factors in motivation, Fromm differs from Freud by recognizing the adaptability of the human organism as it interacts interpersonally and socially. Although Horney continued to accept many Freudian views (e.g., free association, unconscious motivation), she disagreed with some of his views concerning sex and placed greater emphasis on the social milieu as a factor in human motivation.

13. Louis P. Thorpe, *The Psychology of Mental Health,* Second Edition. Copyright © 1960. The Ronald Press Company, p. 288.

FIELD THEORY

When one speaks of field theory in psychology, the work of Kurt Lewin immediately comes to mind.[14] He viewed man as being constantly in a field of force, influenced by elements within this field. Personality development, according to this framework, is the process of adjusting to and maintaining equilibrium in a challenging environment. Man must adapt to the situations that cause physical or emotional imbalance. Failure to respond adequately to these imbalancing forces threatens survival. When one considers the complexity of contemporary society and its inherent stresses, it is easy to appreciate the importance Lewin placed on man's adaptability and resilience.

PERSONOLOGY

H. A. Murray is probably the most widely recognized personologist since his work at Harvard University has had considerable influence on contemporary psychology.[15] Like the field theorists, Murray was aware of the importance of environment on personality. He placed considerable emphasis on various functions and operations of the intellect as integrating forces in individual behavior. Murray is perhaps best known for his development of constructs relating to at least twenty basic human needs. According to his theory, as inner needs motivate the individual, he seeks need satisfaction through interactions with environmental factors that help to determine the direction his need-reduction behavior will take.

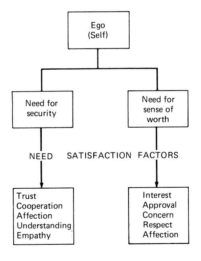

Fig. 5–2. Ego needs and their satisfaction.

LEARNING THEORY

The fundamental emphasis of the learning theory approach to personality development is that one's behavior and personality must be learned. Learning theorists, therefore, differ significantly from those psychologists who stress innate and instinctive qualities as the basic determinants of behavior

14. K. Lewin, *A Dynamic Theory of Personality* (New York: McGraw-Hill Book Co., 1935).
15. H. Murray, *Explorations in Personality* (London: Oxford University Press, 1938).

and personality. Dollard and Miller represent the modern school of learning theory.[16] This group believes that by following certain principles of learning (e.g., reward, punishment, imitation, generalization) one can greatly modify personality. In a sense, learning theorists are environmentalists, for they attempt to discover how learning principles can be utilized in order that some aspect of the environment becomes part of one's personality. It is also important to note that learning theory, perhaps more than other theoretical postures discussed in this section, has been verified by rather precise clinical research. Learning theory cannot only play a role in the development of healthy personality, but also has potential value in the treatment of some emotional problems (e.g., phobias), as recent research has demonstrated.

This discussion of theoretical views of personality and personality development has necessarily been limited. Time and space have permitted no more than a cursory description of a few schools of thought. Hopefully some readers will be encouraged to do additional reading in depth, for the better the grasp one has of personality theory, the greater the likelihood that he will appreciate dynamic behavior and its mental health implications.

THE CONCEPT OF STRESS

Human beings are repeatedly subjected to stimuli which more or less upset their intrinsic attempt to maintain physiological and psychological equilibrium. A state of tension exists until the demands of these stimuli are met and the individual regains a degree of stability. "If a stimulus or some combination of stimuli make too great demands on the organism, however, a state of stress exists. Stress may be either of short or long duration, but the organism must eventually make some adaptation to the stress in order to survive."[17] For example, when pathogenic organisms (stress agents) enter the body and infection develops, normal body functions are disrupted to some extent. In short, a condition of physiological stress exists. Reactions to this situation include increase in white blood cell count, inflammation, pain, increased heart rate, and elevation of body temperature. Naturally, the appearance of specific symptoms, as well as their severity, is dependent upon several factors including the virulence of the infectious agent and the individual's level of resistance. Each physiological response to infection represents an attempt to overcome the stress-producing organisms and helps the body regain a more balanced physiological state. Unless defenses are mobilized to overwhelm the disease organisms, stress intensifies and one's survival is jeopardized. The theoretical work of Hans Selye (*general adaptation syndrome*), which describes human responses to stress in terms of three distinct stages, is discussed at some length in chapter 1.

When stress (severe anxiety) is encountered, the nervous system prepares the person for some type of responsive activity. This general activity occurs whether the forces of stress pose threats to physical or emotional security. Walter B. Cannon is recognized for his pioneering studies of the effects of emotions upon physiological responses.[18] According to his findings, when one's security or sense of personal worth is threatened, responses

16. J. Dollard and N. Miller, *Personality and Psychotherapy: An Analysis in Terms of Learning, Thinking, and Culture* (New York: McGraw-Hill Book Co., 1964).

17. Katz and Lewis, *Abnormal Behavior*, p. 60.

18. W. Cannon, *Bodily Changes in Pain, Hunger, Fear, and Rage*, 2nd ed. (New York: Harper & Row, 1963).

include fear or anxiety or anger and hostility. Under these circumstances, behavior may involve physical or psychological flight, compromise, or defensive reactions. Cannon demonstrated that when a person's emotional or physical safety is endangered marked changes occur in body processes. In some instances functions are inhibited, while in others they are augmented. For example, heart rate accelerates and general blood pressure increases, thus supplying the musculature with increased amounts of blood and oxygen with which to enhance muscular efficiency. Liver function, particularly the release of glycogen, is increased, providing a higher level of blood sugar for energy. Digestion, on the other hand, is inhibited since blood is diverted from digestive organs to the skeletal muscles in anticipation of strenuous muscular activity. In addition, blood coagulation time is decreased to protect the organism from possible blood loss. Vision improves because the pupils dilate and permit more light to strike the retina. Sweat glands also become more active during periods of stress, thereby increasing the body's capability for cooling itself if physical activity ensues. All of these reactions are precipitated by threats to one's psychological or physical security since organ systems and body tissues (e.g., circulatory system) are not capable of distinguishing between threats to physical or psychological well-being.

When basic psychological needs are threatened (e.g., rejection by loved ones), a variety of behaviors may result. Emotional outbursts, withdrawal, and use of adjustive mechanisms such as rationalization, compensation, and projection may be used as stress-reducing techniques. Character disorders (e.g., aggressive antisocial tendencies), psychoneuroses, and psychoses also represent efforts to cope with ego threats.

In the minds of some people stress has a totally negative connotation. Under some circumstances, especially when anxiety-producing forces are intense or prolonged, or when one is unable to cope with them, stress may indeed lead to disintegration of behavior. However, most stresses are relatively minor and can be overcome with a minimum of effort by most stable personalities. Actually, life would prove unbearably drab were it not for many of the stresses we face. Some stress agents are extremely useful, for they encourage increased effort, ingenuity, and initiative that might otherwise lie dormant. In a sense, individuals develop their abilities and grow in self-understanding as a consequence of exposure to stress. In fact, schools capitalize on the stress phenomenon and depend upon it as a powerful pupil motivator. Threats of reprimand, failing grades, isolation, and parent conferences are perceived as stress by some pupils who, to the delight of their teachers, respond with increased effort and improved behavior. Unfortunately, situations such as these pose little, if any, threat to some children and therefore are of limited value as motivators. Those who have learned by repeated school failure and ridicule that they are not expected to achieve academically do not interpret additional failure as stressful.

DIFFERING REACTIONS TO STRESS

Though all people experience stress, individuals' reactions under these circumstances show wide variations. Katz and Lewis have suggested that these differences are the result of individual perceptions of stress-producing situations, variations in stress-coping abilities, and the sources of stress.[19]

19. Katz and Lewis, *Abnormal Behavior*, p. 60.

When stress originates outside of the individual (external stress), there is a greater likelihood that one will appraise the situation realistically than if the stress were of internal origin. That is, a person can be reasonably objective in identifying and responding to social, economic, occupational, and other external factors that create stress for him. Internal stress, on the other hand, defies such objectivity because its causes are frequently obscured by ego-defense mechanisms that preclude a realistic appraisal of the conditions precipitating the stress.

Regardless of the situation one faces, if it is not perceived as threatening to the physical or psychological self, it will not produce stress symptoms. Since each of us perceives and assesses present situations in terms of our past experiences, what is interpreted as an extreme threat by one person may pass practically unnoticed by another. The child once bitten by a dog may experience severe anxiety when approached by a dog even years after the frightening experience. Other youngsters having positive animal experiences would have no reason to perceive this situation as a serious threat to their safety. Any conditions (e.g., age, sex, socioeconomic status) that contribute to individual differences also account for differences in individuals' perceptions of stress.

> In general, that which is new or unexpected, or which requires a new response from the organism, is likely to be interpreted by the organism as a stress situation. There is a certain amount of security in the familiar, even when the familiar pattern brings nothing but unhappiness and self-destruction. This explains, in part, why so many patients with emotional problems find it difficult to give up their neurotic patterns of behavior and assume more rearding patterns; why they often fear success more than failure. If a person has learned to adjust to failure, defeat, unhappiness, and rejection, he may find that success, acceptance, and pleasure, in making demands on his organism for new modes of behavior, become a source of stress. At simpler levels of behavior, the same principle exists. The young bride who is attempting to balance the family checkbook for the first time may find this a very trying ordeal, whereas an experienced accountant would view the same task as a routine matter.[20]

Perception of self is another factor that influences how a person reacts when faced with a threatening situation. When the self is believed capable of overcoming stress-producing conditions, it is likely to respond by moving against or attacking these forces. However, if one's self-perception indicates that he is incapable of coping with agents of stress, compensatory behavior or retreat may result.

While responding to stressful circumstances, the mentally healthy person considers his personal assets and liabilities and assesses his chances of success. It may be necessary for him to alter his goals or in some other fashion compromise his situation. As a result of previous successes and failures in dealing with life experiences, we learn which behaviors to employ or avoid in responding to present circumstances. Children who discover that pouting is an effective technique for getting their own way will usually resort

20. Katz and Lewis, *Abnormal Behavior*, p. 61.

Chapter 5

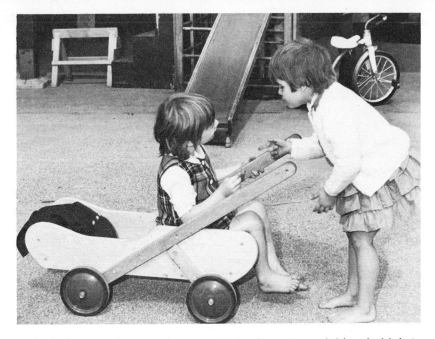

Fig. 5–3. Learning to share and becoming sensitive to the needs of age-mates is a source of anxiety for many primary grade children. (Reprinted by permission of Illinois Department of Mental Health. Photo by Ray Armes, Jr.)

to this behavior as long as it is successful for them. Some children hold their breath or bang their head against the floor, hoping that this will gain them the attention they seek. The wisest way of responding to these stress-coping behaviors is to ignore them; otherwise the technique is reinforced. These and other infantile ways of relieving stress ordinarily give way to more socially acceptable stress-reducing behaviors as children develop.

Schools can assume an important role in helping young people cope with the stresses of life. In fact, many educators consider this to be a basic function of education on all levels. Primary grade teachers, for instances, recognize the need for their pupils to develop attitudes of respect for others. Considerable emphasis is given to sharing, being polite, and respecting the rights of classmates. Though most children negotiate this critical period in their social and emotional development, they often encounter considerable emotional stress in the process. Most of this anxiety stems from their transformation from a self-centered being to one who recognizes and respects the needs of others. As a matter of fact, the school age child is exposed to considerable stress as a consequence of both normal human development and the school itself.

STRESS IN THE CLASSROOM

In spite of the widely acknowledged belief among educators that the initial five years of life are most important to the child's total development, the years between six and twelve are critical in their own right. These are the middle years during which children progress through the elementary grades and prepare for life as responsible adults. To the casual or uninformed observer, the transition from early childhood to adolescence may appear uneventful and orderly. However, the developmental demands of these middle years are the source of stress to virtually all children. Included among the developmental tasks that much be negotiated during this period of life are the following:

1. Control and expression of emotions in socially acceptable ways
2. Development of fundamental intellectual skills (e.g., reading, calculating)
3. Development of positive self-attitudes and successful interactions with peers
4. Growth in autonomy and independence
5. The emergence of a sense of values, conscience, and moral standards
6. Ability to deal with abstract concepts such as truth, honesty, and justice
7. Increasing skills in dealing with anxiety and conflict

For the child first entering school there is no greater demand than that of adjusting to the impersonality of a strange new world. Accustomed to special status in his immediate family, he is suddenly thrust into a group where he has little identity, save a name tag pinned to his shirt. Unlike his out-of-school playmates, the members of this new group are not of his own choosing. Instead of his mother who lovingly met his every need, a new adult has taken her place for several hours a day. He soon discovers that his teacher shows none of the preferential treatment he received at home, but instead treats him no differently from the other children. Little wonder that the first few days in school are characterized by tear-filled eyes, perplexed little faces, withdrawal, and common manifestations of stress. Mere attendance at school is, therefore, anxiety producing, for it marks the first time that many children have been separated from their mothers for extended periods of time. Yet, the discomfort that the child experiences and eventually overcomes is only the first of many steps toward reducing dependency on the home and family. Thus, the stress resulting from impersonality upon entering school serves a useful purpose, even though it is a source of concern to the child.

> Although the child entering school at five or six must relinquish the close affectional relationships with his mother, he can do this without damage if he can replace it with a warm, friendly relationship to a respected adult who will respect him, treat him with the dignity to which he aspires, and enable him to accept a less personalized relation of pupil to teacher and nonsibling peers. Because the school may be the child's first experience with impersonality, it is possible that a school not attuned to his needs may develop in him patterned ways of dealing with the nonpersonal world he senses by adapting repressive impersonality that may easily become a lifelong mode of behaving toward others.[21]

Impersonality in the classroom is usually a temporary source of stress as most children manage to cope with their new situation long before the end of the first year at school. Once he is over this initial emotional hurdle, the child's experiences with school-related stress are not ended. Four general sets of conditions will account for much of the stress he will face during his

21. J. Connor, "The Teacher in a World of Increasing Impersonal Relations," in *Mental Health and Achievement,* eds. E. Torrance and R. Strom (New York: John Wiley & Sons, 1965), p. 177.

remaining school years. Alexander has described these as "(1) conflict conditions, which result because expected standards are not met; (2) socioeconomic conditions, which have an unfavorable effect on various aspects of development; (3) institutional conditions, which prevent normal acquisition of experience; and (4) traumatic conditions, which impair psychological development by causing continuing anxiety."[22]

Conflict conditions The anxiety-producing state resulting from the opposing nature of two or more motives or drives is known as conflict. In Freudian terms, conflict exists when unconscious id drives are in opposition to ego and superego demands. The child whose instinctive id forces demand aggression, for instance, experiences conflict because he has learned at home and in school that such behavior is unacceptable. Rather than focus on specific situations that are compatible with any given personality theories, the present discussion is concerned with three general categories of conflict situations, all of which affect school age children.

Approach-avoidant conflicts are encountered when a motive or behavior has both positive and negative implications. The third grade boy who enjoys school and is highly motivated to achieve knows that he will gain recognition and approval from his teacher and parents for his high level of performance. However, in gaining this desired adult approval, he realizes that he must face the risk of peer rejection. This is not uncommon on the elementary level, where some boys tend to equate high achievement in school with femininity. What children do not realize and need help in understanding is that it is possible to maintain positive peer group relationships while excelling in their schoolwork.

Double approach conflicts occur when one is forced to make a choice between two equally appealing courses of action. This dilemma is less threatening than approach-avoidant conflicts but, even so, is capable of causing considerable stress. Situations of double approach occur, for example, when a child is presented two positive options and is forced to select one, knowing full well that his choice will automatically eliminate the other option. Teachers who are tuned in to the needs of youngsters realize how important conflicts of this type are to child development. When faced with double approach conflicts, pupils begin to realize the importance of assessing options realistically and making sound choices. More important, these choice-making opportunities contribute to the self-discipline that is required to make the best of one's decisions, regardless of the outcome.

Stress that is created when one must select between two equally undesirable choices is the result of double avoidant conflict. The sixth grade boy who is openly challenged to an afterschool fight by the largest boy in his class knows that if he ignores the challenge his friends will call him "chicken." Yet, he fully realizes that if he agrees to fight he will be mauled by the stronger, more skillful challenger. Stress results from the conflict between the motive to preserve his image among his peers and his need to protect himself from certain physical harm. He must either fight or retreat, and in either case, his choice is most unpleasant. One of the few certainties of life is that stress will occasionally be encountered, regardless of what one might attempt to avoid it. Children in particular, because of their limited

22. T. Alexander, *Children and Adolescents: A Biocultural Approach to Psychological Development* (New York: Atherton Press, 1969), p. 287.

repertoire of stress-coping behaviors, need understanding and support in developing techniques of facing stress that are self-enhancing and socially acceptable.

Socioeconomic conditions   Recent progress notwithstanding, most public schools remain essentially middle-class institutions staffed predominantly by faculties and administrators with a middle-class philosophy and providing educational experiences that are most meaningful to middle-class children. There is a plethora of evidence suggesting that children from minority groups and poor families are likely to be poorly prepared to enter and progress in schools with this orientation.

> In general, children and young people who come from poverty backgrounds tend to do less well in school and on intelligence tests, as we have noted. Preschool learning conditions leave many poor children unprepared for entrance into kindergarten or elementary school since the expectations of educators are usually founded upon middle-class norms. Educators, for example, rely heavily on verbal skills, which are not highly valued in disadvantaged homes. Unable to cope with the demands made upon them, many disadvantaged children develop negative feelings toward the school. The fact that schools have not successfully met the challenge of educating such children is indicated by the large numbers of poor children who lag further behind their more affluent counterparts as they advance into higher grades.[23]

In addition to the likelihood of being handicapped in approaching school tasks requiring basic cognitive abilities, disadvantaged children are too frequently handicapped by feelings of inadequacy and depressed self-concepts that are reinforced in many school settings. Not infrequently these children are ridiculed by peers because of their untidy or poor physical appearance as well as because of the difficulty they face in understanding and accepting the new demands of their new environment. Consequently, they may find it difficult to establish group affiliations and friendships that aid in identifying with school. The families of some of these youngsters are quite transient, a factor that further contributes to the difficulty faced in identifying with peers and gaining satisfaction from school. As a rule, parents of disadvantaged pupils show the same tendency as their children in not being able (or willing) to identify with the school. This explains, at least in part, their limited interest in school affairs and their relative disregard for high academic performance. Finally, but certainly not the least significant of the stress factors that socioeconomically deprived children face in schools, is the fact that too many teachers consider them not merely as "different" children, but also as "inferior" children. Where this prejudice exists, it is understandable why poor and minority group pupils are discouraged and frustrated by their school experience.

The foregoing discussion is not intended to suggest that nonmiddle-class individuals should commit themselves to the middle-class life-style. They know from bitter experience that hard work and adherence to pre-

23. Joint Commission, *Crisis in Child Mental Health*, p. 195.

vailing societal patterns have not succeeded in removing them from the poverty-discrimination cycle that has possessed their lives. That schools and other institutions must change in order to respond to this clientele is abundantly clear.

> It would be a mistake, however, to assume that what is required to meet the educational needs of the disadvantaged child is simply more of what has traditionally been provided the average middle- and upper-class child. Certainly, the disadvantaged child, like all children, needs decent physical surroundings and educational facilities, and dedicated, skillful teachers. But he also needs new and imaginative kinds of approaches to education and curricular development; to vocational, social and personal guidance; and to community involvement with the schools. All of these things are necessary, not merely to help the disadvantaged child to compensate for his general academic deficiencies, as judged by traditional measures of performance, but also to respond to his specific life problems and, it should be added, to take maximum advantage of his particular assets and aptitudes, whether they fit traditional middle-class patterns or not. After all, not all of the characteristics of the disadvantaged child represent liabilities, even when these characteristics may pose difficulties within the framework of traditional middle-class oriented educational systems.[24]

Institutional conditions   A third category of stress conditions for children is comprised of factors directly or indirectly related to the organization and operation of the school itself. Naturally, these conditions, above all others, are the ones that professional educators have an opportunity to preserve, modify, or eliminate, depending upon their awareness of them and their influence on learning.

Adult expectations—Not infrequently, parents encourage their offspring to establish goals that they cannot possibly attain. Teachers, it must also be noted, occasionally set pupil goals that are quite unrealistic in terms of the physical and intellectual capabilities of their pupils. One commonly observed tendency is for teachers and parents to view children as miniature grown-ups, fully expecting from them behavior they are incapable of performing. When placed in this position and when they believe they have failed to live up to the expectations of the significant adults in their lives, children feel guilty. These feelings of guilt create anxiety for the youngster because he is not prepared to cope with the situation. Similarly, expectations that are unreasonable in the opposite direction and therefore fail to challenge a child's intellect, imagination, or creative ability are capable of producing stress. Teachers should not always be singled out as the sole cause of unchallenging educational experiences for their pupils. Overcrowded classrooms, inadequate learning resources, and restrictive school philosophies and policies may militate against the type of challenging experiences that teachers realize some of their children need.

24. P. Mussen, J. Conger, and J. Kagen, *Child Development and Personality*, 3rd ed. (New York: Harper & Row, 1969), p. 567.

Competition—Traditional classroom competition is too frequently a source of ego-damaging stress for the school child. Typically, competition is viewed as a process where different individuals strive to outdistance each other in striving for the same objective or to achieve the same objective more efficiently than their competitors. When overemphasized or engaged in on unequal bases, competition may lead to unfortunate consequences.

> Those who argue for inclusion of competitive grading at the elementary level insist that such preparation is necessary for the type of life one can expect to encounter in our society. This misguided premise fails to consider the fact that competition can occur only within a range of uncertainty, that is, the range in which both success and failure are possible. Competition cannot occur where each participant does not have a chance, where the outcome of victory or defeat is predetermined. It is to be noted that life's competitive situations are chosen where one perceives the possibility of success. "Competition" so-called in school is hardly chosen by children but is forced upon them by compulsory school laws, anxious parents, and ill-trained teachers.[25]

When competing individuals possess different learning abilities and show wide variations in physical and psychological capabilities, the competition is clearly unfair. Classroom grouping of pupils is one popular method of creating more equal and beneficial learning experiences. Traditional methods of class grouping of children by chronological age foster wide developmental discrepancies that make for unfair competition and unnecessary stress. All five- or six-year-olds, for instance, are simply not equally ready to enter school. Many children exhibit readiness for school at a younger age. For this reason, some educators have suggested that other developmental ages (e.g., physical, social, emotional) are more appropriate criteria for school entry and grade level placement. To date, these recommendations have received only limited support in the educational community.

Cooperative classrooms, rather than highly competitive settings, encourage children to work together toward group objectives. Instead of being forced to do something for which he is poorly equipped, a child derives satisfaction by being able to contribute that which he is able to do well. In terms of mental health, the positive self-regard that develops from these involvements is of critical importance. When the child must face the task of developing new skills, he then has a backlog of ego-enhancing successes in cooperative group activities upon which he can depend for support. Actually, this is the essence of so-called progressive education, an approach to learning that promotes success, considers individual motivations, and permits children to progress at their own speed. Needless to say, this approach to learning is entirely compatible with the framework of mental health discussed previously in this chapter.

25. R. Strom, "School Evaluation and Mental Health," in *Mental Health and Achievement*, eds. E. Torrance and R. Strom (New York: John Wiley & Sons, 1965), p. 389.

Failure—Just as success begets success, repeated failure generates further failure. Rather than viewing new challenges with eager anticipation, the child who has repeatedly failed in school tasks develops a negative self-concept and frequently withdraws from challenging situations, certain in his own mind that he cannot cope with their demands. So widespread is this situation that some educators believe that education today is largely failure-oriented. Unable to achieve in school, many young people are forced to achieve recognition and identity through withdrawal and delinquency, rather than by feelings of self-worth and social responsibility.

> Very few children come to school failures, none come labeled failures; it is school and school alone which pins the label of failure on children. Most of them have a success identity, regardless of their homes or environments. In school they expect to achieve recognition and, with the faith of the young, they hope also to gain the love and respect of their teachers and classmates. The shattering of this optimistic outlook is the most serious problem of the elementary schools. Whatever their background, children come to school highly receptive to learning. If they then fail to continue to learn at their rapid preschool rate, we may if we wish blame it on their families, their environment, or their poverty, but we would be much wiser to blame it on their experience in school.[26]

The ages between five and ten years are thought to be critical in maintaining the confidence and motivation of youngsters. If by the fifth or sixth grade the child has experienced substantially more failure than success, it is likely that his confidence will disappear, and he will identify with failure throughout his remaining educational career. Thus the elementary years are of extreme importance, and every effort should be made to provide a positive, self-enhancing experience that allows for failure but does not make it a way of life.

Traumatic conditions   Any circumstances that threaten a child's sense of security will undermine his mental health. Strained family relationships, separation or divorce, acute or chronic illness, the presence of a newborn in the family, and loss of a loved one are common traumatic happenings that have an impact on the young. Extreme fear, regardless of its source, is also responsible for stress in this age group. Fear may be the result of factors as diverse as child abuse in the home to intimidation by a classmate. Since fear usually has its origins in conditions outside of the classroom, it is desirable for teachers' knowledge of their pupils to extend beyond their school experience .

Ideally, schools should be more concerned with the primary and secondary prevention of emotional problems than with the treatment of these disorders after they occur. Programs that strive to provide an environment

**MENTAL HEALTH
ROLE OF SCHOOLS**

26. W. Glasser, *Schools Without Failure* (New York: Harper & Row, 1969), p. 26.

which promotes the optimal personality development of all children are termed primary prevention programs. Thorpe suggests that these programs should include the following:

A *democratic philosophy of education* which reflects an atmosphere of academic freedom, initiative, and shared activity and in which pupils and teachers work together cooperatively.

Attention to physical health and growth which includes the giving of periodic health examinations, encouraging teachers to be alert for symptoms of health disability, where possible providing for the services of medical and dental specialists, protecting the child against communicable diseases, and promoting health instruction and practices.

A *comprehensive program of activities* which stresses play and recreation, a variety of scholastic endeavors, activities leading to pupil self-direction, responsibility, and resourcefulness, as well as respect for the rights and property of others, and enjoyable social participation.

Effective methods of study and work which enable the pupil to experience the satisfaction and sense of competence which the mastery of work and study responsibilities brings in its wake.

The *adjustment of tasks to levels of maturity* and to individual capacity, thus promoting the feeling of personal adequacy which comes from achieving desired goals and attaining a sense of personal security.

The *development of a wholesome attitude toward sexual relationships* as well as achieving masculine or feminine identification through healthy boy-girl relationships and association with teachers.

A *consistent and intelligent program of discipline* directed toward healthy psychological adjustment and sound efforts to guide pupils' conduct in harmony with desirable social standards and their own basic needs.

The *presence of one or more adults in whom the pupil can confide,* thus providing a "substitute parent" for the emotionally unstable pupil as well as helping him with the relief of tensions and the solution of disturbing problems.[27]

In summary, virtually everything that contributes to a first-rate educational system promotes the mental health of children and youth. Yet, in spite of our best efforts to provide schools that promote mental health, there are always some school age children who suffer emotional difficulty and therefore place additional demands on the educational system.

Secondary prevention of poor mental health involves both the early recognition of behavioral symptoms and the provision of help before serious disorders develop. Many of the early indications of emotional problems are easily recognized by astute classroom teachers. Caution is the byword in making these observations, for even highly trained observers of child behavior are careful not to base their judgments on single observations or

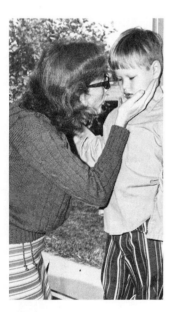

Fig. 5–4. Child mental health is promoted by teachers who are willing to "reach out" to understand their pupils. (Reprinted by permission of Illinois Department of Mental Health. Photo by Ray Armes, Jr.)

27. Louis P. Thorpe, *The Psychology of Mental Health,* Second Edition. Copyright © 1960. The Ronald Press Company, New York.

isolated episodes. Also, as was suggested earlier, one must take into account the circumstances surrounding child behavior, for these conditions often determine the extent to which behavior is indicative of normal or abnormal personality.

The Joint Committee on Health Problems in Education has developed the following guidelines for the consideration of classroom behaviors that may be indicative of early emotional difficulties:

Educational progress
> Failure to achieve in proportion to probable capacity
> Marked disparity in achievement in various areas: e.g., a unique disability or conspicuous talent in writing, spelling, reading or arithmetic as compared to achievement in other subjects
> Gradual deterioration or marked sudden drop in educational achievement
> Poor memory
> Poor retention of material apparently learned
> Poor reasoning ability
> Disorderly and careless work
> Refusal or failure to complete assignments, unrelated to ability
> Meticulous neatness and compulsive orderliness so that work is never finished to a child's satisfaction
> Lack of interest or motivation
> Intense ambition, especially if inconsistent with potential

Physical appearance
> Obesity or underweight
> Restlessness, hyperactivity
> Lethargy, sleepiness, torpidity
> Illnesses that sometimes have psychogenic components: asthma, eczema, etc.
> Poor coordination
> Shambling gait
> Poor posture
> Facial tics or other repetitive mannerisms
> Bladder or bowel control inconsistent
> Lack of personal cleanliness, disorderly appearance
> Compulsive cleanliness and neatness

Speech and language
> Lying
> Fanciful tales
> Foul language
> Disorganized, bizarre content of speech
> Stuttering
> Lisping
> Very low, very high, or very loud voice
> Indistinct speech

Social behavior
> Constant seeking for popularity

Constant seeking for attention
Withdrawal, shyness
Bizarre dress or grooming
Boisterous, noisy behavior
Behavior irritating to other children
Aggressive behavior
Cruelty
Defacement of property
Sexual aggression, exhibitionism, provocation
Immature, babyish behavior
Fearfulness
Temper tantrums
Daydreaming
Inattention
Unhappiness
Promiscuity

Personal symptoms (inward directed)
Isolation from the group
Approach to a new situation in a tense, silent manner
Conviction of inferiority or marked difference from his peers
Expectation of failure
Expectataion of rejection
Fear of loss of affection or attention
Painful confusion about what the child is doing
Unrealistic rationalizations of behavior
Preoccupation with personal problems—inward turmoil
Indications of anxiety
Inability to recognize what is expected

Violations of law
Theft in school or community
Truancy from school
Truancy from home
Fire setting
Traffic violations
Vandalism
Assault[28]

SUMMARY   The individual's state of health is mutually dependent upon both physical and mental well-being. In recent years, increased emphasis has been accorded the mental and emotional aspects of health and their influences on the total state of the organism.

In spite of difficulties encountered in arriving at a singular operational definition of mental health that is acceptable to all authorities, general

28. Joint Committee on Health Problems in Education of National Education Association and American Medical Association, *Mental Health and School Health Services* (Chicago: American Medical Association, 1965), pp. 9–10. Reprinted with the permission of the Joint Committee on Health Problems in Education of National Education Association and American Medical Association.

agreement has been reached on the components of positive mental health and their classroom implications.

Among the forces having impact upon children's mental health, stress in the school setting is of special significance. Stress of this type is usually associated with conflict conditions, socioeconomic factors, institutional forces, and various traumatic events.

Teachers' effectiveness in promoting mental health in the classroom depends upon their awareness of stress-producing situations and their ability to create an atmosphere that facilitates optimal personality development and promotes learning.

Discussion Questions

1. Support or refute the claim that the mental health of children should be a primary concern of teachers.
2. Briefly describe what is meant by the "ecology of mental health."
3. Select one of Jahoda's mental health criteria and explain how schools can encourage its development in children.
4. Explain how a given theory of personality development helps you in understanding mental health.
5. Describe several responses to ego-threat that are likely to be observed in elementary or middle-grade children.
6. React to William Glasser's assertion that American education is largely failure-oriented.
7. What innovations would you recommend for the elementary or middle grades in order to reduce the classroom stress facing socioeconomically deprived children?
8. Discuss the relative merits of competition and cooperation as techniques to encourage learning at a given grade level.

References

Alexander, T. *Children and Adolescents: A Biocultural Approach to Psychological Development.* New York: Atherton Press, 1969.

Cannon, W. *Bodily Changes in Pain, Hunger, Fear, and Rage.* 2nd ed. New York: Harper & Row, 1963.

Carroll, H. *Mental Hygiene: The Dynamics of Adjustment.* 4th ed. Englewood Cliffs, N.J.: Prentice-Hall, 1964.

Connor, J. "The Teacher in a World of Increasing Impersonal Relations." In *Mental Health and Achievement,* ed. E. Torrance and R. Strom. New York: John Wiley & Sons, 1965.

Dollard, J., and Miller, N. *Personality and Psychotherapy: An Analysis in Terms of Learning, Thinking, and Culture.* New York: McGraw-Hill Book Co., 1964.

Fromm, E. *The Sane Society.* New York: Holt, Rinehart & Winston, 1955.

Glasser, W. *Schools Without Failure.* New York: Harper & Row, 1969.

Hall, C., and Lindzey, G. *Theories of Personality.* New York: John Wiley & Sons, 1957.

Jahoda, M. *Current Concepts of Positive Mental Health.* New York: Basic Books, Inc., 1958.

Joint Commission on Mental Health of Children. *Crisis in Child Mental Health: Challenge for the 1970's*. New York: Harper & Row, 1969.

Joint Committee on Health Problems in Education of National Education Association and American Medical Association. *Mental Health and School Health Services*. Chicago: American Medical Association, 1965.

Jourard, S. *Personality Adjustment: An Approach Through the Study of Healthy Personality*. 2nd ed. New York: Macmillan Co., 1963.

Kaplan, L. *Foundations of Human Behavior*. New York: Harper & Row, 1965.

Katz, B., and Lewis, R. *The Psychology of Abnormal Behavior*. 2nd ed. New York: Ronald Press, 1961.

Lewin, K. *A Dynamic Theory of Personality*. New York: McGraw-Hill Book Co., 1935.

Menninger, K. *The Human Mind*. 3rd ed. New York: Alfred A. Knopf, 1937.

Murray, H. *Explorations in Personality*. London: Oxford University Press, 1938.

Mussen, P., Conger, J., and Kagen, J. *Child Development and Personality*. 3rd ed. New York: Harper & Row, 1969.

Riesman, D., Glazer, N., and Denny, R. *The Lonely Crowd*. New Haven: Yale University Press, 1950.

Strom, R. "School Evaluation and Mental Health." In *Mental Health and Achievement*, ed. E. Torrance and R. Strom. New York: John Wiley & Sons, 1965.

Thorpe, L. *The Psychology of Mental Health*. 2nd ed. New York: Ronald Press, 1960.

Chapter 6
THE
HEALTH
STATUS
OF
AMERICAN
YOUTH

How has the concept of health measurement changed significantly during the past several decades?

Why should teachers be concerned with the health status of their students?

How may a health problem influence a child's ability to function effectively in the classroom?

What are the educational, psychological, and social implications of certain health problems of children?

The state of health of the American people has traditionally been determined by employing indexes based upon mortality data. Crude and age adjusted death rates,[1] infant mortality rates, and expectation of life have been most widely used as measures of levels of health. Generally, a decreasing death rate has been interpreted as an indication of the increased health status of a population. However, crude and age-adjusted death rates for the American public have shown little change since 1955. Moreover, analysis of these mortality patterns indicates that mortality rates from chronic diseases and accidents are likely to sustain the death rate near its present level until major advances are made in the control of deaths from these leading killers. The stability of these indexes does not imply that there has been no change in the health status of our population since 1955. It merely serves to remind us of the problems inherent in relying upon mortality statistics to measure health status.

The World Health Organization defines health as "a state of physical, mental and social well-being, and not only the absence of disease." An examination of their definition further underscores other difficulties involved in the measurement of health. Our common indicators measure only the latter part of this definition, that is, the absence (or presence) of disease. Furthermore, reliable and valid statistical indexes are noticeably lacking in our attempts to measure mental and social well-being. Thus, we have

1. A crude death rate refers to the total number of deaths from all causes per 100,000 persons. Thus, this rate does not take into consideration the changing age patterns in a population. However, age-adjusted death rates account for the changing age distribution patterns.

tended to focus our major efforts on measuring the negative component of health (death and illness) rather than on measuring the positive side (well-being).

In recent years, however, the concept of health measurement has changed significantly. Linder discusses this emerging concept rather aptly by stating:

> There is a new interest in the total quality of life rather than merely the length of life, in the positive elements of good health rather than merely the absence of disease and infirmity. As medical science advances, moreover, it becomes increasingly pertinent to know the extent and degree to which new knowledge and techniques are being applied throughout the population. The death rate, and indeed the entire battery of vital statistics that have long been collected by the states and the Federal Government, no longer yield enough information on which to base a sound national health policy.[2]

The development and implementation of the National Health Survey by the National Center for Health Statistics introduced a new dimension into our concept of health measurement.[3] Rather than being concerned merely with the collection and analysis of disease statistics, the Center focused its attention on certain fundamental issues and questions. For example: What impact does illness and injury have on the lives of people? How much disability does ill health cause and to what degree does such disability restrict the normal activity of the individual? What do people do to seek relief from illness? How available are medical and dental care to different segments of the population? Does health and disability insurance adequately cope with the economic impact of illness? Additionally, the survey classified the data into several demographic, social, and economic characteristics in order to more fully assess the influence of race, age, sex, education, income, place of residence, and other variables upon the health status of the American public.

In 1969, the Urban Coalition Health Task Force recommended that in order to more fully assess health status and the health care needs of our population, regular data should be collected in such areas as narcotic addiction and mental retardation, lead poisoning, housing code violations, and rats and vermin, as well as on the expressed needs for medical service with regard to accessibility and personalization.[4]

In summary, one may surmise that health professionals generally feel that the economic and social consequences of health, illness, and poverty need to receive more attention in evaluation of levels of health and health problems. We cannot rely on the mere collection of death and illness statistics to fully understand our health-related problems. There is a great need for our health indicators to be viewed in close relation to economic, social, and demographic variables. For as Austin stated: "The public is becoming

2. F. E. Linder, "The Health of the American People," *Scientific American,* June 1966, p. 21.

3. Linder, *"Health of American People,"* p. 23.

4. Report of Health Task Force of Urban Coalition, "RX for Action" (Washington, D.C., 1969).

more aware of the problems of fragmentation of services, lack of continuity of care, unequal access to service, and rapidly rising costs."[5] Americans, today, consider health to be a fundamental right and not a privilege to be enjoyed solely by the wealthy.

Tremendous progress has been made in the past forty years with respect to the health conditions of infants and school age children. This is reflected in lower mortality rates as well as in changes in the leading causes of death and illness among youth. For example, in 1935 the infant mortality rate was 55.7 per 1,000 live births in contrast to 1972 when the corresponding rate was 16.7. As of 1974, the infant mortality rate had declined even further to 16.5 per 1,000 live births.[6] Of all the children who die before their first birthday, about three-fourths of whom were premature, most do not survive the first month. Approximately 95 percent of these deaths result from postnatal asphyxia, congenital malformations, and other diseases peculiar to early infancy. In addition, the mortality rates of school age children (five to fourteeen years) have declined from 150 per 100,000 in 1930 to approximately 41 per 100,000 population in 1970.[7]

The kinds of diseases that were previously reported by pediatric clinics and hospitals such as rheumatic fever, rheumatic heart disease, osteomyelitis, mastoiditis, pneumonia, streptococcal infections, meningitis, and poliomyelitis have sharply declined. The major group of illnesses that are reported by these same services today are conditions that are of prenatal origin rather than the infectious diseases. The shift is also reflected in the current leading causes of death in children, with accidents, cancer, and congenital malformations accounting for the majority of deaths. Table 6–1 compares the major causes of death by sex among school age population five to fourteen years of age.

MORTALITY OF SCHOOL CHILDREN

Table 6–1. Death and Death Rates for the Six Leading Causes of Death for School-age Children Five to Fourteen Years by Sex, 1970

	Male		Female	
Cause of Death	Number	Rate per 100,000 Population in Age Group	Number	Rate per 100,000 Population in Age Group
1. Accidents	5,695	27.4	2,508	12.5
2. Malignant neoplasms	1,389	6.7	1,040	5.2
3. Congenital malformations	481	2.3	420	2.1
4. Influenza and pneumonia	327	1.6	324	1.6
5. Homicide	215	1.0	145	0.7
6. Diseases of heart	182	0.9	162	0.8
All causes	10,491	50.5	6,356	31.8

Source: Adapted from U.S. National Center for Health Statistics, Facts of Life and Death, 1974, p. 34.

5. C. J. Austin, "Selected Social Indicators in the Health Field," American Journal of Public Health 61, no. 8 (1971): 1507.

6. U.S., Department of Health, Education, and Welfare, Monthly Vital Statistics Report: Provisional Statistics, vol. 23, no. 12, HRA 75–1120 (Rockville, Md.: National Center for Health Statistics, 1973), p. 3.

7. U.S., Department of Health, Education, and Welfare, Monthly Vital Statistics Report: Summary Report, vol. 22, no. 11. HRA 74–1120 (Rockville, Md.: National Center for Health Statistics, 1974), p. 5.

The progress in child health over the past several decades has resulted from a multiplicity of factors such as the improvement of environmental sanitation, the development and application of new antibiotics and immunization agents and diagnostic and surgical techniques, the availability and utilization of health services, and the implementation of health education programs. The continuing National Health Survey will undoubtedly provide further insight into the health of school age children and provide youth workers with continuing data on children's illness, hospitalization and medical and dental care, as well as on other related health matters.

ACUTE CONDITIONS AMONG SCHOOL CHILDREN

The National Health Survey found that there was a high incidence of acute illness among children.[8] Children between six to sixteen years of age experienced a rate of about 2.5 episodes a year of acute illness per person. Respiratory conditions were the chief cause accounting for approximately 61 percent of all acute illness. These acute conditions resulted in an average of 4.4 days lost per child from the classroom during the school year. Studies relative to the cause of absenteeism in school vary in their findings, but typically figures such as those shown in figure 6–1 have been reported in the literature. School administrators generally report 4 to 5 percent of their total enrollment as being absent each day. Epidemics of measles have at times raised the daily absenteeism principally in the primary grades to as high as 50 to 75 percent.

Fig. 6–1. Days lost from school associated with acute conditions among children six to sixteen years of age per year by condition group. (Adapted from U.S., Department of Health, Education, and Welfare, *Acute Conditions, Incidence and Associated Disability, United States, July 1972–June 1973,* Government Printing Office, 1975, p. 18.)

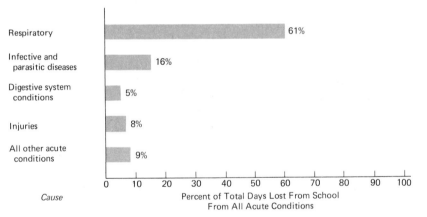

CHRONIC CONDITIONS AMONG SCHOOL CHILDREN

For children under seventeen years of age, approximately fourteen million chronic conditions are reported annually, with about one out of five children reporting at least one chronic condition. Table 6–2 summarizes the prevalence rates for chronic conditions among children. Hay fever, asthma, and other allergic conditions, as well as sinusitis, bronchitis, and other respiratory diseases, were found to account for almost half of all the chronic conditions reported in the National Health Survey. However, the Survey also disclosed that of the total fourteen million children with chronic disorders only six out of ten had received medical attention within the pre-

8. U.S., Department of Health, Education, and Welfare, Health Resources Administration, *Acute Conditions: Incidence and Associated Disability, United States, July 1972–June 1973* (Washington, D.C.: Government Printing Office, 1975), p. 19.

Table 6–2. Prevalence Rate for Selected Chronic Conditions Reported in Children Under the Age of Seventeen Years

Chronic Condition	Rate per 1000 Children
Hay fever, asthma, and other allergies	74.3
Sinusitis, bronchitis, and other respiratory diseases	34.2
Paralysis and orthopedic impairments	26.3
Hearing impairments	06.5
Speech defects	08.8
Heart disease	04.2

Source: Adapted from U.S., Department of Health, Education, and Welfare, Public Health Service, *Health of Children of School Age* (Rockville, Md.: National Center for Health Statistics, 1964), p. 4.

vious year, while 28 percent had not received such attention for more than a year, and 10 percent had never sought medical attention.

Higher prevalence rates of chronic illness were reported for children in higher income families than for those in lower income families. This finding probably can be accounted for as the result of more frequent physician visits and the greater financial access to medical care by the high-income group, thereby having specific chronic health conditions verified by clinical examination. On the other hand, the serious and visible chronic health problems such as paralysis, blindness, speech defects, and orthopedic impairments were more prevalent among the lower income groups.

HANDICAPPING CONDITIONS

Although precise figures are not available on the number and variety of handicapping conditions found in school age children, various estimates have been reported by the Children's Bureau. Table 6–2 illustrates the estimated prevalence of children in our population who have handicapping conditions. Stewart suggested that at least one-third of these handicapping conditions could be prevented or successfully corrected by comprehensive medical care prior to age six years and that continuing care up to age eighteen years would prevent or correct 60 percent of these conditions.[9]

While morbidity surveys such as the National Health Survey and others possess certain limitations with respect to the validity and reliability of the data, nevertheless, they do provide valuable information on the health status of our population by which health professionals may formulate priorities for planning and evaluating our health programs. Furthermore, the inherent implications that may be suggested by the analysis of the data in these surveys aid in understanding the strengths and weaknesses contained within our child health care system. As Haggerty so aptly stated:

> In summary, the strengths of the present health care system for children in the United States are, for the advantaged: (1) combined curative-preventive services, (2) continuity from office to hospital, (3) free choice from reasonably well-trained pediatricians, and (4) the high degree of technical skill of subspecialists providing care for rare diseases in the hospital . . .
> The most important major weaknesses of the health care of

9. W. H. Stewart, "The Unmet Needs of Children," *Pediatrics* 39 (1967): 157–160.

children in the United States are: (1) inadequate care for the disadvantaged, (2) manpower problems, (3) increasing costs, and (4) lack of knowledge of diseases and lack of prompt application of what knowledge we have.[10]

SELECTED MAJOR HEALTH PROBLEMS OF CHILDREN

It is not our intention to describe in detail all of the health-related conditions and problems that afflict children. However, we have selected certain major health conditions that we feel are of importance to elementary teachers in aiding them to understand the more common health problems that they will most likely observe in their classrooms. Elementary teachers are in a strategic position for making health observations as they see the child daily over a considerable part of the school year. Therefore, they are in a unique position to detect deviations from normal with respect to the child's health and behavior. What the teacher detects and does about these observations may significantly influence a child's progress and adjustment in the classroom. The importance of teacher observation in the health appraisal process will be more fully discussed in chapter 8.

DENTAL PROBLEMS AND DENTAL HEALTH

Dental health is a significant part of every child's total well-being. There are instances where deviations in dental health are closely interrelated with other factors affecting growth and development of children. The association of poor dental health with sickle cell disease and abnormalities in the eruption of teeth in children with cleft palate and other facial defects have been well documented.[11] Furthermore, a child in school who has a toothache or some other dental problem may be irritable, inattentive, and disinterested in classroom activities until he receives relief from the condition.

Dental abnormalities including caries (dental decay) make up the single most common health problem of children and adults. The average child at age five years has 0.36 carious teeth; at age ten years, five carious teeth; and by age fifteen years he has eleven carious teeth. About 100 million adults have at least half of their teeth either decayed, missing, or filled, and various estimates report that about 20 percent of the adult population are completely without teeth. The onset of poor dental health often begins in early childhood, with poor dental hygiene being practiced in combination with poor diet and failure to receive adequate dental care.

The National Health Survey has indicated that 86 percent of white and 94 percent of nonwhite children under age five years have never visited a dentist.[12] Whereas in the age group five to fourteen years, 80 percent of the whites but only 46 percent of nonwhites have had some dental care. Dental care was also shown to bear a relationship to family income. In families with income under $2,000, 58 percent of the children in the age group five to

10. R. J. Haggerty, "Present Strengths and Weaknesses in Current Systems of Comprehensive Health Services for Children and Youth," *Supplement to American Journal of Public Health* 60, no. 4 (1970): 77–78.

11. J. B. Richmond, and L. Weinberger, "Program Implications of New Knowledge Regarding the Physical, Intellectual, and Emotional Growth and Development and the Unmet Needs of Children and Youth," *Supplement to American Journal of Public Health* 60, no. 4 (1970): 34.

12. U.S., Department of Health, Education, and Welfare, Children's Bureau, *The Nation's Youth,* Publication no. 460 (Washington, D.C.: Government Printing Office, 1968), p. 43a.

fourteen years had not been to a dentist, but for the same age group in families with an income of $10,000 and over, only 6 percent had not been to a dentist. Thus, as was also noted in chapter 2, the child living in a poverty environment is much less likely to receive dental care than his more affluent peers. When the child of poverty does receive dental care, he is much more likely to be treated by extractions than by the filling of cavities due to the total neglect of his dental health.

The efficacy of fluoridated water supplies in the prevention of caries has been amply determined. Most studies indicate that children who have consumed fluoridated water from birth through the developmental period of their teeth will experience a reduction in dental decay by as much as 65 percent in comparison to those children residing in communities that do not have a fluoridated water supply. Community water fluoridation reduces the cost of dental care for children by lowering the hazard of tooth loss as well as by keeping the cost of dental treatment at a sufficiently low level, thereby making it possible for families to maintain optimum dental health.

Teachers should be alert to obvious indications of poor dental hygiene. Any child with grossly neglected teeth should be referred for dental examination and treatment. Some school systems employ dental hygienists who work under the supervision of a dentist and assist the classroom teacher in the total dental health education program. Teachers should also promote positive dental health by encouraging children to take care of their teeth through controlling plaque properly, brushing, eating nutritious foods, and having regular dental examinations.

NUTRITIONAL PROBLEMS

Hunger and malnutrition exist widely in many areas in the United States.[13] Undoubtedly, many of the estimated 27 million persons living under poverty conditions are financially unable to purchase adequate nutritious foods. Inadequate nutrition may lead to poor physical growth, impaired ability to learn, as well as to needless discomfort and distress. Furthermore, as noted earlier, a hungry child in the classroom is not likely to be overly receptive to or interested in the educational activities enjoyed by his well-fed peers.

It seems paradoxical that hunger and malnutrition should exist in a prosperous nation. Millions of Americans are simply too poor to feed their families properly. A sufficient income for food, however, is not the only answer as people must be educated in the selection of proper foods. Poor and nonpoor alike must be reminded that a proper diet is a basic determinant for maintaining adequate health status. President Nixon in his opening remarks before the White House Conference on Food, Nutrition, and Health stated:

> We see, then, that the problem of hunger and malnutrition is, really, two separate problems. One is to ensure that everyone is able to obtain an adequate diet. The second is to ensure that people actually are properly fed, where they have the ability to obtain the adequate diet. On the one hand, we are dealing with problems of income distribution. On the other hand, with problems of education, habit, taste, behavior, person preferences—

13. *White House Conference on Children: 1970; Report to the President* (Washington, D.C.: Government Printing Office, 1971), p. 160.

the whole complex of things that lead people to act the way they do, to make the choices they do.[14]

Nationwide concern over the nutritional status of school children has been increasing. Consequently many communities have since initiated studies to determine the nutritional status of their children. One such representative study conducted in Baltimore, Maryland, involving 59,000 school children in grades one to three found that 40.7 percent of the children from low-income families had iron deficiency anemia.[15] Furthermore, undernutrition was observed among the children in the lowest school grades. Of serious concern are the undetected detrimental effects that undernutrition plays on the learning ability, mental capacity, and behavior of these school children.

Nutritional studies have also focused on the problem of overnutrition with respect to the presence of obesity in children. Huenemann in her survey of California teenagers found that 6 percent of the boys and 5 percent of the girls in her sample were obese as determined by body fat content.[16] Other findings indicated that the obese children consumed less food, their diets were lower in nutrient value, and they were much more likely to skip meals and to snack less frequently than the nonobese children. Most characteristic, however, was the finding that obese children while eating less than their normal peers were also relatively physically inactive.

Findings from a study conducted at the University of Washington indicate that the control of excessive weight gain during infancy and childhood might help prevent overweight during adolescence.[17] Furthermore, it was observed that obese children had been introduced to solid foods earlier in infancy than those of normal weight, and many of the parents of obese children reported using food as a reward for acceptable behavior in their children.

Obesity may be influenced by the presence of a genetic factor. Although there is insufficient evidence to properly assess the exact role that a genetic factor may play in obesity, accumulating evidence tends to indicate that a hereditary factor does exist.[18, 19]

It is apparent that psychological, cultural, genetic, familial eating patterns, physical activity, and dietary practices all exert some influence in the development of childhood obesity. To criticize a child by saying that "he is fat because he eats too much" may indeed be erroneous. The relative importance of each of the ecological factors in producing childhood obesity must be determined on an individual basis.

14. *White House Conference on Food, Nutrition, and Health* (Washington, D.C.: Government Printing Office, 1970), p. 8.

15. J. B. Saratsiotis, and J. Gordon, "Nutritional Status of Primary School Pupils in Baltimore," *HSMHA Health Reports* 86, no. 4 (1971): 305.

16. R. L. Huenemann, "A Study of Teenagers: Body Size and Shape, Dietary Practices and Physical Activity," *Food and Nutrition News* 37, no. 7 (1966): 4.

17. "Overfeeding in Infancy Seen Factor in Adolescent Obesity," *Pediatric Herald*, September–October 1971.

18. "Obesity in Some People May Be Inherited," *HSMHA Health Reports* 80, no. 2 (1971): 131.

19. P. S. Peckos, "The Teenage Obesity Problem—Why?" *Food and Nutrition News* 42, no. 506 (1971): 1.

Comprehensive health education programs in elementary and secondary schools offer an excellent opportunity to make nutrition education available to all children. Health education programs provide the opportunity for making nutrition education exciting and relevant to the needs and interests of school children. Learning experiences can be arranged so that a progression occurs from the simple to the complex, permitting the student to gradually evolve his own ideas and concepts. Many of the same subject topics can be found in the different grade levels, but the learning experiences should be geared to the abilities and needs at each level in order to avoid repetition of identical experiences and to provide for increased depth of understanding and potential for application to one's daily living. For example the New York State Curriculum Guide contains the following statement:

> . . . students through the grades can develop the idea of nutrition as a part of the total interaction of man with his environment. In the early elementary grades, children can find out that people eat many kinds of foods. Older elementary pupils can study the role of food in the history of man—its effects on politics, war, revolutions, exploration. They can explore some of the factors which determine what people eat. In junior high school, students can delve into some of the factors which affect nutritional health—including the availability of food, enrichment and fortification programs, advertising, and the propaganda of the food faddist. In senior high school, students can explore the problems of malnutrition in developing countries and in the United States; and they can evaluate programs which attempt to improve the nutritional health of people.[20]

The nutritional status of children should be very much the concern of not only the parents, but also of the classroom teacher. A child's diet is crucial to growth and development. Teachers can help by developing meaningful educational programs and learning experiences. Furthermore, teacher-nurse and teacher-parent conferences can be valuable in helping to understand and deal with individual nutritional problems in the classroom.

SKIN CONDITIONS

Rashes, blisters, and sores are very common among elementary school children. Some skin conditions may be contagious, be indicative of a communicable disease, be due to an allergy, or be an indication of poor nutritional status.

Scabies is a highly infectious skin disorder caused by a small parasite, the itch mite, which travels in the skin, forming burrows about 1/8 inch in length. The skin eruptions are found most frequently between the fingers and on the forearms but may involve the entire body. Marked itching is typical of the disorder and may be suspected by the presence of scratch marks, sores, and scabs on the body that are due to infection. Infected children should be excluded from the classroom as they may infect their class-

20. J. Sinacore, and G. Harrison, "The Place of Nutrition in the Health Education Curriculum," *American Journal of Public Health* 61, no. 11 (1971): 2288.

mates through close contact. Under proper treatment the child may return to school within two days. Unfortunately, a social problem is often involved since whenever the disease exists all members of the family need to be screened for the presence of scabies. Generally, the disorder is uncommon in families where cleanliness is stressed but at times may occur even in the best of homes. Cooperation of the family is required since clothing, bedclothes, rugs, and furniture often need to be properly cleaned and laundered.

Pediculosis (lice) is a skin disease characterized by infestation of the scalp, of the hairy parts of the body, or of clothing with adult lice, larvae, or nits (eggs). Lice are small gray insects which commonly lay their eggs in the hair, particularly at the nape of the neck and near the ears. The disease is transmitted by direct contact with an infected person or by indirect contact with their personal belongings such as clothing and headgear. Unless this condition is identified early, a child with pediculosis may infect many classmates since the disease is highly contagious. Pediculosis may be suspected when the teacher observes a child persistently scratching the head and the presence of red marks at the hairline. Closer inspection often reveals the presence of the louse itself, a grayish insect approximately 1/8 inch in length and the whitish eggs attached to the hair shaft. It has been said that "the child's head looks like someone sprinkled salt all over the scalp."

When a case occurs in the classroom, the infected child should be excluded from school, and the hair of all the other children should be examined. Effective treatment involves not only the child with pediculosis, but many times also the family since they are also likely to be infested with lice. Personal cleanliness is essential, as is the proper laundering of clothes, in order to destroy both the nits and lice. A child under treatment generally can return to school in one or two days.

Ringworm of the scalp (tinea capitis) is also highly contagious and may become epidemic among elementary school children. This particular fungus infection occurs chiefly in childhood and is rarely observed after the onset of puberty. Generally, the infection begins as a small papule (blister), spreads, and leaves scaly patches of baldness. The infected hairs become brittle and break easily. When one or more cases are detected in school, all children should be screened with a filtered ultraviolet light (Wood's light) which causes the infected hairs to emit a green fluorescence. Children with ringworm of the scalp should be excluded from school until they receive medical treatment.

Impetigo is a condition in which the staphyloccocci grow in the epidermis and form small blisters. Eventually the blisters become ulcerated and are covered with yellow crusts or scabs that characteristically expose an oozing surface. The initial infection usually occurs on the lower part of the face that is more likely to be touched or fingered by the child. Impetigo may spread rapidly among elementary school children through contaminated objects such as toys, pencils, and other items that have been touched by the infected child. Children with impetigo should be excluded from school until proper medical treatment can be obtained.

VISUAL CONDITIONS

Although the eye is anatomically nearly complete at birth, vision develops only gradually. At one year of age visual acuity is approximately 20/100; by

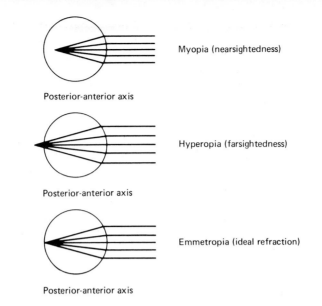

Myopia (nearsightedness)

Posterior-anterior axis

Hyperopia (farsightedness)

Posterior-anterior axis

Emmetropia (ideal refraction)

Posterior-anterior axis

Fig. 6–2. In myopia the anterior-posterior axis of the eye is too long, and the parallel light rays focus in front of the retina. In hyperopia the axis is too short: thus the parallel light rays reach the retina before coming to a focus. The emmetropic eye represents an ideal state since the parallel light rays focus directly on the retina.

two years, 20/70; and by six years, 20/20. Approximately 80 percent of children are born with hyperopia (farsightedness) and 5 percent with myopia (nearsightedness). The eyes of the newborn are normally hyperopic, and as the child grows, the eyes also grow and develop. However, some eyes do not grow enough and the hyperopia remains; some eyes grow to normal size, while others continue to grow and myopia results.

In myopia, the eyeball is too long with respect to the anterior-posterior axis. Thus, the parallel rays of light focus in front of the retina, and the resultant image is blurred (fig. 6–2). The exact cause is unknown; however, there appears to be a genetic factor involved in the condition.

Myopia appears to progress during the adolescent years regardless of the amount of close visual work performed by the child. Eye exercises and increased vitamin consumption do not improve visual acuity for the myopic child. The problem of the nearsighted child is simple. He does not see well with respect to distant vision. Since the child has good near vision, he does not have any discomfort with respect to near visual tasks. Observant teachers may notice that the child tends to squint when viewing distant objects.

In order for the child to obtain a focus on the retina, a concave lens is utilized to diverge the rays of light. This type of lens is referred to as a minus lens because it decreases the refracting power of the eye.

Hyperopia results when the eyeball is too short with respect to the anterior-posterior axis; thus the point of focus for parallel rays of light is behind the retina. In order for the child to obtain a clear image, some degree of accommodation (focusing of the eye for near vision by contraction of the ciliary body) is necessary for distant vision, and a greater amount is required for close work. Children with normal visual acuity do not have to accommodate for viewing distant objects; however, the hyperopic child must continually accommodate to obtain a correct focus. Since children have a great power of accommodation, hyperopia only presents a problem in extreme cases. If a child presents such visual symptoms as excessive blinking or rubbing of the eyes, he should be referred for an eye examination.

Strabismus or cross-eyes may be caused by hyperopia because viewing objects for close work requires convergence (bringing two eyes inward in looking at a near object) as well as accommodation. Since the hyperopic child must accommodate continuously, there is a tendency for him to over-converge. Because children are normally hyperopic, visual activities requiring close work, particularly in the lower elementary grades, should be of brief duration. This may explain in part their lack of interest in activities requiring prolonged periods of near vision.

Another refractive condition of the eye is astigmatism in which certain irregularities in the curvature of the surfaces of the cornea or lens occur. In this condition the degree of blurring will depend upon the deviation of the curvature from normal.

Sometimes a teacher may observe a child with an eye that deviates or turns inward or outward. A deviation that is apparent is referred to as a tropia, while an inapparent deviation is called a phoria. Screening tests only screen for latent strabismus or phoria. Children with strabismus suppress the image in the deviating eye so as not to see double. Consequently, vision in the unused eye may be suppressed. If suppression continues for a period of time, amblyopia (lazy-eye blindness) may result. Corrective procedures must be instituted as soon as strabismus is detected. No child should be allowed to reach school age with strabismus since the feeling of being different and the possible humiliation from the ridicule of peers may create personality difficulties.

Classroom teachers should be familiar with signs of eye difficulties in their pupils since children seldom complain of blurred or double vision. Eye difficulties should be suspected when a child exhibits one or some combination of the following symptoms:

1. Attempts to brush away a blur, frowns, or rubs the eyes excessively.
2. Shuts or covers one eye; tilts or thrusts the head forward when looking at near or distant objects.
3. Has difficulty in reading or other work requiring close use of the eyes.
4. Holds books or small objects close to the eyes.
5. Blinks more than usual or is irritable when doing close work.
6. Is unable to participate satisfactorily in games requiring distant vision.
7. Shows undue sensitivity to light.
8. Has red-rimmed, encrusted eyelids or swollen and watery eyes.
9. Complains of nausea, dizziness, or headache following close visual work.
10. Complains of pain in the eye or surrounding tissue.

Teacher observations combined with periodic screening tests for visual acuity may detect many of the common eye problems of children. When such problems do occur, they should be referred to the school nurse or other designated person in order that the necessary care for the child is undertaken.

HEARING PROBLEMS

Incidence of hearing loss in the school population has been variously estimated at from 5 to 10 percent. The great majority of these children will respond to medical treatment if the condition is detected during the early stages. Approximately 1 percent of these children will have a permanent hearing loss that will be of a handicapping nature.

The child with a handicapping hearing loss will usually have difficulty in keeping up with his peers in his schoolwork, and his lack of success may cause him to lose interest in school. Furthermore, he may be regarded as being slow, dull, or mildly retarded by his peers and the teacher. Consequently, because of his difficulties in his social relationships and school, he may exhibit antisocial tendencies and become a behavior problem.

If the hearing problem is particularly severe, his speech will almost always be affected. Thus, the hearing loss may have serious effects on the child's ability to express himself as well as produce problems in understanding and comprehending the speech of other children and adults.

The early detection of hearing impairment is important since the earlier a loss is detected, the more readily it responds to treatment and correction. School children should receive audiometric screening tests on a periodic basis to detect problems before they become chronic and irreversible.

From a medical viewpoint there are three major types of hearing impairment: poor conduction of sound to the sense organ, abnormality of the sense organ or its nerve, and hearing loss that results from some injury or failure of function in the central nervous system.

Peripheral hearing loss may be classified as either conductive, sensory-neural, or mixed. Conductive hearing loss may be caused by many factors such as impacted wax in the ear canal, congenital malformations of the ear or canal, bacterial or fungus infections of the canal, and otitis media (middle-ear infection). Generally the defect occurs in either the outer ear or the middle ear.

Loss of hearing caused by some abnormality or disease of the inner ear is referred to as a sensory-neural loss. Exposure to certain drugs, allergens, infectious agents, and noise, as well as advancing age, can lead to a degeneration of sensory cells and nerve fibers which results in a sensory-neural loss. Mixed hearing loss is a combination of conductive and sensory-neural hearing loss.

Hearing impairments that cannot be explained by abnormality of the sense organ or auditory nerve are called central hearing loss. In this broad classification the difficulty lies somewhere in the central nervous system. Many different types are included in this category such as sensory aphasia (word deafness), phonemic regression (failure to understand words), and psychogenic dysacusis (nonorganic deafness).

Conductive hearing loss if found early can often be arrested and improved. Sensory-neural hearing loss may sometimes be helped medically if it has not been present in the child for any considerable length of time. Central hearing loss requires the combined efforts of the otologist, neurologist, psychiatrist, psychologist, and educator.

In summary, only the physician can determine the cause of deafness. The teacher however should be concerned with certain signs and symptoms that may indicate hearing loss. A child may be suspected of having a hearing problem if he has any of the following symptoms:

1. Fails to respond to the calling of his name.
2. Tilts the head to one side so that the better ear is toward the speaker.
3. Frequently does not follow oral directions.
4. Mispronounces common words.
5. Requests to have words repeated or gives irrelevant answers to simple questions.
6. Speaks in a monotone, speaks too loud or soft, omits *s, sh, ch,* or *j* sounds, and/or substitutes one vowel sound for another.

The early identification of children with hearing loss of any degree and an understanding of how impaired hearing may affect a child's mental, social, and emotional well-being are fundamental to the provision of special educational services. In spite of all the efforts that may be undertaken to restore hearing to a normal level, there will always be some children who will continue to have a significant hearing loss. Generally, these children will require educational adjustments or services such as preferential seating, speech reading, auditory training, speech correction, or the use of a hearing aid. Some may also require placement in a conservation-of-hearing class or in a school for the deaf.

LEARNING DIFFICULTIES DUE TO MINIMAL BRAIN DYSFUNCTION

A child with minimal brain dysfunction (MBD) is often unable to learn in the ordinary school situation. This child often has difficulty with language, writing, reading, spelling, arithmetic, and memory. One estimate indicates that about 5 percent of American school children have learning disabilities due to slight irregularities of brain function.[21]

Children with MBD may be classified into subgroups according to the predominant symptom. Examples include hypoactive (underactive), hyperkinetic (overactive), and developmental dyslexic (language disturbed) disturbances. Often teachers may observe a child printing upside down and backward, copying symbols in reverse, or having difficulty reading and spelling simple words. Problems of a perceptual nature can often be improved and corrected with special educational and psychological help.

COMMUNICABLE DISEASES

While modern man has made considerable progress in the control of communicable diseases from a mortality point of view, much still remains to be accomplished with respect to morbidity. Table 6–3 lists reported cases of specified notifiable diseases in the United States for the year 1973.

Jekel has identified a number of ecological factors that are detrimental to our efforts in controlling communicable diseases.[22] Among the critical factors are the following: population explosion, trend toward urbanization,

21. U.S., Department of Health, Education, and Welfare, National Institutes of Health, *Learning Disabilities Due to Minimal Brain Dysfunction,* no. 71-154 (Washington, D.C.: Government Printing Office, 1973), p. 6.
22. J. F. Jekel, "Communicable Disease Control and Public Policy in the 1970's—Hot War, Cold War, or Peaceful Coexistence?" *American Journal of Public Health* 62, no. 12 (1972): 1573.

Table 6–3. **Reported Cases of Specified Notifiable Diseases in the United States, 1973**

Disease	Cases	Disease	Cases
Chicken pox	182,927	Tuberculosis (new, active cases)	32,882
Diphtheria	228		
Hepatitis, serum	8,451	Syphilis	87,469
Hepatitis, infectious	50,749	Gonorrhea	842,621
Measles (rubeola)	26,669	Poliomyelitis (paralytic)	7
Mumps	69,612		
Measles (German)	27,804	Salmonellosis	23,818

Source: Adapted from U.S. Public Health Service, *Annual Supplement to Morbidity and Mortality Weekly Report*, Atlanta: Center for Disease Control, July 1974.

increasing mobility of the population, declining levels of acquired immunity, resistance of the host to antibiotics and other drugs, new circumstances such as the purchase of pet turtles and ducks infected with *Salmonella* organisms, and apathy of the public concerning the risk of contracting communicable diseases.

Of particular concern is the declining immunization levels of children that have been observed in several studies. The United States Immunization Survey found in 1972 that only 63 percent of children age one to four years had received three or more doses of poliomyelitis vaccine.[23] Outbreaks of diphtheria and measles have occurred in many states recently due to the declining levels of adequately immunized children. Unfortunately, many parents rely on the fact that many states require children to be immunized upon entering school and wait until their children reach school age before giving them the necessary protection.

As noted earlier in this chapter, respiratory diseases including the common communicable diseases of childhood are the chief causes of acute illness in children. Diseases of the respiratory tract follow a characteristic pattern, as observed in figure 6–3.

The incubation period refers to the stage in which the pathogenic agent multiplies in the host without producing any symptoms. Generally, an infectious respiratory disease is not communicable during this period, although evidence indicates that chicken pox and measles may be transmitted to susceptible individuals during the last two or three days of its incubation stage.[24] Hence, the child may transmit these diseases to classmates while in an observable "healthy" state.

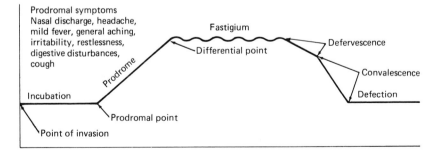

Fig. 6–3. Course of an infectious respiratory disease. (From C. L. Anderson, *School Health Practice*, ed. 5, C. V. Mosby Co., 1972.)

23. "Survey Finds Need for Emphasis on Immunization," *American Medical News*, 8 October 1973, p. 1.

24. C. L. Anderson, *Community Health*, ed. 5 (St. Louis: C. V. Mosby Co., 1972), p. 139.

The prodromal point refers to the first observable signs and symptoms in the host. Symptoms during this period are nonspecific and resemble those of the common cold, that is, watery eyes, nasal discharge, headache, and other general indications of ill health. During this stage, the child is highly communicable and from a public health point of view represents a threat to others as he is often perceived of as having "just a cold," whereas he may be spreading measles or any other respiratory disorder to susceptible hosts. The prodromal period lasts for one or two days, terminating at the differential point where specific signs and symptoms appear indicating a specific disease. For example, in measles rubeola, the child may exhibit a fever, have inflamed eyes, and have Koplik's (white) spots on the buccal mucosa inside his mouth. This is the point at which a physician can make a specific diagnosis.

During the fastigium the disease is at its height, and the body is mobilizing its full powers to fight the infection. Even though the disease is highly communicable during this period, the child is generally restricted to bed and only exposes those individuals who are serving his nursing needs.

In the defervescence period the severity of the disease begins to decline. Secondary complications such as pneumonia may arise because his body defenses have been weakened by fighting the original infection.

Convalescence refers to the recovery period, and defection represents the stage in which the child has cast off the organisms. Both of these stages may overlap to some degree.

Appendix A contains a summary of communicable diseases for teachers which gives early signs and symptoms, incubation period, method of transmission, control of cases, and other information concerning diseases of significance to school age children.

SELECTED CHRONIC DISEASES

While many chronic diseases could be selected for inclusion in a textbook for elementary teachers, we decided to delimit this section to sickle cell anemia, epilepsy, and cystic fibrosis because of interest expressed by former elementary majors in these particular disorders. Individuals interested in other chronic disorders may refer to appropriate health education textbooks.

SICKLE CELL ANEMIA

This particular disorder is a hereditary blood disease caused by abnormal hemoglobin in the red blood cells. The defect lies in the hemoglobin molecule in which one amino acid, valine, is substituted for another, glutamic acid, causing the hemoglobin molecules to become rigid and assume a sickled appearance. Rather than possessing the normal disc shape, the red cells of individuals with this disease have distorted sickle or crescent shapes when their oxygen supply becomes low.

Sickle cell anemia is presently an incurable illness which may be serious at any age and is often fatal during childhood. Typically, symptoms begin to appear between the ages of two and four years. Signs and symptoms such as colic, distention of the abdomen, poor appetite, frequent illnesses and infections, pains in the joints, and anemia may occur. Unfortunately these symptoms are often associated with other illnesses and may not be recognized as signs of sickle cell anemia.

During the acute sickle cell attack (crisis), the cells take on their crescent shape and begin to cluster in some of the capillaries, causing blood clots to form. This can be very painful to the patient and may serve as a forerunner to serious complications that may result in death. Blood clots that form in the lungs, kidneys, and brain may be quite serious. Infections such as a sore throat or cold as well as oxygen deprivation following exercise may trigger an acute crisis.

The hereditary transmission of sickle cell anemia is similar to that of other autosomal recessive traits. If both parents possess a trait (carriers), the children born to such parents have a one in four chance of having sickle cell anemia, one in two of being a carrier, and one in four of having neither the trait nor sickle cell anemia.

In the United States, the sickle cell trait has been reported to be found in approximately 7 to 13 percent of the black population in different geographic areas of the country. Sickle cell anemia is estimated to affect about 25,000 to 50,000 persons. Individuals who are carriers for the trait are generally unaware that they have abnormal hemoglobin since it rarely produces a problem except under unusual circumstances such as flying in unpressurized aircraft, diving to deep underwater areas, undergoing anesthesia, or living in extremely high altitudes.

Teachers should be aware of the fact that children with sickle cell anemia may be absent from school for prolonged periods because of repeated crises. In school, these children often fatigue more easily and may not be able to engage in activities of a strenuous nature. Alert teachers should also recognize that children with sickle cell anemia will require special attention and encouragement to foster successful school performance.

EPILEPSY

The word *epilepsy* stems from the ancient Greek word for seizure. Epilepsy, however, is not a disease but is a symptom of some underlying pathological condition that exists within the central nervous system. The seizure itself is produced by a chemical disturbance in the brain wave pattern observed on the electroencephalogram (EEG).

Various estimates by voluntary and professional associations suggest that there are approximately two million persons with epilepsy in the United States, with about one in fifty children being afflicted. The exact number is difficult to determine since often parents themselves are unaware of the condition, particularly if their child has the petit mal or psychomotor type of epilepsy.

There are several major classifications of epilepsy. Depending upon the part of the brain in which the abnormal electrical discharge occurs, various symptoms may result. The individual may exhibit a blank stare (often mistaken for daydreaming) or rapid blinking of the eyelids that is sometimes accompanied by small twitching movements on one part of the body. Usually these signs of petit mal epilepsy last less than a minute and may occur many times during the day. In psychomotor epilepsy, the child may display inappropriate or purposeless behavior such as chewing motions or smacking of the lips.

Most commonly the child may have an epileptic seizure (grand mal epilepsy) characterized by a warning cry, unconsciousness, and some of the following signs: jerking, tongue biting, loss of bladder and bowel control, and extreme tiredness afterward.

If teachers suspect that a child in their classroom has epilepsy, it is important that they consult the health personnel in their school for appropriate action. Any child with epilepsy should be under medical supervision as most cases of this disorder can be controlled or eliminated by medication.

CYSTIC FIBROSIS

Cystic fibrosis, one of the most common chronic disorders of children, is an inherited disease that affects the exocrine or external secreting glands of the body. It is estimated that anywhere from 2 to 20 percent of the population may be carriers and that one of every 3,000 newborn infants is afflicted.

In cystic fibrosis, the mucus-producing glands produce an abnormal, thick, sticky mucus that tends to accumulate in various parts of the body and interferes with other normal body funtcions such as breathing and digestion. In addition, other abnormalities are found in the glands that secrete sweat, saliva, and tears in that their secretions contain abnormally high amounts of salt.

Most of the deaths from cystic fibrosis occur from progressive damage to the respiratory system. Colds and other respiratory diseases pose a considerable threat to the child. About 20 percent of the afflicted children are now surviving to adolescence. Hopefully with our advancing medical knowledge of cystic fibrosis, early detection and prompt treatment of the disorder, and the development of newer drugs the outlook for afflicted children will improve in future years.

SUMMARY

In order to effectively meet the educational and health needs of children, it is essential that schools secure the necessary information concerning their physical, mental, and social condition. Teachers should assume the responsibility for knowing the health status of each pupil as revealed by inquiries of parents, pupils, and school nurses, from observation and screening by school personnel, by health examinations by medical personnel, and by familiarity with pertinent data on the child's health record. Informed teachers are in a more advantageous position to adjust the school program to the students' needs and encourage parents to obtain the necessary follow-through recommended by the physician and/or dentist and psychologist.

Discussion Questions

1. Does the World Health Organization present an adequate definition of health? What are the advantages and disadvantages of utilizing their definition?
2. What are the major causes of mortality and morbidity of school age children?
3. Discuss the various factors that have accounted for the progress in child health during the past several decades.
4. Why is dental health considered to be a part of every child's well-being?

5. Why should the nutritional status of school children be of concern to educators? to parents? to the community?
6. Discuss some of the major skin conditions that afflict school children.
7. What are some of the common visual and hearing problems of children?
8. How can a classroom teacher suspect the presence of a visual and/or hearing problem in a child?
9. What is minimal brain dysfunction? Why does a child with MBD often have difficulty with learning in the regular classroom?
10. What ecological factors appear to be detrimental in our efforts to control communicable diseases?
11. Discuss the course of an infectious respiratory disease.
12. What is sickle cell anemia? How is it transmitted? Why may a teacher need to adapt her program for children with this disorder?
13. Discuss the different types of epilepsy that occur in children.
14. What is cystic fibrosis?

References

Anderson, C. L. *Community Health,* ed. 5. St. Louis: C. V. Mosby Co., 1972.

Austin, C. J. "Selected Social Indicators in the Health Field." *American Journal of Public Health* 61, no. 8 (1971): 1507.

Haggerty, R. J. "Present Strengths and Weaknesses in Current Systems of Comprehensive Health Services for Children and Youth." *Supplement to American Journal of Public Health* 60, no. 4 (1970): 37–78.

Huenemann, R. L. "A Study of Teenagers: Body Size and Shape, Dietary Practices and Physical Activity." *Food and Nutrition News* 37, no. 7 (1966): 4

Jekel, J. F. "Communicable Disease Control and Public Policy in the 1970's —Hot War, Cold War, or Peaceful Coexistence?" *American Journal of Public Health* 62, no. 12 (1972): 1573.

Linder, F. E. "The Health of the American People." *Scientific American,* June 1966.

"Obesity in Some People May Be Inherited." *HSMHA Health Reports* 80, no. 2 (1971).

"Overfeeding in Infancy Seen Factor in Adolescent Obesity." *Pediatric Herald,* September–October, 1971.

Peckos, P. S. "The Teenage Obesity Problem—Why?" *Food and Nutrition News* 42, no. 506 (1971).

Report of Health Task Force of Urban Coalition, "Rx for Action." Washington, D. C., 1969.

Richmond, J. B., and Weinberger, L. "Program Implications of New Knowledge Regarding the Physical, Intellectual, and Emotional Growth and Development and the Unmet Needs of Children and Youth," *Supplement to American Journal of Public Health* 60, no. 4 (1970): 34.

Saratsiotis, J. B., and Gordon, J. "Nutritional Status of Primary School Pupils in Baltimore." *HSMHA Health Reports* 86, no. 4 (1971): 305.

Sinacore, J., and Harrison, G. "The Place of Nutrition in the Health Education Curriculum." *American Journal of Public Health* 61, no. 11 (1971): 2288.

Stewart, W. H. "The Unmet Needs of Children." *Pediatrics* 39 (1967): 157–160.

"Survey Finds Need for Emphasis on Immunization." *American Medical News,* 8 October 1973.

U.S., Department of Health, Education, and Welfare. Children's Bureau. *The Nation's Youth,* Publication no. 460. Washington, D.C.: Government Printing Office, 1968.

U.S., Department of Health, Education, and Welfare. Health Resources Administration. *Acute Conditions: Incidence and Associated Disability, United States, July 1972–June 1973.* Washington, D.C.: Government Printing Office, 1975.

U.S., Department of Health, Education, and Welfare. *Monthly Vital Statistics Report: Provisional Statistics,* vol. 23, no. 12, HRA 75–1120. Rockville, Md.: National Center for Health Statistics, 1973.

U.S., Department of Health, Education, and Welfare. *Monthly Vital Statistics Report: Summary Report,* vol. 22, no. 11, HRA 74–1120. Rockville, Md.: National Center for Health Statistics, 1974.

U.S., Department of Health, Education, and Welfare, National Institute of Health, *Learning Disabilities Due to Minimal Brain Dysfunction,* no. 71–154. Washington, D.C.: Government Printing Office, 1973.

White House Conference on Children: 1970; Report to the President. Washington, D.C.: Government Printing Office, 1971.

White House Conference on Food, Nutrition and Health. Washington, D.C.: Government Printing Office, 1970.

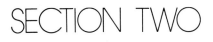

SECTION TWO   PROGRAMS OF SCHOOL HEALTH

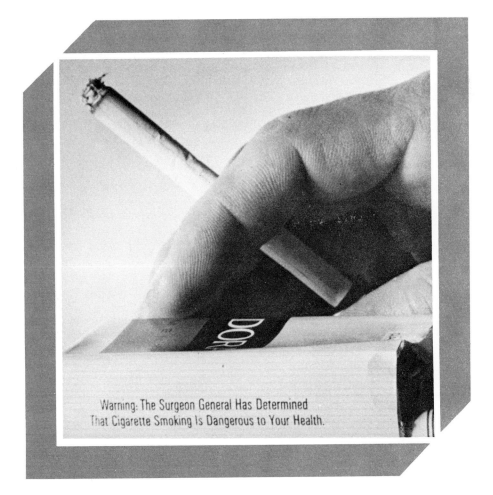

Warning: The Surgeon General Has Determined That Cigarette Smoking Is Dangerous to Your Health.

Chapter 7
SCHOOL HEALTH: RATIONALE AND ISSUES

What are generally recognized as the goals of health education?

How is the school administrator's orientation toward crises related to the importance he places on the school health program?

What are the major components of a comprehensive school health program?

What are some of the main challenges facing school health education in the 1970s?

How does the school health coordinator's role augment the efforts of classroom teachers?

School health programs are by no means a recent arrival on the educational scene. Initial concern, expressed in the early 1800s, focused on the relationships between environmental conditions in schools and the health of school children. Horace Mann, the father of American public schools, discussed school hygiene in his initial report to the Massachusetts Board of Education in 1837. Six years later, Mann recommended that elementary and secondary school curricula include instruction about physiology and hygiene. In 1850 Massachusetts became the first state to require these studies in its public schools. During the next half century, the temperance movement and developments in public health provided impetus to concern for the health of school children. Means reports that by 1890 thirty-eight states and territories had passed legislation requiring the teaching of physiology and hygiene in public schools.[1] Though these pioneering efforts were limited in many ways, they nonetheless provided a foundation for contemporary school programs.

In spite of its one-and-three-quarter-century history, school health has not developed as rapidly or as fully as one might expect. Incredible though it seems, most states have not yet established certification requirements for teachers assigned health teaching responsibilities. The obvious result of this inaction is that individuals with virtually no special preparation are pres-

1. R. Means, *A History of Health Education in the United States* (Philadelphia: Lea & Febiger, 1962), pp. 50–56.

ently teaching health in our schools. For example, in one Midwestern state, where elementary and secondary school health instruction was mandated in 1971, less than 15 percent of those teachers responsible for health instruction met what were considered minimal standards for health education. Poor teacher preparation has played no small part in the disappointing development of health education in schools. The historic School Health Education Study (SHES) gathered information on the health education experiences provided in 1,101 elementary and 359 secondary schools across the nation.[2] Levels of student health information were deficient, and a surprisingly large number of the students sampled held dangerous misconceptions regarding health. In short, the SHES research team concluded that school health education still suffered from the attitudes of benign neglect that had handicapped it for decades.

> The response by school administrators and teachers. . . . revealed a marked deficiency in the quantity and quality of health education in both the elementary and secondary schools. The problems confronting school personnel included: failure of parents to encourage health habits learned at school; ineffectiveness of instruction methods; parental and community resistance to discussions of sex, venereal disease, and other controversial topics; insufficient time in the school day for health instruction; inadequate preparation of the staff; indifference toward and lack of support for health education on the part of some teachers, parents, administrators, health officers and other members of the community; inadequate facilities and instructional materials; student indifference to health education; lack of specialized supervisory and consultative services. . . .[3]

WHAT IS HEALTH EDUCATION?

Educational experiences concerned with matters of physical and mental health are conducted in many different locations including migrant labor camps, industrial plants, outpatient clinics, and schools. Regardless of the setting in which it is implemented, the target audience, or the specific topic of concern, the basic process of health education is essentially the same. Naturally, the pedogogical method and goals will differ, depending upon these variables.

In general, professional health educators agree, at least philosophically, on the ingredients of operational definitions of health education. One group of leaders in the field has defined health education as "the process of providing learning experiences which favorably influence understandings, attitudes, and conduct in regard to individual and community health."[4]

Willgoose views health education as "the sum of experiences that favorably influence practices, attitudes, and knowledge relating to health."[5]

2. E. Sliepcevich, *School Health Education Study: A Summary Report* (Washington, D.C.: School Health Education Study, 1964).
3. Sliepcevich, *School Health Study*, pp. 42–43.
4. Joint Committee on Health Problems in Education of the National Education Association and the American Medical Association, *Health Education* (Washington, D.C.: National Education Association, 1961), p. 7.
5. C. Willgoose, *Health Education in the Elementary School* (Philadelphia: W. B. Saunders Co., 1969), p. 30.

A somewhat broader, yet compatible, description of health education has been offered by the President's Committee on Health Education. In its view, health education "embraces those processes of communication and education which help each individual to learn how to achieve and maintain a reasonable level of health appropriate to his particular needs and interests, and to be motivated to follow personal and community health practices which contribute to his state of health and well-being—a positive concept going well beyond the mere absence of disease or infirmity."[6]

For the purposes of this discussion, health education is considered as that multidimensional process designed to favorably influence the health knowledge, attitudes, and behavior of individuals and groups. Upon closer examination, this rather simplistic description of health education reveals that it is an exceedingly complex and challenging undertaking. Education about health is *multidimensional,* for at least two reasons: (1) because the health needs of any audience are seldom, if ever, explained in unidimensional terms, a point made clear in the earlier discussion of ecology and health; and (2) because a variety of educational approaches and methodologies are necessary to serve the health needs of a group. The term *designed process* is of special significance, for it underscores the fact that health teaching should be planned and purposeful, rather than haphazard and aimless. Finally, the concept that health education transcends the mere acquisition of knowledge emphasizes its ultimate concern with behavior modification. In summary, successful health education experiences are dependent upon accurate need identification, intelligent planning, use of appropriate learning experiences, and process outcomes that result in behavioral change.

Promoting the health of young people involves school activities and programs that extend beyond the traditional classroom. All of these related and mutually supportive endeavors are elements of what is generally recognized as the total, or comprehensive, school health program. It consists of three interrelated components: health instruction, healthful school living, and school health services. The first of these, health instruction, has already been described in some detail and is emphasized in chapter 10. A brief description of school health services is in order, at this point, but is discussed at length in chapter 8. This component of the total program encompasses those procedures employed by physicians, nurses, dentists, and other school health service personnel to appraise, protect, and promote optimum health of students and school personnel. The third essential ingredient of the total health program, healthful school living, is described in chapter 9. Its attention focuses on all of those environmental considerations including school safety, organization of the school day, and school sanitation that influence social, emotional, and physical health.

These three program components are delineated here solely for discussion purposes. While each consists of somewhat diverse activities and may involve different personnel, they all overlap and coordinate their efforts to prevent health problems, detect departures from sound health, and correct remediable disorders. In actual practice, all three program thrusts should

THE COMPREHENSIVE SCHOOL HEALTH PROGRAM

6. President's Committee on Health Education, *The Report of the President's Committee on Health Education* (New York: The Committee, 1973), p. 13.

be planned and implemented in a coordinated manner so that they are clearly identifiable as a single health program (fig. 7–1).

PROGRAM ADMINISTRATION

Local boards of education are responsible for the organization and administration of school health programs. In many states, legislation requires that local school districts develop health programs. Typically, these statutes suggest minimal guidelines that are well within the capability of most school systems. Unfortunately, either unintentionally or by design, too many school administrators interpret these minimal recommendations as guidelines for an optimal program of health. This posture quickly stifles the development of quality school health programs.

One would be remiss in failing to acknowledge that some school districts approach the question of a comprehensive program with vigor and enthusiasm. Almost without exception, these school systems excel in other aspects of the curriculum. As far as health is concerned, these superior systems base their programs on local need, interest, and involvement, and far surpass the minimal requirements established at the state level.

Figure 7–2 represents an effective structure for planning and conducting the school health program. The chief administrator of a school and the board of education establish school policies, including those related to the health program. Ultimate responsibility for implementing policies rests with the superintendent of schools, but is often delegated to his administrative staff and building principals.

At the administrative level, consultative services may be available from the local health department and similar community groups. For instance, the board of education or administrative council may formulate policy concerning school closure during epidemics of certain communicable diseases only after conferring with local health authorities. The input of these consultants need not be restricted to policy determination, however. Frequently they are called upon to apprise school officials of local health problems or concerns that have implications for conjoint school-community health programs.

Fig. 7–1. Comprehensive school health program.

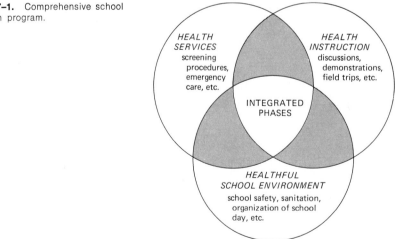

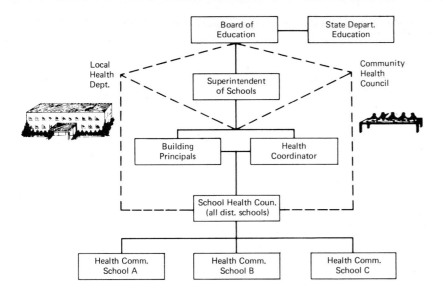

Fig. 7–2. Organization of the school-community health program.

One way to develop support and encourage input from all areas of the school system is to organize a district health council, consisting of key administrative personnel, health service representatives, teachers, curriculum specialists, and other appropriate individuals who serve as a sounding board to influence districtwide decisions and facilitate the coordination of a comprehensive effort. On an individual school basis, it is recommended that a small health committee be formed. This group provides impetus to the ongoing program while addressing itself to health concerns or issues that may be unique to their particular school.

CONCERN FOR CHILD HEALTH

No other objective of American education has been so frequently pronounced but so seldom pursued as the health of children. Philosophically, few educational leaders disagree with the claim that the health of children and youth should be a priority concern of schools. Yet, only recently have we witnessed sustained efforts by states and individual school systems to address themselves to the health needs of young people. This reluctance is difficult to explain, for concern with child health has an unusually rich heritage. While it is not our purpose to dwell upon this history, highlights of the past are useful if one is to appreciate contemporary school health programs.

Perhaps the most influential early event recognizing health as a major aim of American education was the 1918 statement of the Commission on the Reorganization of Secondary Education, a group appointed by the National Education Association.[7] Their pioneering report recognized health as one of seven major concerns of education.

In 1938, the Educational Policies Commission issued its classic statement that described the health-educated person as (1) an individual who understands the basic facts concerning health and disease, (2) one who pro-

---

7. U.S., Department of the Interior, Bureau of Education, *Cardinal Principles of Secondary Education,* Bulletin 1918, no. 35, (Washington, D.C.: Government Printing Office, 1918).

tects his own health and that of his dependents, and (3) a person who works to improve the health of his community.[8] Reaffirming its conviction that schools must be concerned with child health, the Educational Policies Commission stated, in 1959, that the elementary school curriculum should include the essentials of safety and personal health.[9] More recently, a joint committee of the National Education Association and American Medical Association adopted a resolution urging all schools to develop balanced health education programs. This position is supported by the American Academy of Pediatrics which claims that freedom from disabling disease, whether organic or psychosocial, is a major factor contributing to children's optimal school performance.[10]

The National Congress of Parents and Teachers has also been a vigorous advocate of health education in schools. In 1970, this organization once again spoke out in support of comprehensive school health programs and urged that they be given higher priority at the local, state, and national levels. Like other influential groups that are supportive of school health, the Parent-Teacher Association (PTA) has consistently pointed out that: (1) the health status of children is closely related to their receptivity to learning; (2) a child's successful health education experience will ultimately reflect upon his performance in the total school program; (3) children of school age are most receptive to educational experiences that encourage the development of positive health attitudes and behaviors; and (4) no other social institution, including the family, has assumed responsibility for a comprehensive educational program based upon child health needs and interests.

A 1974 policy statement of the American Public Health Association further indicates the importance that national authorities place on comprehensive school health education programs.

> The American Public Health Association supports the concept of a national commitment to a comprehensive, sequential program of health education for all students in the nation's schools, kindergarten through the twelfth grade.[11]

NEW IMPERATIVES FOR SCHOOL HEALTH

Modern preventive medicine including health education reflects the same basic educational commitments as those expressed by Mann and other school health pioneers. Contemporary affairs, however, have created new health issues and problems that are by-products of American life during the last half century. Many health concerns of previous years (e.g., vitamin deficiency diseases, poliomyelitis, smallpox) are of decreasing significance and

8. National Education Association and American Association of School Administrators, Educational Policies Commission, *The Purpose of Education in American Democracy* (Washington, D.C.: Educational Policies Commission, 1938).

9. National Education Association and American Association of School Administrators, Educational Policies Commission, *An Essay on Quality in Public Education* (Washington, D.C.: Educational Policies Commission, 1959).

10. American Academy of Pediatrics, *Report of the Committee on School Health of the American Academy of Pediatrics* (Evanston, Ill.: The Academy, 1966).

11. American Public Health Association, "Proposed Policy Statements," *Nation's Health* 4, no. 10 (October 1974): 10.

should not receive the instructional emphasis they once deserved. Today's health teacher is in a brand-new ball game. How effectively this contest is waged will depend greatly on the extent to which schools and individual teachers recognize contemporary health problems and accept the challenges they pose.

BIOMEDICAL REVOLUTION

Those readers born in the post-1950 era may have difficulty appreciating that we are indeed caught up in a revolution in the biological and medical sciences. New knowledge in the health sciences is accumulating at an unprecedented rate. For example, total joint replacements, organ transplantations, and other surgical procedures, considered unlikely as recently as twenty-five years ago, are rapidly becoming commonplace. The efficacy of previously unavailable therapeutic agents is demonstrated, and their benefits are quickly made available to the public.

Social welfare health programs provided by state and federal agencies are not only widely available today, but are also in a more or less constant state of flux. Researchers publish a continuous flow of findings that add to our understanding and management of health affairs.

While most Americans have benefited directly or indirectly from these and other biomedical advancements, the gains have not been without cost. One unfortunate and too-seldom recognized outcome is that an information gap has developed between health scientists and the lay public. This is a far more serious development than many are willing to admit, for the health of a nation is dependent upon more than the sophistication of its medical knowledge and hardware. Consumers who utilize much of this information and technology must be at least reasonably well informed if their involvement is to be effective. Unfortunately, efforts to keep lay people abreast of rapid changes in the health sciences have been feeble, at best. Consequently, consumers face a dilemma that complicates their health decisions

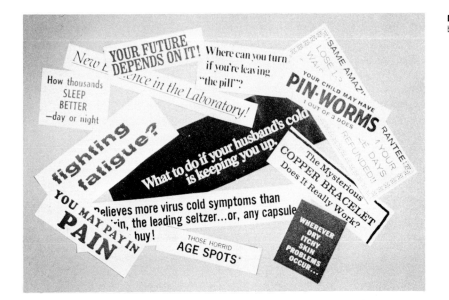

Fig. 7–3. Advertising claims can be confusing to consumers.

and often prevents them from utilizing available information and services that promote optimal health.

While mass media, advertising, and the popular press have proved effective as conveyors of health information, their role in confounding the consumer must also be recognized. Conflicting information and misleading or erroneous reports create an atmosphere of uncertainty that is difficult for the public to resolve. Education faces the task of helping individuals sift through this information to separate fact from fiction and sound health practices from fads. For without a firm foundation of sound health information, it is doubtful that consumers will share the benefits of modern health and medical sciences.

CHANGING AGE-COMPOSITION OF POPULATION

A second major development that necessitates a shift in emphasis for health education is the changing age-composition of our population. Most significant in this regard is the increasing proportion of senior Americans. One of every ten citizens is presently age sixty-five years or older. Figure 7–4 reveals the extent to which the proportion of this age group to the total population has increased in recent decades.

Gains in the control of communicable diseases that once claimed the lives of many infants and children enable more of the young to survive the early years of life and live to be old. Naturally, this trend has contributed to the increase in average life expectancy. Concomitant with this trend has been the emergence of health problems characteristic of an aging population. Cardiovascular illnesses, cancer, and chronic disablers such as arthritis have assumed greater prominence today than in former years.

Table 7–1. Leading Causes of Death by Rank in United States, 1900 and 1973

	1900				1973		
Rank	Cause of Death	Deaths per 100,000 Population	Percent of all Deaths	Rank	Cause of Death	Deaths per 100,000 Population	Percent of all Deaths
	All causes	1719.1	100.0		All causes	942.1	100.0
1	Pneumonia and influenza	202.2	11.8	1	Diseases of heart	359.5	38.2
2	Tuberculosis	194.4	11.3	2	Cancer	168.4	17.9
3	Gastritis, etc.	142.7	8.3	3	Vascular lesions of central nervous system	102.3	10.9
4	Diseases of heart	137.4	8.0	4	All accidents	54.8	5.8
5	Vascular lesions of central nervous system	106.9	6.2	5	Pneumonia and influenza	29.1	3.1
6	Chronic nephritis	81.0	4.7	6	Diabetes mellitus	17.4	1.8
7	All accidents	72.3	4.2	7	Cirrhosis of liver	16.0	1.7
8	Cancer	64.0	3.7	8	Arteriosclerosis, general	15.9	1.7
9	Diseases of early infancy	62.6	3.6	9	Diseases of early infancy	14.8	1.6
10	Diphtheria	40.3	2.3	10	Bronchitis, asthma, emphysema	14.4	1.5

Source: 1973 data: *Vital Statistics Report, Annual Summary for the United States, 1973* (HRA) 74–1120, vol. 22, no. 13 (Rockville, Md.: National Center for Health Statistics, 1974).
Note: Rates for 1900 apply to death-registration states only.

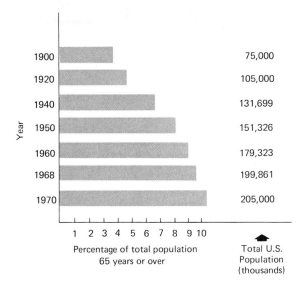

Year		Total U.S. Population (thousands)
1900		75,000
1920		105,000
1940		131,699
1950		151,326
1960		179,323
1968		199,861
1970		205,000

1 2 3 4 5 6 7 8 9 10

Percentage of total population
65 years or over

Fig. 7–4. Percentages of total United States population age sixty-five years or more for selected years.

HEALTH INSULTS

Health authorities now recognize that one's health status during childhood and adolescence is related to the health problems he will encounter in later life. Viewed as "insults" to well-being, these negative episodes (i.e., serious illnesses and injuries) appear to have a cumulative effect upon health in later life. School health programs should, therefore, show concern with the avoidance of behaviors in childhood that may lead to difficulties in adulthood.

Nutrition, physical and emotional fitness, physical trauma, and illness history during childhood are widely recognized as factors which can have great impact on the individual's adult status. For example, the American Academy of Pediatrics has reported that the salt intake of children can predispose them to high blood pressure in later life.[12] Likewise, cigarette smoking, a habit that frequently begins in the elementary grades, can develop into a lifelong habit that significantly increases the risks of lung cancer, emphysema, and cardiovascular disease during adulthood. Additional evidence has demonstrated that overweight children are more likely to become overweight adults than are their age-mates who fail to manifest this childhood tendency.

In summary, elementary and secondary schools find themselves in a unique position to encourage health practices having lifelong implications. Increasingly, educators view the school's position not simply as opportune, but as critical, since no other institution, apart from the family, devotes as much time to educating the young.

OTHER IMPERATIVES

Environmental quality, mental health, drug abuse, and sexual behavior are among the other concerns that have been surfaced, complicated, or intensified by recent social, economic, and technological trends. Seldom are the solutions to contemporary health problems simple, ready-made, or univer-

12. Committee on Nutrition, American Academy of Pediatrics, "Salt Intake and Eating Patterns of Infants and Children in Relation to Blood Pressure," *Pediatrics* 53, no. 1 (January 1974): 115–121.

sally acceptable. Clearly, the substance of modern health education is complex, dynamic, and in many instances controversial. The magnitude of the challenge notwithstanding, schools must assume increasing responsibility for helping individuals in identifying, understanding, and coming to grips with these and other emergent health concerns.

BASIC ISSUES IN SCHOOL HEALTH

Many elements of the school curriculum including health education are involved in issues that to some extent affect their status in the total school program. How relevant is a particular curriculum offering? Can a given subject be taught most effectively by traditional methods or does it lend itself to individualized instruction? Should some areas of study be afforded priority status in the curriculum?

In some instances, the views that evoke these questions and the issues they involve represent divergent philosophies. Often they reflect preferences imposed by austerity budgets, space limitations, and similar operational considerations. The issues germane to health education are neither more numerous, nor more complex than those facing other school subjects. Most of the significant health-related issues are closely related to the school's attitude or general orientation toward health instruction, curriculum saturation and scheduling, mandated programs, teacher preparation, and controversial subject matter.

CRISIS PREVENTION OR CRISIS INTERVENTION?

Health behavior and decision making are greatly influenced by one's acceptance or rejection of the belief that health problems can be averted by whatever means are available to him. This applies to individuals making daily decisions affecting their personal well-being and to institutions like the school that care about the welfare of their clients. On the one hand, there are those who become concerned about health problems only when they face a health crisis. At that point, and not until then, do these crisis-oriented individuals show concern for their plight and attempt to resolve the problem. Prior to that time they appear oblivious to or are unconcerned with health risks capable of precipitating the problem. This posture is incompatible with modern-day health education.

On the other hand, when individuals or institutions do not wait for a health crisis to develop before taking positive, preventative action, they manifest an orientation of prevention. This position characterizes the health-educated person and is based on the belief that by taking reasonable measures one may reduce the risks that might otherwise lead to health problems. This tendency to engage in risk-reduction behavior does not mean that an obsessive preoccupation with potential health threats is desirable. It does mean, however, that reasonable measures (e.g., fluoridation, annual health checkups) should be taken to promote optimal health.

Clearly, these two different health orientations and the behaviors they encourage do not exist in pure forms, but are influenced by such variables as the availability of resources, one's recognition of health hazards, and willingness to accept risk. Poverty and the inaccessibility of medical personnel and facilities prevent large segments of the population from seeking preventive health care. Lack of information stands in the way of others, even though finances and health resources are not precluding factors for them.

Inability or unwillingness to think in preventive terms is not uncommon in our public schools. Naturally, efforts to promote health by preventing health problems require time, special effort, patience, and, most critical of all, funds. Regardless of the magnitude of these demands, superintendents, principals, and classroom teachers who support health education will take the time, make the effort, exercise the necessary patience, and locate the resources required for health instruction.

During the early 1970s, I had occasion to speak with several school officials concerning the question of student abuse of drugs. Though none of the school districts were experiencing a serious drug abuse problem, each school administrator recognized that the potential for a serious drug problem existed in his school. When the proposal was made to develop and implement a comprehensive drug education program in grades kindergarten through twelve, the administrators reacted in ways that were not altogether unexpected.

Relatively few were receptive to the suggestion, but even in the face of rigid budgetary restrictions and crowded programs, were willing to try a preventative educational program. Their concern and willingness to take action exemplified the orientation that is basic to health education. Most of the other leaders reacted in a very different way. They claimed that since their schools were not in the grips of a widespread drug abuse problem it would be impossible to justify a drug education program—that is, until a well-defined crisis developed. This reluctance was expressed even though each of the administrators recognized the societal drug problem and the likelihood that it would one day infiltrate their schools.

A major obstacle to the development of comprehensive school health education programs is the failure of some educational leaders to identify prevention as a means of saving lives and money, avoiding misery and disability, enhancing learning and human development, and conserving human resources.

THE SATURATED CURRICULUM

Administrators and classroom teachers are often apprehensive when recommendations are made to teach additional subject matter. This concern is understandable, for in most schools hardly enough time exists to meet existing curriculum demands. Suggestions to reorder educational priorities are usually doomed, for this would threaten the traditional curriculum framework. There is, however, a more realistic approach that has proved quite workable.

Elementary teachers, regardless of the school, are usually involved in health teaching, perhaps more than many of them realize. To add meaning and continuity to this instruction requires not the addition of a new subject, but better individual and grade level planning. The point is, that in elementary schools health instruction can be readily integrated with the existing curriculum. For instance, emphasis on community helpers in kindergarten provides many opportunities to acquaint children with doctors, the school nurse, and other health workers as the class learns about their community and its resources. Abundant opportunities exist for the inclusion of health instruction in language arts, social studies, music, and virtually every phase of the elementary grade curriculum. Experience has shown that elementary school teachers are generally willing to integrate their health instruction, but to do so effectively requires awareness, skill, and a good grasp of fundamental health concepts.

MANDATING HEALTH INSTRUCTION

Several states have mandated the teaching of health in the elementary and secondary grades. Since programs of this type are required by state law, districts are obliged to conduct them according to guidelines set forth by the state education agency. Usually the guidelines and the state-developed curriculum materials to implement them are sufficiently flexible to allow school districts to develop programs that meet local needs while satisfying state education requirements.

Opponents of mandated programs contend that these laws impose restrictions and hardships on school districts and deprive them of local control of their programs. What they are reluctant to admit is that without a state mandate many schools would not include health instruction for all students. Regardless of their specific arguments against health education mandate, school administrators somehow are able to incorporate health education into the total school program.

The following excerpt is taken from the education law that requires health instruction in the schools of Illinois:

> The health education program at the elementary level should place strong emphasis on the health guidance of elementary school children. Many of the health education experiences of primary-age children should be planned around the regular school programs and activities of daily living in the school, home, and community. While some of the most effective learning experiences for the elementary school child should result from his living in an environment that promotes good health and safety, the elementary school program should also provide a planned curriculum composed of specific units of instruction for particular grade levels. These units of instruction should be clearly related to the comprehensive health education curriculum plan for the school system.
>
> Health education should be part of the regular formal instruction offered in the elementary school. In addition, special attention should be given to opportunities for incidental instruction in health and safety education when appropriate situations arise during the school day.[13]

Obviously, to require that schools teach health education is but one step toward encouraging quality programs. Preservice and in-service educational programs are essential to develop the competencies that teachers need in the classroom. Training of this type requires support by local administrators, willingness on the part of classroom teachers, and considerable funding, ordinarily from state sources. By and large, experience has demon-

13. Office of Superintendent of Public Instruction, *Guidelines for Implementing the Critical Health Problems and Comprehensive Health Education Act* (Springfield, Ill.: 1970).

strated that health education mandates can effectively improve the quality of health instruction to a greatly expanded audience.

CONTROVERSIAL SUBJECT MATTER

Controversy is as essential to the vitality of schools as it is to other democratic institutions, provided that it allows for free exchange of divergent opinions and ultimately contributes to the mission of school. It is manifest at national, state, and local levels of education and involves such issues as busing, open classrooms, arbitration, tracking, and teacher tenure. Additionally, elements of the curriculum, including some health topics, have demonstrated an ability to generate controversy. Family life, nutrition, drug abuse, and communicable disease instruction are among these. While space does not permit a lengthy discussion of each of these instructional areas, teachers should at least be aware of some of the ways they can cause controversy. This is not to suggest that these topics should be avoided. Rather, it is more often an indication that they need to be included in the instructional program.

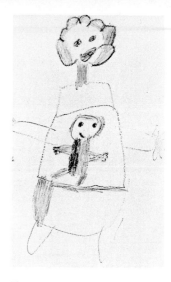

Fig. 7–5. Indications of healthy sexuality in crayon drawing of kindergarten pupil. Expectant mother's smile reflects her attitude toward having a child. Happy expression on face of fetus indicates positive feelings also.

Family life education The teaching of family life education including sex education has probably stirred more public emotion than any other single curriculum entity. A few poorly informed groups, moved largely by emotionalism, insist that the teaching of sex education in schools is evidence of a conspiracy to undermine our morality and contribute to the eventual collapse of American society. Notwithstanding the unreasonable views of these vocal groups, most parents believe that somewhere, somehow, their children should receive family life education.

Controversy emerges when the source of this instruction is discussed. Should the family provide this experience? How involved should schools, churches, or community agencies be in these efforts? Basic responsibility for family life education rests with the family, whose efforts should be reinforced and supplemented by the church and school. Most agree that the American family has not truly accepted this basic responsibility. In all fairness, the track record of most schools and churches in this regard is not much better. All need to work closely to develop effective programs. Prior to the actual planning of units of study in family life education, teachers need to be cognizant of community sentiments toward and perceptions of the school's role in family life education.

Concern is frequently expressed about the competency of classroom teachers to deal with family life understandings. This is a valid issue, for relatively few elementary grade teachers have special training in the area. Those with some knowledge of the field recognize that it is far more complex than many other subjects taught in school. Unfortunately, instruction is often limited to the anatomy and physiology of sex. For untrained teachers, this may well represent their total concept of family life education. Unfortunately, they may fail to recognize that the psychological, sociological, and emotional aspects of family life deserve emphasis also.

A considerable amount of parental discontent can be generated when sophisticated concepts, generally related to sexual physiology, are introduced at what parents consider too early an age. It really makes little difference whether the teacher responsible for this has had special training or not. The teacher's sincerity and desire to provide a good learning experience are seldom issues either. Parents insist, and justifiably so, that in family life education, as in other studies, pupil readiness be considered before instruction is provided.

In the absence of a well-planned and sequential family life education program, it is difficult to appreciate how much or how little children understand and what prior educational experiences they have had. As a consequence, many fundamental understandings, basic to the learning of advanced material, are overlooked. Teaching about family planning and contraception, for instance, somehow does not make much sense unless young people appreciate the roles of the family and its various members in society. Yet, some schools plunge headlong into the topics of contraception and abortion without first providing some understanding of the family unit. This and similar crash programs, at any grade level, are ill-advised, are indicative of poor planning, and almost always succeed in arousing a degree of public concern.

Regardless of the particular issue that one may raise concerning family life education in schools, much of the opposition is a by-product of Victorian attitudes and the social stigma that still shrouds sexual matters. To imply that these negative influences can be dealt with easily and quickly would mislead the reader. Curriculum planning that involves parents, religious leaders, educators, and representatives of other interested community groups can effectively resolve many of the problems that might otherwise preclude community support for school family life education programs.

Nutrition education Unlike the emotionally charged issue of whether or not family life should be included in the school curriculum, the study of nutrition is much less likely to arouse public sentiment. There are, however, at least two major areas of nutrition that can evoke controversy. One of these concerns dietary sources of protein. Some groups, for religious and other reasons, choose not to include animal flesh in their diets. Instead, they prefer to rely upon vegetables for their protein intake.

Meat is generally recognized as our best source of complete proteins.[14] Vegetable products (nuts, whole grains, etc.) are eaten instead of animal protein by some people. Their decision is clearly a personal one, but criticism by the teacher may be provocative. To avoid a possible confrontation with parents, the teacher would be wise to emphasize in the instruction those vegetables products known to be good sources of protein. If the teacher is unaware of the different beliefs represented in the class, she runs the risk of stepping on toes and arousing the ire of both students and parents. This is a case in point of the importance of knowing your students well.

In spite of research to the contrary, many organic gardeners and natural food fanciers are convinced that the safety and quality of our food supply have suffered because of unwise use of pesticides, overprocessed foods, and widespread use of food additives. Diets consisting of organically grown or natural foods, while tending to be more expensive and harder to find than other foods, are nutritious. Actually these beliefs are not likely to undermine the nutritional status of those who hold them. When teachers are not able to respond to their claims with reliable information, however, they are not acting in the best interest of the rest of the class.

14. Complete proteins contain the amino acids that are essential to life, but which the body cannot synthesize.

Drug abuse education   Instruction concerning the use and abuse of drugs should be included in the elementary grades. In fact, these early grades are perhaps more critical than others when one considers the impact of learning on attitude development. The approach should be positive and matter-of-fact, rather than negative and emotional. Children need to learn about drug safety in the home. They should recognize that medicines must be stored safely and used responsibly. A study of how common drugs (antibiotics, insulin, etc.) have helped mankind is another area of possible study. These basic, yet essential, understandings emphasize to the young that the responsible use of most drugs can benefit mankind in many ways. Perhaps the most worthy aim of elementary school drug education is to help children develop respect for drugs of various types. Those who insist that the primary grades are too soon to engage in drug education are usually unaware of the several facets of the topic.

Too frequently, the initial instruction focuses on the street "drug scene," and on the dramatic and emotional aspects of this form of drug abuse. One consequence of this shortsighted approach is that it really does not help individuals to deal responsibly with drugs in a society that is largely drug-oriented.

Little, if any, evidence exists to support the assertion that overemphasis on illicit drugs encourages young people to engage in drug experimentation. One should recognize that this complaint may be registered in schools with a limited perspective on education about drugs.

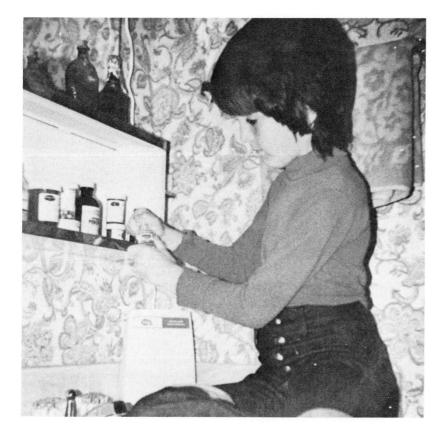

Fig. 7–6. Accidental poisoning from common household medications is a hazard faced by children.

Communicable disease education Understandings involving the germ theory of disease causation, as well as disease transmission, immunization, and therapy, fall under the rubric of communicable disease education. Generally, this body of knowledge arouses no controversy. Nonetheless, the astute classroom teacher recognizes that scientific views on this subject are frequently in conflict with the teachings of Christian Science. Parents who hold these beliefs may prefer (but usually do not) to have their children excluded from class when the germ theory of disease causation is discussed. The principle of voluntary exclusion on religious grounds is recognized in many states, and its implications extend beyond curriculum considerations. For example, immunization requirements for school attendance in some states may be waived if a family objects because of religious beliefs, or if they believe the requirement is a violation of their constitutional rights.

To avoid unnecessary conflict related to school communicable disease policies and instruction, teachers should be aware of existing practices in their states and school systems.

TEACHER PREPARATION

In general, the various states do not require the completion of a college health education course for teacher certification at the elementary level. Typically, certification requirements specify that one must hold at least a baccalaureate degree, has taken a prescribed number of professional education credits, and has successfully completed a supervised student teaching experience.

The individual's readiness to teach art, music, science, social studies, language arts, and other subjects included in the elementary school curriculum is largely dependent upon the required and elective courses studied in an undergraduate program. Many elementary teachers have never completed a health education course at the college level. Those having completed a course specifically dealing with health education at the elementary grade level are even fewer in number.

In a sense, therefore, you and others who are taking the course for which this text has been written are a privileged minority. You, perhaps more than others in your school, will understand what health education is all about. Moreover, your orientation to this field of study may even establish you as a health education resource person in your school.

Whether or not one's future as a teacher finds him in a position of leadership, he should encourage the development of in-service health education programs for his teaching colleagues. Some states, usually those with a health education mandate, have funds available for teacher in-service education. New York State school systems have successfully tapped college and university departments of health education for assistance in conducting in-service programs of this type. In one particular upstate New York school system, I taught a six-week health course for elementary grade teachers. All costs were absorbed by the state education department, and those completing the course were awarded two hours of graduate credit. Incentives of this type make an in-service education experience attractive to teachers, but more important, such a course equips them to do a more effective job of teaching health in the classroom.

PROGRAM COORDINATION

Teamwork is absolutely essential to the management of a quality school health program. Cooperation is needed to integrate the activities of the three major thrusts that comprise the total program. Additionally, planning must extend beyond the school and take into account community agencies and organizations whose activities may augment school health education efforts. To say the very least, cooperation of this magnitude requires time and talent. When these are lacking, program fragmentation, duplication, and unrelatedness are bound to occur.

Unfortunately, the smooth and efficient operation that typifies a well-integrated school and community effort is not created by administrative fiat. Leadership, whether it consists of a full-time health coordinator or of a school health coordinating committee, must be provided.

Large districts that include one or more secondary schools and several elementary units often employ a health coordinator. The individual selected for this position should be an experienced and fully certified health educator who can either devote full time to coordination or divide time between classroom teaching and program leadership. Naturally, the degree of leadership required in different school systems varies considerably. The following summary includes those coordinating functions that are common to most:

1. Structure a coordinated overall health program for the school.
2. Furnish the staff with all necessary information regarding the total school health program.
3. Serve as the line of communication between the school, the home, the health department, and other sources in the community that contribute to child health.
4. Develop a plan for keeping health records.
5. Arrange for school health services.
6. Provide procedures by which classroom teachers observe and report departures from normal child health.
7. Assist teachers in assessing health needs of pupils and in interpreting policies and procedures to be followed in the event of pupil injury and illness.
8. Provide specific procedures for effective referrals and follow-ups.
9. Arrange for in-service health preparation for the teaching staff.
10. Obtain and distribute to the teachers recommended health instruction materials.
11. Arrange for the coordination and progression of health instruction from grade to grade.
12. Provide for health counseling.
13. Provide leadership in the promotion of healthful school living.
14. Provide leadership in the promotion of safety practices and sanitation in the school.
15. Arrange for periodic evaluations of the overall school health program.[15]

15. C. L. Anderson, *School Health Practice,* 5th ed. (St. Louis: C. V. Mosby Co., 1972), p. 99.

Experience has demonstrated that program leadership is usually most effective when vested in a single professional. Smaller school districts or those operating on severely restricted budgets may find it impossible to employ such a person. In these cases, a health coordinating committee may assume some of the leadership functions.

The curriculum integration function of the health coordinator or co-ordinating committee is considered of paramount importance. Elementary grade educational experiences need to be planned sequentially, with a gradual sophistication of concepts and subject matter as children progress through the grades. Teacher involvement in this process is vital because of their understanding of students' readiness, needs, concerns, and interests, as well as of the teachers' familiarity with other facets of the total elementary and middle school curricula. Regardless of their special credentials, teachers simply do not have the time, energy, and experience to provide first-rate program leadership. When they are used extensively on coordinating committees, they should be provided released time from their classroom responsibilities.

SUMMARY

Educators have been concerned with the health of school age children for well over a century. Early interests focused on healthful conditions in the school environment, but eventually broadened to include what is now recognized as the health instructional program.

Health education is described as a multidimensional process, the purposes of which include teaching reliable health information and developing positive health attitudes and behaviors. Contemporary programs of school health consist of health instruction, health services, and healthful school living, all of which are organized and implemented as a single comprehensive program.

Education about health must reflect the dynamic character of the nation's health. Implications of the biomedical revolution, changing age-composition of the population, the concept of health insults, environmental quality, mental health, and drug abuse are enumerated as topics deserving of consideration.

Among the attitudinal and operational forces that impede effective programs are orientation of crisis intervention, crowded curricula, controversial subject matter, and inadequate teacher preparation in the health sciences.

Program coordination is of paramount importance and can be realized in one of several ways, depending upon the availability of funds, size of the school district, and extent to which school and community leaders desire an effective total school and community effort.

Discussion Questions

1. What are the advantages and disadvantages of school health programs having a state mandate?
2. Describe an innovative classroom learning experience that involves elements of the health services program.
3. How can one justify the inclusion of chronic disease concepts in the elementary and middle school program?

4. Support or refute the claim that schools should avoid becoming involved in family life education.
5. Comment on trends to indicate that the content of health instruction today should be somewhat different from that of fifty years ago.

References

American Academy of Pediatrics. *Report of the Committee on School Health,* Evanston, Ill.: American Academy of Pediatrics, 1966.

American Public Health Association. "Proposed Policy Statements." *Nation's Health* 4, no. 10 (October 1974): 10.

Anderson, C. L. *School Health Practice.* 5th ed. St. Louis: C. V. Mosby Co., 1972.

Committee on Nutrition, American Academy of Pediatrics, "Salt Intake and Eating Patterns of Infants and Children in Relation to Blood Pressure." *Pediatrics* 53, no. 1 (January 1974): 115–121.

Joint Committee on Health Problems in Education of the National Education Association and American Medical Association. *Health Education.* Washington, D.C.: National Education Association, 1961.

Means, R. *A History of Health Education in the United States.* Philadelphia: Lea & Febiger, 1962.

National Education Association and American Association of School Administrators. *An Essay on Quality in Public Education.* Washington, D.C.: Educational Policies Commission, 1959.

National Education Association and American Association of School Administrators. *The Purposes of Education in American Democracy.* Washington, D.C.: Educational Policies Commission, 1938.

Office of Superintendent of Public Instruction. *Guidelines for Implementing the Critical Health Problems and Comprehensive Health Education Act.* Springfield, Ill.: 1970.

President's Committee on Health Education. *The Report of the President's Committee on Health Education.* New York: The Committee, 1973.

Sliepcevich, E. *School Health Education Study: A Summary Report.* Washington, D.C.: School Health Education Study, 1964.

U.S., Department of the Interior, Bureau of Education. *Cardinal Principles of Secondary Education,* Bulletin 1918, no. 35. Washington, D.C.: Government Printing Office, 1918.

Vital Statistics Report, Annual Summary for the United States, 1973 (HRA) 74–1120, vol. 22, no. 13, Rockville, Md.: National Center for Health Statistics, 1974.

Willgoose, C. *Health Education in the Elementary School.* Philadelphia: W. B. Saunders Co., 1969.

Chapter 8
SCHOOL
HEALTH
SERVICES

What are the basic components of school health services?

Why is the classroom teacher considered to be the key person in the appraisal process?

What are the objectives of the health appraisal?

School health services represent one aspect of a comprehensive school health program and are interrelated with the areas of health education and healthful school living. While the areas may be categorized with respect to a delineation of the basic functions contained within each area, in essence they are all designed to maintain, promote, and preserve the health of the school child. In addition, all of the major components provide an essential educational function within the total health program.

School health services refer to the procedures conducted by teachers, physicians, nurses, dentists, psychologists, counselors, and others to appraise, protect, and promote the health of students and school personnel. Such procedures are designed primarily (1) to appraise the health status of students and school personnel; (2) to counsel pupils, parents, and others concerning appraisal findings; (3) to encourage the correction of remedial defects; (4) to assist in the identification and education of handicapped children; (5) to help prevent and control diseases; and (6) to provide emergency service for students with an injury or sudden illness.

Parents or guardians have the primary responsibility for the health care of their children. School personnel should respect this responsibility and should consult with the parents concerning conditions related to the health of their children. School health services are primarily designed to encourage parents to devote attention to their children's health and to acquaint them with health problems of which they might be unaware. Consequently, these services should also facilitate and encourage parents to utilize the medical and other health services within the health care delivery system.

One of the major problems concerning parental responsibility occurs when the parent appears to be acting irresponsibly with respect to the health of his or her child. When evidence of child neglect and abuse is present, the school must be the child's advocate and defender. Some states have now made the physician and school legally responsible for reporting instances of child abuse.[1]

HEALTH APPRAISAL

The term *health appraisal* refers to a series of procedures designed to assess the physical, mental, emotional, and social health status of individual pupils and school personnel through the use of health histories or inventories, teacher and nurse observations, screening tests, and medical, dental, and psychological examinations. The proper functioning of the health appraisal process is dependent upon the cooperation of parents, teachers, health educators, psychologists, physicians, dentists, and other personnel engaged in the conduct of the health service program. In order to work together cooperatively, these personnel must also be able to communicate effectively across professional channels. The inability of schools to establish proper lines of communication may result in friction and misunderstanding. Thus, when a child's physician fails to communicate his medical findings to the school, the school may feel the need for a medical examination to be conducted within the school settings.[2] In a similar manner, the physician may feel the need to duplicate certain screening procedures which had been performed by school personnel since the schools did not transmit the results to his office.

Health appraisals in most states are required by statute. A majority of state laws mandate what the schools are to require concerning basic immunizations for the school child as well as emergency care procedures. In general the courts have recognized the importance of school health services and have ruled fairly consistently in favor of the school in terms of litigations brought against certain segments of the program.[3]

The major objectives of health appraisals are as follows:

1. To locate pupils in need of medical or dental treatment.
2. To identify pupils who are poorly adjusted and in need of special attention at school or of treatment by a psychiatrist, psychologist, or child-guidance clinic.
3. To locate pupils with defects requiring modified programs of education as, for example, the mentally retarded, partially sighted, hard-of-hearing, and others.
4. To identify pupils who may need a more thorough examination than that provided in school, for example, X-ray examinations, examination by specialists, and other examinations.
5. To inform school personnel and parents concerning the health status of children.
6. To encourage parents to recognize and accept the responsibility when necessary for obtaining the necessary health care for their children.

1. *School Health: A Guide for Physicians* (Evanston, Ill.: American Academy of Pediatrics, 1972), p. 3.
2. Joint Committee on Health Problems in Education of the National Education Association and the American Medical Association, *Health Appraisal of School Children* (Washington, D.C.: National Education Association, 1961), p. 7.
3. D. F. Miller, *School Health Programs: Their Basis in Law* (Cranbury, N.J.: A. S. Barnes & Co., 1972), p. 47.

7. To aid pupils with health problems to compensate or make adjustments for their condition.
8. To provide an educational experience for children, parents, teachers, and other school personnel.
9. To provide the basis for classification in a modified modern program of physical education.

Ideally, health appraisals of children should start as early as possible, preferably during the preschool years so that remedial treatment or special educational procedures can be undertaken before the child enters school. The health appraisal program should be a continuous process throughout the school and college years. The program should be based on accepted standards and adapted to a particular community. The extent and nature of the program will be influenced by many factors such as local policies, variety and availability of health professionals, and community resources and agencies. Likewise, the degree of involvement in the health service program by the elementary teacher will also be determined by these same general factors.

APPRAISAL TECHNIQUES

Many different kinds of appraisals can be performed by school personnel ranging from nondiagnostic techniques by parents and teachers to medical and laboratory tests performed by health professionals.[4]

HEALTH OBSERVATIONS

The classroom teacher is in a unique position to observe departures in the child's physical, mental, emotional, and social health status since she is with the child more hours of the day than any other adult, with the exception of his parents. Because the teacher is familiar with the child's usual appearance and behavior patterns, she can easily observe deviations from health.

Teacher observations should also supplement other techniques for assessing pupil health. They are especially helpful in detecting the initial onset of a variety of communicable diseases that commonly are found among elementary school children. The teacher may note pupils with signs and symptoms of the common cold, skin infections, sore throats, headaches, vision and hearing problems, emotional disturbances, and other departures from good health. In addition to observing the child's appearance and behavior, the teacher should give consideration also to pupils' verbal complaints of ill health. However, teachers must be aware of the fact that the responsibility for observing children for possible indications of illness does not present them with an opportunity to make a diagnosis of the child's condition.

If the teacher suspects that a pupil has a communicable disease, it is important that the child be separated from his classmates and a place be available in the school building for the child to rest while arrangements are made for him to be sent home. If a school nurse is not available, either the teacher or principal will need to contact the parents to make the necessary plans for getting the child home.

Whenever appropriate, the teacher should consult with the school nurse concerning observations of pupils that she suspects need attention.

4. D. Oberteuffer, O. Harrelson, and M. Pollock, *School Health Education* (New York: Harper & Row, 1972), p. 294.

When a nurse is not available, the teacher might decide to telephone the child's parents to discuss his health problem or arrange for a school or home conference. Sharing observations with others such as the parents, school nurse, physician, guidance counselor, and psychologist can be quite useful in terms of selecting the proper action for an appropriate referral.

Table 8–1 presents some signs of conditions and examples of behavior that might provide clues to physical and emotional problems of children.

Table 8–1. Some Possible Indications of Physical and Emotional Departures from Health

School Performance	*Skin and Scalp*
Failure to achieve	Patches of very dry skin
Marked deterioration in work	Rashes or sores
Poor memory	Numerous pimples, blackheads
Very careless work	Nits on hair
Lack of interest	Bald spots
Poor reasoning	Frequent scratching
Compulsive neatness to the	
point that assignments	*Teeth and Mouth*
are never completed	Irregular teeth
	Bad bite
General Appearance	Inflamed or bleeding gums
Very thin or overweight	Cracked lips, especially
Radical changes in weight	at corners of mouth
Unusual gait or limp	Dental caries
Uncleanliness	
Very pale or flushed	*General Behavior*
Poor posture	Constant need for attention
Lethargic, unresponsive	Docile, apathetic, lethargic
Facial tic	Unusually timid, fearful
	Aggressive, cruel
Eyes	Excessive daydreaming, inattentive
Crossed or turned out	Destructive
Squint, frown, scowl	Temper tantrums
Holding book too close	Cries easily
Inflamed, watery	Depressed and unhappy
Frequent styes	Restless, hyperactive
	Slurred speech, stuttering, lisping
Ears	
Discharge	*Behavior at Play*
Turning head to hear	Easily fatigued
Asking to have things repeated	Breathless after moderate exercise
	Lack of interest
Nose and Throat	Very clumsy
Persistent mouth breathing	Poor coordination
Frequent colds	Extremely excitable
Enlarged glands in neck	Difficulty playing with others
Nasal discharge	

Source: *Looking for Health*, Metropolitan Life Insurance Company, 1974, p. 28.

HEALTH RECORDS

Cumulative health records generally provide information on such items as the child's previous illnesses or medical conditions, immunizations, teacher observations, screening-test results, findings of medical, dental, and psychological examinations, and follow-up procedures. Such health records provide cumulative data on the child's health during the elementary and secondary school years.

Teachers can utilize the information contained in the health record to gain a better understanding of the health status of their students. However it is also imperative that teachers realize the privileged nature of information that might be found in the child's folder. The code of ethics of the medical, dental, and nursing professions does not permit the release of any type of health information to other people without the consent of a parent or guardian.[5]

In addition to the cumulative health record, every school should maintain a complete card index file on each student for emergency reference. The card should be filled out at the beginning of the school year and kept up to date. The pupil emergency information card should be kept in the principal's office or the health room. A sample form indicating the type of information is shown in figure 8–1.

Fig. 8–1. Pupil emergency information card.

Name of pupil _____

Home address _____ Telephone _____

Name of father _____ Business telephone _____

Name of mother _____ Business telephone _____

Name of responsible adult who will assume responsibility for the child if parents cannot be

reached _____

Address _____ Telephone _____

Physician of choice   (1) _____ (2) _____

Telephone _____ Telephone _____

Dentist of choice _____

Telephone _____

Hospital of choice _____

Telephone _____

Special health conditions of child, if any _____

_____

If you and the physician of choice as indicated above cannot be reached in an emergency, and if in the judgment of the school authorities immediate medical and/or hospital attention is indicated, do you authorize responsible school authorities to send your child (properly accompanied) to an available hospital or physician?

Yes _____ No _____

_____
Signature of Parent or Guardian
Date _____

Children that have special health problems such as epilepsy, diabetes, allergic reactions (including asthma), heart defects, and perceptual defects should be known by the teacher. Some schools identify the pupil emergency cards with a special marking to alert school personnel to a particular medical condition in case an emergency should arise. Also, some children are now wearing the identification symbol recommended by the American Medical Association to identify their specific medical condition in case of sudden illness.

5. A. Nemir, *The School Health Program* (Philadelphia: W. B. Saunders Co., 1970), p. 336.

SCREENING TESTS

Screening tests are considered to be preliminary evaluation of the state of development and function of various body organs. These tests are performed by trained teachers, nurses, technicians, or parental volunteers. The function of these tests is to screen out those children needing further examination and diagnosis by specialized health service personnel. Screening procedures utilized within the school setting should be in accord with standards recommended by the local medical society, health department, or other appropriate community physicians. Generally, physicians would not support a screening program involving tests that have not achieved general medical acceptance for school purposes.[6]

The screening tests that are most often employed in the school include procedures for measuring height and weight and for determining acuity of vision and hearing. Screening tests should reinforce teacher and nurse observations and are of value if they lead to remedial care when a health deviation is detected. The purposes of all screening tests are to secure a better understanding of the student, to help him attain greater physical effectiveness, and to increase his knowledge with respect to healthful living.[7]

Tests for measuring height and weight that provide information concerning growth were discussed in chapter 4. Therefore this discussion will be limited primarily to acuity tests for vision and hearing.

Vision screening Approximately one of every four school age children has an eye problem that requires referral to appropriate health personnel in the community.[8] Vision screening as applied in the school context should not provide definitive diagnosis of a child's visual problem, but should serve as the basis for referral to visual practitioners within the community.

The standard test of visual acuity is the Snellen Chart which is read at a distance of 20 feet. Various modifications of the test have been developed such as the Illiterate E for children who are not familiar with the alphabet.

The National Society for the Prevention of Blindness recommends referring children who cannot read the 20/30 line in the third grade and below; and the 20/20 line in the fourth grade and above.[9] Also children who consistently exhibit signs of visual disturbance regardless of the results of the Snellen Test should be referred (see chapter 6 for teacher observations). Generally, all failures on the Snellen Test should be rescreened to reduce overreferrals within the vision screening program. However, referral criteria should be established following consultation with medical professionals in the local community.

The Snellen Test in combination with teacher-nurse observations should identify most children needing a complete eye examination. Additionally other tests may be utilized that include the "plus" or convex lens test for

6. Joint Committee, *Health Appraisal of School Children*, p. 17.
7. "Suggested School Health Policies," Prepared by the National Committee on School Health Policies of the National Education Association and the American Medical Association (Washington, D.C.: National Education Association, 1966), p. 13.
8. *Vision Screening in Schools* (New York: National Society for Prevention of Blindness, 1975).
9. *Vision Screening of Children* (New York: National Society for Prevention of Blindness, 1971).

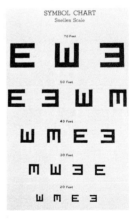

Fig. 8–2. Snellen Chart.

hyperopia, tests of ocular muscle imbalance (latent or manifest strabismus), and tests of color vision. Several studies have indicated that as the complexity of a screening examination increases so does the likelihood of obtaining false or excessive referrals. As a result, negative community feedback stemming from unnecessary referrals may create problems in some schools. Since there are wide differences of opinion as to which tests should be employed in a school screening program, the decision should be established locally, utilizing the knowledge, experience, and judgment of the school administrator, physician, nurse, health educator, and practitioners who might examine the referred child. It is particularly important that ophthalmologists be consulted in relation to the medical aspects of the program.[10] Ideally, vision screening should begin well before the child enters school. Many specialists feel that this should be accomplished by age four years. Since vision disorders increase in frequency with age, school vision screening programs should begin during kindergarten or first grade and be repeated annually.[11] Generally, however, visual screening is recommended at two- to three-year intervals. Also, these examinations may be profitably combined with instruction on the eye and vision. Ideally, all health services conducted in the school have an educational component.

Hearing screening The sound frequencies most commonly tested in screening programs are those found within the speech range from 500 to 3,000 cycles per second (cps). These are the frequencies that are most commonly affected by middle ear disease that is common in childhood and associated with upper respiratory infections.

There are two methods of testing a child with an electronically produced pure tone: the sweep test and the threshold test. In the sweep test,

Fig. 8–3. Audiometer used by specially trained audiologist in conducting hearing examinations.

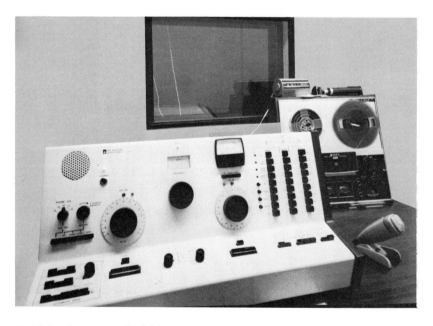

10. *Vision Screening of Children*, p. 3.
11. *School Health: A Guide for Physicians*, p. 84.

the audiometer is preset at an intensity of 25 decibels (ISO), and the various frequencies of 250, 500, 1,000, 2,000, 4,000 and 8,000 cps are scanned. A child who fails to hear two or more tones in either ear is administered the sweep test at a later date since he may have an inflammation of the eustachian tube due to a respiratory infection. If the child fails to pass the screening test at a later date, he is administered the threshold test. In this test the child is presented a tone at gradually decreasing volume levels in order to measure the lowest volume that the child can hear. A normal threshold is called zero, and abnormal thresholds are measured from this standard in decibels of loss. Threshold testing is considered to be the most accurate test for hearing acuity. It is used for diagnostic purposes and to validate screening tests.[12]

Generally, hearing screening is not usually conducted by the elementary teacher but by specially trained personnel such as audiologists, nurses, volunteers, and technicians. Appropriate referrals are based on the results of the threshold test, observations of the teacher and nurse, and complaints of the child (see chapter 6 for teacher observations). Fortunately only a few of the children referred for medical evaluation of their hearing problem have serious disorders. It is recommended that hearing screening be done at least biennially in the elementary grades and at least once in four years in high school. Those children found to have hearing handicaps should be tested every year.[13]

Other screening tests　In some circumstances local medical personnel may recommend other screening tests such as skin tests for tuberculosis, urinalysis, blood tests, and others. Screening for sickle cell disease and trait has also been included in some school programs because of the high prevalence rates in blacks. Most of these screening tests however require the services of skilled medical technicians.

MEDICAL EXAMINATIONS

Most authorities agree that pupils should have a minimum of four periodic medical examinations: upon entrance in school and at approximately the fourth, seventh, and tenth grades, with additional examinations being conducted whenever observation might indicate the necessity for such an examination. Preferably the medical examination should be conducted by the student's personal physician since a more thorough medical examination can be made in the physician's office, and the continuity of medical care can be more efficiently maintained. The physician should also have a summary of teacher and nurse observations and the results of the child's screening tests.

Basically the objectives of the school medical examination are as follows:

1. To provide information that will assist in promoting healthy growth and development in the child.
2. To discover defects that might interfere with learning and to initiate correction of those that are remediable.

12. V. Eisner, and L. Callan, *Dimensions of School Health* (Springfield, Ill.: Charles C Thomas, 1974), p. 62.
13. *School Health: A Guide for Physicians*, p. 85.

3. To encourage family and educational adjustment of those disabilities that cannot be corrected.
4. To provide a learning experience for children and parents with respect to health protection.
5. To suggest improvement in health behavior when it is necessary and to encourage elimination of undesirable practices.[14]

Most of these objectives can be more effectively met when the school medical examination is performed in the family physician's office with the child's parents present. Within this context, the physician can administer the necessary therapy since parental authorization is available. Examinations conducted in the school setting by school physicians have been increasingly under criticism since the Yankauer studies were completed.[15, 16, 17, 18] The major conclusion reached by these studies was that school medical examinations generally disclosed few previously unknown health problems in pupils and that the examination was valueless from a case-finding standpoint. Eisner and Callan believe that the classroom teacher should become the focus of case-finding efforts and that the pupils' behavior and functioning should assume the primary indicators of health.[19] Thus, school physicians would then be able to devote their primary efforts with the children who had been identified as having medical problems.

DENTAL EXAMINATIONS

It may be assumed that most children need dental care since dental disease is the commonest pathological condition of childhood. Consequently some individuals feel that dental inspection conducted in the school is a waste of time since all children need care semiannually, and that the effort should be focused on encouraging periodic visits to the family dentist. Others, however, feel that dental health inspection provides a proper educational experience and offers an inducement for the child to visit a private dentist for needed care. Also, in schools in high socioeconomic areas where children receive good dental care, the schools' screening program can be used to locate children with inadequate dental care early and to refer them to their dentist before the decay process becomes extensive. In low-income areas where a large amount of dental disease can be anticipated, screening would enable the schools to screen out those children that need emergency dental care.[20]

14. American Medical Association, *Report of the Fifth National Conference on Physicians and Schools* (Chicago: American Medical Association, 1955), p. 27.
15. A. Yankauer and R. Lawrence, "A Study of Periodic School Medical Examinations: I. Methodology and Initial Findings," American Journal of Public Health 45 (1955): 71–78.
16. Ibid. "II. The Annual Increment of New Defects," American Journal of Public Health 46 (1956): 1553–1562.
17. Ibid. "III. The Remediability of Certain Categories of Defects," American Journal of Public Health 47 (1957): 1421–1429.
18. Ibid. "IV. Education Aspects," American Journal of Public Health 51 (1961): 1532–1540.
19. Eisner and Callan, *Dimensions*, p. 51.
20. Eisner and Callan, *Dimensions*, p. 65.

These basic considerations need to be carefully assessed within the local community in order to determine the formulation of the dental screening program and should be critically evaluated by appropriate groups concerned with dental health.

PSYCHOLOGICAL, PERSONALITY, AND INTELLIGENCE TESTING

A wide variety of psychological, personality, and intelligence tests are available for use with school children. Tests of these types are usually administered by psychologists, counselors, and social workers and sometimes by classroom teachers. Findings of such tests should be interpreted to classroom teachers and recorded on the child's cumulative health record. Decisions as to which tests should be utilized and how referrals are to be handled should be in accordance with local school policy and determined by appropriate community and school personnel.

Indications of emotional problems in children may be observed by teachers; however, it is important to remember that children differ in temperament, ability, and adaptability and should not be expected to conform to a particular mode of behavior.[21] Table 8–1 provides some possible indications of emotional departures from health, while the guidelines discussed in chapter 5 present a more detailed list of classroom behaviors indicative of emotional problems.

The follow-up of health conditions and problems identified through the appraisal process is an important part of school health services. Health counseling should accomplish the following:

HEALTH COUNSELING AND FOLLOW-UP PROCEDURES

1. Give pupils as much information about their health status as revealed by health appraisal as they can use to good advantage.
2. Aid in interpreting to parents the significance of health conditions and to encourage them to obtain needed care for their children.
3. Motivate pupils and their parents to seek needed treatment and to accept desirable modifications of their school programs.
4. Promote each pupil's acceptance of responsibility for his own health in keeping with his stage of maturity.
5. Contribute to the health education of pupils and parents.
6. Obtain for exceptional pupils educational programs adapted to their individual needs and abilities.[22]

Health counseling may involve many different school and community health personnel: the physician, school nurse, counselor, social worker, teacher, and principal. Follow-up is ordinarily the responsibility of the health service personnel in the school, usually the school nurse. However, when limited services are available the classroom teacher frequently assumes the responsibility for making parents or the child's guardians aware

21. *Looking for Health* (New York: Metropolitan Life Insurance Co., 1969), p. 23.
22. C. C. Wilson, ed., *School Health Services* (Washington, D.C.: National Education Association and American Medical Association, 1964), pp. 111–112.

of the health needs of their children. Of particular concern in the follow-up process are children who for financial reasons are unable to utilize the normal channels for receiving medical care. Consequently, school personnel need to be aware of existing community agencies that provide services for indigent or medically indigent children.

EMERGENCY CARE

Every school should have a well-planned program related to emergency care procedures. This is especially important since the teacher is acting *in loco parentis* ("in place of the parent") with respect to her relationship with the child. Thus, the teacher has moral and legal responsibility to render emergency care for a pupil who becomes sick or injured in the classroom (see chapter 9 for discussion of liability).

School administrators should provide written policies and procedures to be followed in emergency situations involving injury or illness. Such policies should be developed in consultation with proper medical and legal authorities. Furthermore, the written procedures need to be known by all school employees. The school has a responsibility for the following: (1) giving immediate emergency care in case of an accident or sudden illness, (2) notifying parents or guardians, (3) getting the child home or to some other place of safety, and (4) guiding parents, whenever necessary, to sources of treatment.

GIVING IMMEDIATE CARE

Ideally all school personnel, teachers, maintenance personnel, bus drivers, teacher aides, clerical staff, and others should be qualified to administer basic first aid. However, few school administrators require training in emergency care procedures as a prerequisite for employment by their school district. Therefore, it would appear advisable that each school have several persons on their staff available in the building that have received proper first-aid training.

First-aid supplies should be strategically located within the school where they will most likely be used. The number and contents of first-aid kits should be determined with the advice and consent of the school medical consultant.

Only emergency care and not medical treatment is to be rendered by teachers and other school personnel. Under no circumstances should they diagnose a child's condition or illness or administer medication unless directed to do so by a physician. Information concerning the illness or injury and what was done should be entered on the pupil's cumulative health record. In addition, in the case of an accident, it is imperative that teachers fill out the necessary accident report forms.

NOTIFYING PARENTS OR GUARDIANS

Parents must be notified of their child's sudden illness or injury. The information contained on the pupil emergency information card (fig. 8–1) includes the telephone number of the parents or a responsible adult who will assume responsibility for the child if the parents cannot be reached. It also includes the names of several physicians acceptable to the parents who may be called if conditions permit, as well as authorization to send their child to an available hospital.

If the child is sent home, he should be accompanied by a responsible adult, preferably a parent or guardian. The child should not be left at home alone until a reliable person accepts the responsibility for the child.

GUIDING PARENTS

When the parents are called regarding the child's sudden illness or injury, the member of the school staff should be prepared to guide uncertain parents in their decision concerning what is to be done for the child. Therefore, school personnel need to be alert to the treatment facilities that are available in their community.

Detailed information on the communicable diseases likely to be observed in school children is presented in Appendix A. Included in the information are early signs and symptoms, incubation period, method of transmission, control of cases, and other information concerning diseases of significance to school age children.

Control of communicable diseases is the legal responsibility of the local health department, and this agency is responsible for initiating the necessary policies and procedures for the prevention and control of disease. In areas that are without the services of a local health department, the school may obtain counsel and guidance from the state health department and the local medical society. State or local health departments can provide school personnel with information concerning diseases that are legally reportable, regulations concerning isolation, quarantine, and exclusion from school, as well as information regarding signs and symptoms on specific diseases.

The classroom teacher can aid in the program by observing children for possible departures from health and taking the appropriate action when she suspects that a child should be sent home. Policies regarding exclusion and readmission of the child need to be disseminated to all school personnel and parents. Parents also need to be aware of the importance of keeping their sick child at home.

Teachers also can play an active role by conducting planned units on communicable disease in their educational program. Students should also learn how diseases are prevented and controlled as well as how immunizations provide protection.

Immunization against certain communicable diseases such as diphtheria, tetanus, whooping cough, poliomyelitis, measles, and mumps should be encouraged by school personnel. Parents, teachers, administrators, and other school personnel should be aware of the state statutes, state board of health regulations, and school district requirements concerning immunization. Generally, state statutory provisions relating to immunizations either (1) identify the specific diseases for which a child must be immunized or (2) authorize the state health department to mandate the regulations that it feels necessary for the proper protection of the general public.[23]

Health services as a division of the school health and safety program consists of the cooperative activities of teachers, physicians, dentists, nurses,

COMMUNICABLE DISEASE PREVENTION AND CONTROL

SUMMARY

23. Miller, *School Health Programs,* p. 103.

counselors, administrators, and other personnel which are designed to conserve, protect, promote, and improve the physical, mental, and social health of the child. School health services are primarily designed to appraise the physical and emotional health status of pupils and school personnel; to counsel pupils, teachers, parents, and others for the purpose of helping students obtain needed treatment or for arranging school programs in keeping with their abilities; to help prevent and control disease; and to provide emergency care for pupils with an injury or sudden illness. Parents should assume their fundamental responsibility for the health care of their children, with encouragement when necessary from school personnel. Additionally, all aspects of health services provided by the school should have an accompanying educational component.

Discussion Questions

1. Define school health services.
2. Why is the classroom teacher in a unique position to observe departures from health?
3. What are possible indications of physical and emotional departures from health?
4. What are the recommended criteria for referring a child with a visual problem?
5. Discuss the difference between a sweep check and a threshold hearing-screening examination.
6. What are the basic objectives of the school medical examination?
7. Why is health counseling an important aspect of the school health service program?
8. Discuss the basic components of the emergency care program in the school.
9. What is the role of the classroom teacher in communicable disease control?

References

American Medical Association. *Report of the Fifth National Conference on Physicians and Schools.* Chicago: American Medical Association, 1955.

Eisner, V., and Callan, L. *Dimensions of School Health.* Springfield, Ill.: Charles C Thomas, 1974.

Joint Committee on Health Problems in Education of the National Education Association and the American Medical Association. *Health Appraisal of School Children.* Washington, D.C.: National Education Association, 1961.

Looking for Health. New York: Metropolitan Life Insurance Co., 1969.

Miller, D. F. *School Health Programs: Their Basis in Law.* Cranbury, N.J.: A. S. Barnes & Co., 1972.

Nemir, A. *The School Health Program.* Philadelphia: W. B. Saunders Co., 1970.

Oberteuffer, D., Harrelson, O., and Pollock, M. *School Health Education.* New York: Harper & Row, 1972.

School Health: A Guide for Physicians. Evanston, Ill.: American Academy of Pediatrics, 1972.

Suggested School Health Policies. Prepared by the National Committee on School Health Policies of the National Education Association and the American Medical Association. Washington, D.C.: National Education Association, 1966.

Vision Screening of Children. New York: National Society for Prevention of Blindness, 1971.

Vision Screening in Schools. New York: National Society for Prevention of Blindness, 1975.

Wilson, C. C., ed. *School Health Services.* Washington, D.C.: National Education Association and American Medical Association, 1964.

Yankauer, A., and Lawrence, R. L. "A Study of Periodic School Medical Examinations: I. Methodology and Initial Findings." *American Journal of Public Health* 45 (1955): 71–78.

Ibid. "II. The Annual Increment of New Defects." *American Journal of Public Health* 46 (1956): 1553–1562.

Ibid. "III. The Remediability of Certain Categories of Defects." *American Journal of Public Health* 47 (1957): 1421–1429.

Ibid. "IV. Education Aspects." *American Journal of Public Health* 51 (1961): 1532–1540.

Chapter 9

HEALTHFUL
SCHOOL
LIVING

What is an ecological view of healthful school living?

Who is responsible for a safe and healthful school environment?

What school factors influence the health of students and teachers?

How can "living safety" be part of a school environment?

What constitutes a Program of Emergency Controls in an elementary school?

A school building, like a community, can be well planned by a team of farsighted experts, be designed by the lowest bidding construction company, or be some type of temporary shelter. Schools, as well as communities, can be described within a continuum from being an organized, warm, healthful environment to being a disorganized, run-down "penal colony."

Like a community, a school can suffer through periods of overcrowding, financial problems, natural disasters, international problems, epidemics, racism, vandalism, radical politics, mismanagement and credibility gaps. In addition, students reflect the tensions, pressures, and value systems of a given community.

AN ECOLOGICAL VIEW OF HEALTHFUL LIVING

Traditionally, healthful school living has been thought of as being dependent upon the environmental factors within the school. For example, healthful school living has been defined as follows:

> . . . living within a school where all environmental conditions, every social relationship, and every curriculum experience is carried on with due attention to health. . .[1]

However, the impact of the crises in food production, population, energy, and cost-of-living increases has had considerable influence on our schools.

1. Joint Committee on Health Problems in Education of the National Education Association and the American Medical Association, *Healthful School Environment* (Washington, D.C.: National Education Association, 1969), p. 7.

In light of these problems, healthful school living can be defined in an ecological context: healthful school living involves the sociological, personal, hereditary, and ecological factors of the school and community.

The many ecological factors illustrated in figure 9–1 are well beyond the scope of this book and probably of several others. This chapter will discuss several of the major factors within the school milieu that affect the health of students and faculty.

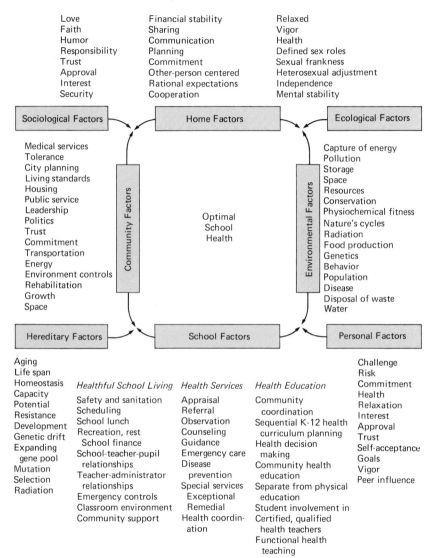

Fig. 9–1. An ecological view of healthful school living.

Sometime during the day, the railing in the stairwell next to Mrs. Swanson's room was broken. Jeff Washington, a student from another fourth grade class, was carrying a load of books down the stairs on an errand to the school library. Jeff stumbled, reached for the broken railing, fell, and was injured.

RESPONSIBILITY FOR HEALTHFUL SCHOOL LIVING

The key question in the scene just described is this: Who was responsible for the incident? The answer from a moral standpoint would be this: Anyone noticing the broken railing should have done something to ensure the welfare of others. A number of different questions arise from this incident. Indeed, some of these questions might be asked by the attorney representing the family of the injured student. A list of the questions that should be asked concerning this accident include the following:

1. How was first aid administered?
2. Did anyone report the broken railing?
3. Was the report of the broken railing in writing?
4. Did the janitor get the work order to repair the railing?
5. Why did not the school district appropriate enough money for such repairs?
6. If the railing could not have been repaired, why was not some type of warning or protection device put up?
7. Did other members of the faculty know the railing was broken?
8. Is not Mrs. Swanson responsible because the railing was just outside of her room?
9. Could the teacher having the student perform the errand be held responsible?
10. When was the facility last inspected?

Responsibility for the health and safety of school children belongs to other persons in addition to the faculty and staff of a given school building. In addition to school personnel, this responsibility rests with state and local governments, school boards, administrative personnel, members of the community, and educational pressure groups. Along with most state mandates that children must attend school six hours a day for one hundred eighty days a year, state boards have gone to great lengths to ensure the health and safety of students by establishing detailed guidelines and standards for the operation of public and private educational facilities. Figure 9–2 outlines responsibility for healthful school living.

The people of a state or district have control and responsibility for

Fig. 9–2. Outline of responsibility for healthful school living.

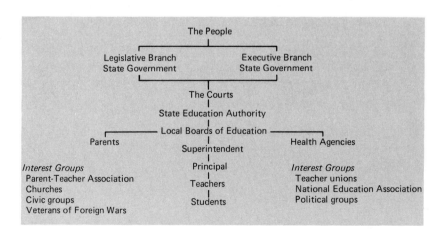

what occurs in their schools. Poorly prepared school officials, overcrowding, tight budgets, and poor facilities usually reflect the interest and will of the citizens of a given community concerning the quality of their schools. As indicated in figure 9–2, special interest groups and organizations can take an active role in formation of school policy. In fact, a small, vocal, and sometimes misguided minority can have an enormous influence on local school districts. In summary, school officials and employees have the immediate responsibility, while the people have the ultimate responsibility, for healthful school living.

Healthful organization of the school day requires careful coordination of the safety program, health services, health instruction, student services, classroom environment, and teacher-administrator relationships. Figure 9–3 lists those aspects of the school organization that may influence the health of students and teachers.

When placed within the context of the broader ecological problems of school planning and administration, the task of protecting the health of students is a staggering one. Some of the physical problems dealing with sanitation, health services, remedial programs, overcrowding, and facilities can be at least partially solved through financial support, qualified personnel, and administrative effort. Other problems dealing with mental health, teacher-administrator relationships, cost effectiveness, accountability, motivation, and student success will require further research, as well as financial and administrative support.

ORGANIZATION OF THE SCHOOL DAY

Fig. 9–3. School day factors that influence the health of students.

Safety Factors

Safety to and from school
Safety patrols
Hall traffic flow
Playground supervision
Classroom safety rules
Physical education safety
Fire prevention
Busing
Accident records

Health Services

Appraisals
Remediation
Counseling
Emergency care
Prevention of disease
Health of teachers

Scheduling

Overcrowding
Tracking
Recreation time
Movement
Teacher breaks
Supervision
Open classroom
Teacher preparation time
Remedial programs
Special interest groupings
Evaluation
Play and recreation
Intramurals

Sanitation and Housekeeping

Dust control
Microorganism control
Storage
Clutter
Waste disposal
Inspections

School Classroom Environment

Heating and ventilation
Lighting and visual fields
Noise control
Facilities and equipment

Food Services

Quality
Space
Time allotment
Supervision
Movement

Teacher-administrator

Communication
Input
Support
Cooperation
Democratic/autocratic

Classroom Environment

Motivation
Approval
Trust
Reward
Guidance
Positive reform measures
Tension
Interest
Positive reinforcement
Negative reinforcement
Goals
Organization
Competition
Conflict
Grading
Tracking
Class size
Valuing
Methodology
Teacher competency
Direction
Student input

School Milieu

Tight-ship concept
Open campus
Student input
Counseling
Parental input

THE FACILITY

One of the positive side effects of the huge increase in school construction during the 1960s was an innovative approach to design and construction of educational facilities. Many school facilities were planned around new curricula concepts, educational objectives, and special needs of communities and students. It was not uncommon for school districts to develop carefully researched thirty-year building construction plans. These plans took into consideration the early purchase of land to save costs, zoning trends, population shifts, and economic predictions. This type of planning has resulted in functional learning facilities that include modern educational concepts at optimal cost. Many districts, however, have continued to operate on a wasteful "crisis-to-crisis" school construction plan. The results of this shortsighted planning are expensive facilities, ill conceived for changing teaching methods and sometimes overcrowded by the time the doors of the facility open for the first time.

Although long-range planning is of great value, the planning of school facilities is becoming an increasingly difficult task. Population shifts, rapid inner-city decay, energy crises, spiraling inflation in building construction, and rising costs in education present seemingly impossible planning problems for the nation's communities.

The following factors[2] are indicative of carefully planned elementary and middle school facilities:

1. Children should be able to walk less than one-half mile to school.
2. The school should be integrated.
3. The school grounds should be a minimum of 10 acres, with one additional acre for every 100 pupils.
4. The school grounds should be away from dangerous traffic flow patterns, railroads, airports, and water hazards.
5. The grounds should have adequate drainage.

Fig. 9–4. Multipurpose area in a typical classroom.

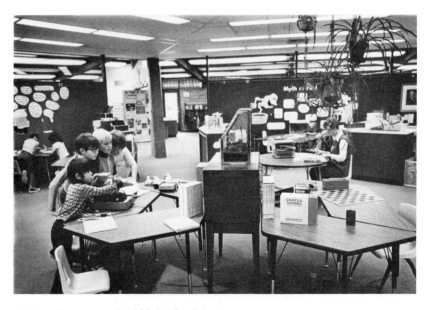

2. Joint Committee, *Healthful School Environment,* p. 149.

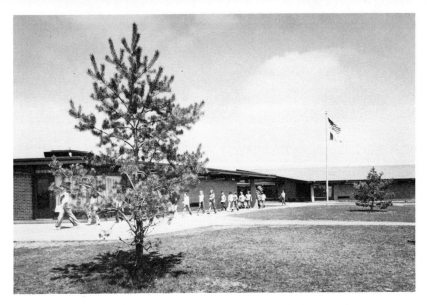

Fig. 9–5. A modern elementary school.

6. The grounds should be landscaped to include sound-intercepting trees and shrubs and aesthetic beauty.
7. Adequate off-street parking should be provided for employees and visitors.
8. The loading zones and traffic patterns should be carefully planned.
9. The facility should be located in a quiet residential area.
10. The area should be utilized for park and adult activities.

Elementary school facilities seem to fall into three categories: (1) the traditional multistory, self-contained classroom structure, (2) the open classroom structure with a center resource area and movable partitions between group areas, and (3) the modified structure containing open classroom areas, self-contained areas, rooms with movable partitions, center resource area, and multipurpose rooms. Further research is needed to determine the most effective type of school building. For example, Sugden found that although student needs were being met and greater interaction occurred between teachers and among teachers and students in an open type structure open structures were found to be noisy, hard to heat, difficult for students who need a more structured environment, and very difficult to manage when overcrowding occurred.[3] It has been suggested that the modified, single-story building using some closed rooms as well as some open classroom areas, combined with a resource center and a separate multipurpose area, may be the preferred approach to modern elementary school construction.[4, 5]

Preplanning and continual evaluation are necessary for achieving maximum potential from any elementary school facility. Some teachers prefer

3. John H. Sugden, "How Effective Are Open Plan Elementary Schools?" *American Schools and Universities* 45 (1973): 18–20.
4. Sugden, "Open Plan Elementary Schools," 45: 18–20.
5. Phillip R. Rittelmann, "How Schools Contribute to the Energy Crisis," *American School Board Journal* 160 (1973): 49–52.

Fig. 9–6. One type of open classroom.

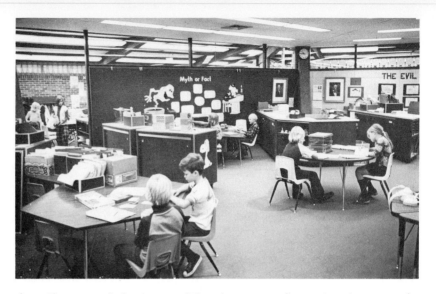

the self-contained classroom, while others argue the merits of team teaching and open classroom approaches. The loss of identity, constant compromise, long planning meetings, and personality conflicts sometimes consequent in team teaching are some of the reasons given by teachers preferring the self-contained classroom. Teachers advocating the open classroom and team teaching approaches prefer the released time to develop new materials and learning activities, share ideas, and teach in their special areas, and they argue that in the long run better teaching occurs. In addition, the team teaching approach can be less traumatic to the beginning teacher. It has become apparent that in order to accommodate the individual differences and needs of teachers and students several different classroom structures are needed. The sense of well-being as well as the health of school children and personnel can be dependent upon the organization, assets, and limitations of a given elementary school facility.

SCHOOL HOUSEKEEPING AND HEALTH

Good housekeeping needs a well-trained, well-equipped maintenance staff and the cooperation of students and teachers. Good housekeeping practices protect the health of students and provide learning experiences in regard to sanitation, dangers of clutter, storage procedures, waste disposal, and cleanliness. Disease prevention, accident prevention, and the aesthetic qualities of cleanliness and order are the primary objectives of school housekeeping. By way of example, clutter accounted for forty-three teachers receiving reportable injuries in a Midwestern school district in 1971.[6]

Many diseases are transferred because of improper use of drinking fountains, poor food-handling procedures, and lack of personal cleanliness. For example, most childhood diseases are transmitted by direct or indirect contact with discharges from the skin, nose, and throat or from fecal contamination.[7] Maintenance personnel should be trained to handle machines

6. "If You Don't Want to Get Injured, Don't Get Near a School," *American School Board Journal* 158 (1971): 31–33.
7. Abram S. Benenson, ed., *Control of Communicable Diseases in Man* (Washington, D.C.: American Public Health Association, 1970).

and chemicals capable of controlling health hazards such as dust, pathogens, and fecal contamination throughout the school building.[8,9] The major factor in disease control, however, is to guide the students toward the proper use of drinking and eating utensils, to prefer and maintain personal cleanliness, and to take the necessary precautions against the spread of communicable disease.

THE SCHOOL LUNCH PROGRAM

In 1946, the Seventy-Ninth Congress of the United States passed Public Law 396, the National School Lunch Act. This law was passed to aid national security by improving the nutrition of our nation's youth. In addition, it helped support the price of farm produce by absorbing some of the surplus food supplies. The program was supplemented by the Special Milk Program established under the Agricultural Act of 1954 and the Child Nutrition Act of 1966 which established the School Breakfast Program.[10] Standards were established and special programs for the disadvantaged were put into operation.

At the present time the program operates on a school district reimbursement basis. It remains to be seen whether this federally subsidized lunch program can continue with the disappearance of food surpluses and the continuing rise in food costs. Smolensky and Bonvechio suggest that the school lunch program, in addition to providing one-third of the daily nutrient requirements of children, can also provide an educational experience in food selection and sound principles of nutrition.[11]

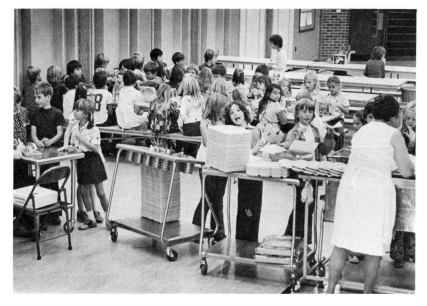

Fig. 9–7. A typical school lunchroom.

8. "Twenty Steps to Programmed Washroom Maintenance," *Nation's Schools* 84 (1969): 106–107.

9. David E. Smally, "New Cleaning Techniques Free Floors From Dirt," *American School Board Journal* 148 (1964): 38, 42, 44.

10. Phyllis Agran, "The National School Lunch Program," *Journal of School Health* 39 (1969): 440–442.

11. Jack Smolensky, and Richard L. Bonvechio, *Principles of School Health* (Boston: D. C. Heath & Co., 1966), p. 97.

The School Lunch Program consists of Type A, B, or C lunches. The Type A Lunch includes the following foods:

1. One-half fluid pint of whole milk as a beverage
2. Two ounces of lean meat, poultry, fish, or cheese or one egg or one-half cup cooked dry beans or peas, or four tablespoons of peanut butter or the equivalent of these
3. Three-fourths cup of two or more vegetables or fruits or both
4. One or more portions of bread or muffins or other bread made of wholegrain cereal or enriched flour
5. Two teaspoons of butter or fortified margarine.

The Type B lunch consists of two-thirds as much food as the Type A lunch, with supplements from home. The Type C lunch consists of one-half pint of whole milk.[12]

State and federal guidelines have been established concerning operation of the school lunch program. These guidelines include the training of personnel, food-handling procedures, preparation and storage regulations, menu planning, cleaning rules, and waste disposal. School lunch programs are complex and require extensive outlays of money in terms of equipment, supplies, and personnel.

The following guidelines were established for the scheduling of school lunch periods:

> Scheduling should include time for handwashing, for securing food, and for eating leisurely. An allowance of 20 minutes at the table is advised in elementary schools . . . an additional 10 minutes is desirable for handwashing and passing to and from the lunchrooms. Insofar as possible, 11:30 should be the earliest hour to serve and 12:30 the latest, with younger pupils served first. . .
>
> When staggered dismissals are not used, one or more shifts may accommodate the number to be served according to the seating capacity of the dining area. Three shifts are the maximum possible within desirable time limits.[13]

School lunchroom supervision has an effect on the length of the lunch break and the type of activities students may pursue after eating. In addition, supervision of the lunchroom has become a factor in negotiation between teacher organizations and school district officials. A research study during the 1970–1971 academic year found that of 170 school districts 74.7 percent (127 districts) contained negotiated lunchroom provisions for elementary teachers. It was also found that in 127 elementary school districts the typical lunch break was 30 minutes. Approximately 75 percent of the districts surveyed indicated the teacher's lunch break was duty free.[14]

12. U.S. Department of Agriculture, Consumer and Marketing Services, *The Type A Lunch Pattern* (Washington, D.C.: Department of Agriculture, 1969).
13. Joint Committee, *Healthful School Environment,* p. 133.
14. National Education Association, Research Division, "Teacher Lunch Periods: An Item of Negotiation," *National Education Association Research Bulletin* 50 (1972): 38–40.

The school lunch program can also be utilized as a learning experience in nutrition. Smolensky and Bonvechio suggest the following learning activities:

1. Supervised handwashing practice, with instruction on the why of personal cleanliness
2. Proper food selection
3. Student planning of menus
4. Demonstrations and explanations on the storage of lunches and food
5. Encouraging students to try new foods on "taste days"
6. Encouraging table manners, serving, passing, noise levels, etc.[15]

THE PHYSICAL ASPECTS OF THE CLASSROOM

Heating, ventilation, lighting, and noise can have a direct influence on the comfort of students and teachers. Although the temperature of a classroom may not have an influence on learning, very few teachers or students enjoy an environment suffering from the terrible toos: too hot, too stuffy, too noisy, too cold, too dark, too dull, too bright, or too long.[16]

Bedell recommends that schools carefully consider heat and air distribution systems, space required for heating and cooling units, fuel selection, and operating costs.[17] Although the classroom teacher probably will never have input into the planning of a school's heating and ventilation system, the teacher can usually control the temperature and air movement in a classroom.

It has been recommended that classroom temperatures vary from 65° F to 76° F, depending upon the age and activity levels of the class. While normal winter classroom temperatures should be below 70° F, primary students may need a slightly warmer room temperature.[18]

The comfort level in a classroom can change rapidly. Teachers need to be alert for environmental changes that occur because of temperature change, activity, clothing, crowding, sunlight, time of day, humidity, stress, and air movement. Air movement may be the most important factor in classroom comfort. A fan or breeze from a window can be the deciding factor between class progress and chaos on unseasonably hot, humid days. Man's ability to perspire allows for quick changes in temperature; however, air movement is required to quickly evaporate perspiration and thereby cool the body. The minimum recommendation for air movement in the classroom is not less than 15 cubic feet of air per minute, per person.[19]

Traditionally, classroom lighting was thought of in terms of the amount of footcandles of illumination needed for halls, for reading, and for study. Today, school designers are more concerned with reflection, glare, natural light, and costs.[20] Controlling reflection factors and light sources will aid in the visual aspects of learning; however, a more important element might

15. Smolensky and Bonvechio, *Principles*, pp. 96–98.
16. Burdette P. Hansen, "A Study of the Effects of Room Temperature On Learning," *Research in Education* 2 (1966): 11.
17. Robert K. Bedell, "Heating Systems Provide Spark for School Environment," *Nation's Schools* 86 (1970): 58–59.
18. Joint Committee, *Healthful School Environment*, pp. 190–192.
19. Joint Committee, *Healthful School Environment*, p. 192.
20. Frederich G. Knirk, "Acoustical and Visual Environments Effect Learning," *Audiovisual Instruction* 15 (1970): 34–35.

be the *visual field* of a classroom. A classroom visual field involves the following elements:

1. Colorful and functional bulletin boards and displays
   a. Motivational and informational
   b. Posters, charts, diagrams, and mobiles carefully arranged
   c. Special projects, art work, unit goals, and individual projects
2. A room free of clutter and debris
3. Outside visual distractions kept to a minimum
4. Study areas, time-out areas, and equipment and resource centers arranged to limit visual distractions
5. Bright, stimulating colors

Noise can also influence the learning environment, the health of students, and perhaps the sanity of the teacher.[21] Sound-absorbing materials, furnishings, and acoustical tile can reduce distracting sound levels and improve the environment needed for study and communication. Acceptable classroom noise levels are 40 decibels or less.[22] Since 40 decibels are only 25 decibels below average factory noise, a classroom is not intended to be a quiet place.[23] It has been pointed out, however, that continuous, prolonged exposure to noise levels of as low as 80 decibels can produce permanent hearing loss. Also, noise can contribute to those health problems dealing with tension, cardiovascular disease, gastrointestinal disorder, and vascular headache.[24]

Fig. 9–8. An ideal classroom visual field. Note the color charts and other displays, the study areas, the special equipment, and study resources such as books and magazines.

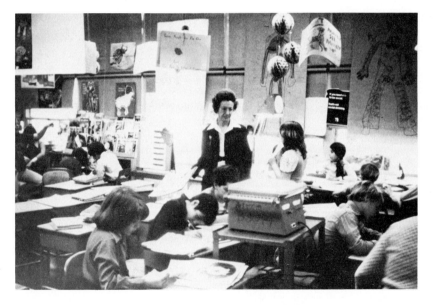

21. Robert A. Baron, *The Tyranny of Noise* (New York: St. Martin's Press, 1970), pp. 36–60.
22. Joint Committee, *Healthful School Living,* p. 40.
23. Theodore Berland, "The Medical Consequences of Noise Pollution," mimeographed (Springfield, Ill.: Environmental Protection Agency, 1970).
24. "How Today's Noise Hurts Body and Mind," *Medical World News* 10 (1969): 42–47.

Accidents continue to be the number one health problem of elementary school children. Accidents account for more deaths in the age group five to fourteen years than do the combined causes of death for all diseases.[25] The number of deaths in 1972 for this age group was 17,431, with 8,186 deaths occurring as a result of accidents. Annually, boys account for 69 percent of the accidental deaths in the five-to-fourteen-years age group. A more important statistic is that for every death occurring as a result of an accident there may be five or six children facing life with some degree of permanent disability. Table 9–1 indicates the accidental death rates among elementary school children.

Table 9–1. Accidental Deaths of Children Ages Five to Fourteen Years in 1970

Cause	Frequency Ages 5–14 yrs.	Frequency All Ages
All accidents	8,203	114,638
Motor vehicles	4,159	54,633
Falls	100	16,926
Drowning	1,550	7,860
Associated with fires	609	6,718
Suffocation, ingested objects	50	1,600
Poisoning by liquids and solids	70	3,000
Firearms	350	1,600
Poisoning by gases and vapors	40	1,000
All other types	1,885	28,501

Source: National Center for Health Statistics.
Note: Death from all causes for ages five to fourteen years were 16,847; from cancer, 2,429; and from congenital anomalies, 901.

Motor vehicle accidents annually claim the lives of over 4,000 elementary school children of whom 1,900 are pedestrians. In addition 550 are killed in pedacycle accidents. In most cases, the child was not following basic pedestrian or bicycle safety rules.

Approximately 38,000 reported school jurisdictional accidents occurred during the 1971–1972 school year. It has been estimated, however, that 800,000 school injuries occur annually. In general, boys have the most accidents. The injury rate in physical education is higher than in any other class. Accident rates are almost as high as in physical education for unsupervised play and play areas, and the highest rates of all occur during classroom recess-type games.

In addition to the moral responsibility, prevention of accidents is a legal and financial obligation. Since one of every thirty-three students suffers a serious injury during a school year, the school district must absorb the costs of law suits, insurance, substitute teachers, and property damage. For example, Babigan and Licht found that one large school district lost over $500,000 through accident-related costs.[26]

Major aspects of a safe school environment include careful planning and supervision and sequential kindergarten through sixth grade safety edu-

PLANNING FOR A SAFE SCHOOL ENVIRONMENT

25. *Accident Facts* (Chicago: National Safety Council, 1974). Unless otherwise noted, all safety statistics cited are drawn from this source.
26. George R. Babigan, and Kenneth Licht, "What Are Accidents Costing Your District?" *American School Board Journal* 157 (1970): 27–28.

cation curriculum planning. As might be expected, the principal usually has the major responsibility for the safety program; however, teachers and staff must take an active role in developing and maintaining a safe school environment. The cooperation of all school personnel and staff are necessary in planning for a safe school environment, and many factors are involved, as the following list indicates:

1. Trained leadership
2. Teacher-student safety committees
3. Careful record keeping
4. Supervision of play areas, halls, and lunchrooms
5. Emphasis on safety in all classroom and student activities
6. Planned movement of classes and groups
7. Safety patrol, crossing-guard system
8. Motor vehicle flow, parking patterns, and bus unloading and loading
9. Pedacycle safety programs
10. Special plans for physical education safety procedures
11. Special planning for all field trips
12. System of inspections
13. Carefully planned fire safety programs
14. Emphasis on clutter-free classrooms, halls, and play areas
15. System of safety campaigns
16. Disaster plans
17. Safety planning for all play areas
18. Cooperative programs with local safety-oriented organizations
19. Planned sequential kindergarten through sixth grade safety education units
20. First-aid and emergency-care procedures

Florio suggests the following objectives for a safe school environment:

1. To create and make effective use of school safety organizations, particularly student patrols
2. To safeguard children in crossing streets on the way to and from school
3. To institute measures designed to protect children using the school bus
4. To eliminate hazards in the school building and on the school grounds and to induce children to behave safely on school property
5. To conduct efficient fire drills
6. To make maximum use of accident reports, especially in planning the safety program.[27]

A PROGRAM OF EMERGENCY CONTROL

In a Program of Emergency Controls the emphasis is on prevention of accidents, with the overlying philosophy of having students, teachers, and staff live safety. A Program of Emergency Controls involves the following six major safety areas:

27. A. E. Florio, and George T. Stafford, *Safety Education* (New York: McGraw-Hill Book Co., 1969), p. 94.

1. Safety education through safe living
2. Fire safety
3. First-aid organization
4. Record keeping
5. Cooperative programs with community organizations and agencies
6. Civil defense and disaster planning

SAFETY EDUCATION THROUGH SAFE LIVING

Safety education includes instruction in living safely and participation in formal safety lessons. The major topics of elementary school safety education include the following: safety in the home, in the community, at work, and during recreation; first-aid and emergency-care of the sick or injured; motor vehicle safety; pedestrian safety; pedacycle safety; fire prevention; poison prevention and/or treatment; safe use of firearms; water safety; and current safety topics. The philosophy of safety education through safe living is applied through student involvement in planning and maintaining a safe school environment.[28] Student involvement may well be the most effective learning activity in safety education and can take place through (1) junior safety councils, (2) safety patrols, (3) classroom safety activities, and (4) schoolwide safety activities.[29]

The junior safety council could be a committee from the student council and to ensure greater student participation should include other room representatives. The activities of this organization could be as follows:

1. Taking part in the planning of all school safety activities
2. Developing special subcommittees on hall, playground, pedacycle, and classroom safety problems and other problem areas
3. Developing safety rules to be posted throughout the school building
4. Organizing schoolwide campaigns on an appropriate safety topic each month
5. Planning special field trips to observe safety programs in action throughout the community

Safety patrols have proved to be effective in reducing injuries. Many schools have expanded their traffic patrol program to include hall, playground, lunchroom, fire drill, and bus patrols. Patrols should be made up of fifth and sixth graders only. This activity can provide leadership training, prevent accidents, provide positive recognition, and develop special safety skills. Ideally, a safety patrol program should be organized and run by students in a manner similar to a student council organization. When students are involved in traffic and bus patrols, the following rules must be considered:

1. Parental permission must be obtained.
2. Children must *not* direct traffic.
3. Children acting as patrol leaders must stand on the curb, never in the street.

28. Herbert J. Stack, ed., *Safety for Greater Adventure: The Contributions of Albert W. Whitney* (New York: New York University Center for Safety Education, 1953).
29. Florio and Stafford, *Safety*, pp. 94–121.

4. Protective coloration should be required.
5. All children in patrols must receive training and supervision.[30]

Students should be involved in formulating safety rules for each classroom activity. At times, this could simply involve asking for safety suggestions prior to beginning an activity. For more complex and potentially hazardous activities, student groups or individuals could be assigned to develop and post the safety rules. Teachers could also appoint a standing safety committee to monitor and make safety suggestions.

It is important to have all students participate in a safe-living program. Since the safety patrol and junior safety council activities involve only a few students at a time, schoolwide activities should be developed. Schoolwide participation could include planning and implementing safety poster campaigns, organizing safety slogan contests, posting safety rules, taking part in community safety campaigns, and participating in room competition for the fewest number of injuries for a given school term.

Fig. 9–9. A typical safety patrol.

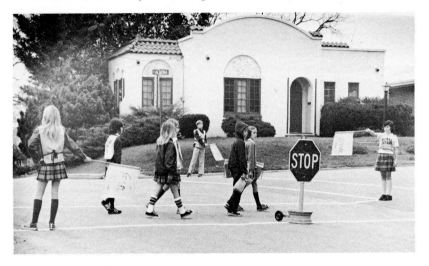

FIRE SAFETY

All schools need a carefully prepared fire protection and evacuation plan. During 1972, approximately 20,500 school and college fires occurred, costing a total of $87,000,000 in damage. The building principal, or a designated individual or committee, must be in charge of the fire-safety program. The local fire department should be sought for assistance in organizing this program.

Suggestions for a fire protection program include the following:

1. All buildings constructed of fire-resistive materials
2. Careful storage of all school materials, especially volatile chemicals
3. Building designed for maximum traffic flow
4. Exit doors equipped with panic bolts
5. Well-lighted hallways with easily visible exit signs

30. National Commission on Safety Education, *Policies and Practices for School Safety Patrols* (Washington, D.C.: National Education Association, 1966).

6. Fire extinguishers properly maintained and inspected
7. Extra extinguishers in all shops, laboratories, and work areas
8. Fire alarm system connected to the local fire department
9. Fire doors strategically placed
10. All school areas free of clutter, debris, and dust

In addition consideration should be given to evacuating the school facility in the event of a fire.

Suggestions for a fire evacuation program include the following:

1. Careful training of *all* school personnel
2. Posted evacuation routes in all rooms
3. Assigned personnel to check that all school areas are cleared
4. A minimum of five fire drills per year
5. Emphasis on school fire safety in early fall
6. Established exit rules that include no talking, single file, no pushing, and walking only
7. Fire drills that are announced, unannounced, and obstructed at unusual times
8. Planned analysis and discussion periods following each exit or disaster drill
9. Rooms given designated areas in which to assemble outside of the building where roll call can be taken
10. Coordination with the local fire department
11. No one may reenter the building until an appropriate reentry signal is given
12. Designated first aid and communication station
13. Designated area for the meeting of fire drill monitors
14. *All* students and personnel participate in each drill

FIRST AID ORGANIZATION

Haag suggests that at least 50 percent of all school personnel have recent training in first aid.[31] In order to handle victims of accidents or sudden illnesses, each school building should have a first-aid room equipped with essential first-aid supplies. All school personnel should know what to do at the scene of an accident; have instruction in the first aid necessary for burns, fractures, shock, poisoning, stoppage of breathing, wounds, bleeding, seizures, drug problems, sudden illness, and choking; and know when and how to move or transport victims. Schools also need written procedures for supervising other children when an accident or sudden illness occurs.

RECORD KEEPING

The National Safety Council has indicated that accident reporting and record keeping are the foundation for school safety planning, and after years of careful research have recommended that an accident report have as a minimum the following content:

1. Name
2. Address
3. School

31. Jessie H. Haag, *School Health Program* (Philadelphia: Lea & Febiger, 1972), p. 118.

4. Sex
5. Age
6. Grade/special program
7. Date and time of accident; day of week
8. Nature of the injury
9. Part of the body injured
10. Degree of the injury
11. Number of days lost
12. Cause of the injury
13. Jurisdictional classification of the accident
14. Location of accident
15. Activity of the victim
16. Status of the activity
17. Supervision
18. Agency involved (apparatus, equipment, etc.)
19. Unsafe acts
20. Unsafe mechanical-physical conditions
21. Unsafe personal factors
22. Corrective action taken or recommended
23. Property damage
24. Description (paragraph form)
25. Date of report
26. Report prepared by (signature)
27. Witness's signature
28. Principal's signature[32]

The National Safety Council suggests the following criteria for distinguishing between a reportable accident and a recordable accident:

1. A *reportable* accident is:
    a. Any school jurisdictional accident which results in any injury to a pupil and/or property damage
    b. Any non-school jurisdictional accident which results in injury causing restriction to the pupil
2. A *recordable* accident is any accident which results in:
    a. Pupil injury severe enough to cause loss of one-half day or more of school time
    b. Pupil injury severe enough to cause the loss of one-half day or more of pupil activity during non-school time
    c. Any property damage as a result of a school jurisdictional accident[33]

Florio suggests that accident records serve as the basis for safety education curriculum planning and the organization of a safe school environment.[34] In addition, records provide data concerning the location of hazard-

32. *Student Accident Reporting Guidebook* (Chicago: National Safety Council, 1966), p. 29.
33. *Accident Reporting,* p. 3.
34. Florio and Stafford, *Safety,* p. 129.

ous areas, the type of supervision at the time of an accident, the names of accident-repeating children, and the names of careless teachers. Such records can be utilized in eliminating dangerous activities, practices, and equipment.

Permission slips from parents for field trips, special events, patrols, and all extracurricular activities should be considered an important part of a record-keeping system. Although the permission slip does not free the teacher from liability when teacher negligence contributes to an injury, a permission slip does prove that the parents are aware of the child's participation and have approved of the activity.

Included in a record-keeping system is a system of notification of parents. If a child is injured or ill, the parents or guardians must be notified as soon as possible. As discussed in chapter 8, this becomes very important when a child needs prompt medical attention. Law suits have occurred when school authorities have taken a child to a medical facility without parental approval. Also unless an extreme emergency exists, physicians are very reluctant to treat a minor without parental permission. On file in the school building should be the parent's or guardian's phone numbers for home and work and the names and addresses of other adults who could assist in locating an injured child's parents or guardians.

On file with each student's medical record and parental notification card should be a card stating any known sensitivity to drugs and bee stings and other allergens. Also noted on this emergency card should be the existence of any known health limitation such as heart disease, epilepsy, diabetes, and other handicaps the school personnel should be aware of in order to protect the student.

COOPERATIVE PROGRAM WITH COMMUNITY ORGANIZATIONS

It is important to realize that a school health and safety program is only a part of the community health and safety program. Community agencies and authorities must be contacted in the planning and supervision of a safe school environment. A cooperative school-community safe school environment is outlined in Figure 9–10.

Figure 9–10. A Cooperative School-Community Program for a Safe School Environment

Agency/Organization	Cooperative Program
Police department	Traffic control, security, large crowd control, protection, evacuation, transportation of victims
Fire department	Fire inspection, planning drills, natural disaster plans, training
Medical facilities	Transportation, treatment, training
Community services	Planning, maintenance, traffic flow, zoning, space, finance, construction
Voluntary community agencies American Red Cross Civil Defense	Training of personnel, planning, supervision, support
Service organizations Parent-Teacher Association Clubs	Manpower, funds, support, equipment, supervision, preschool programs

CIVIL DEFENSE AND DISASTER PLANS

During the late 1950s and the era of the Cuban missile crisis of the early 1960s, a plan for a safe school environment would have included what to do in case of a thermonuclear attack. At the present time, the detente between the world's nuclear powers seems to preclude the specter of children practicing how to avoid a sudden burst of light, shock waves, and radiation from a nuclear bomb. However, it is necessary to develop disaster plans for such natural phenomena as flash floods, hurricanes, tornadoes, violent storms, and earthquakes. For example, around seven hundred tornadoes occur each year in the United States. Emergency plans should include drills, training of students and school personnel, development of warning systems, and development of shelter systems. The United States Weather Service, civil defense agencies, fire departments, and police departments should be consulted in the development and supervision of school civil defense and disaster plans.

LIABILITY IN ELEMENTARY SCHOOL EDUCATION

The health and safety of students is both a moral and a legal responsibility of school personnel. The teacher has the following legal responsibilities:

1. To foresee and prevent unsafe situations, equipment, facilities, and practices
2. To be professionally qualified to supervise and lead student activities
3. To be prepared to act prudently if an accident does occur
4. To know the laws regarding liability of the state or territory in which they are employed

At some point during their careers, even the most skilled and safety-conscious teachers will be unable to avoid the experience of having an accident occur in their classroom. The scope of modern teaching strategies includes such activities as field trips, laboratory-type experiments, use of special equipment, and emphasis on independent work. These activities add to the probabilities of accidents occurring. In layman's terms, a teacher can be held liable and answerable for financial claims and damages if in a court of law it can be proved that the teacher contributed to the cause or causes of an accident.[35]

The purposes of liability laws are to protect and compensate the innocent victim of an accident by forcing citizens to eliminate those conditions and actions which might be damaging to others. An informed teacher is aware that the chances for a lawsuit have increased because of the following factors:

1. Trends in modern teaching strategies
2. Student unrest
3. Overcrowding in schools
4. A lawsuit-conscious public well aware of a current pattern of large financial settlements
5. A salary scale that is large enough to attract suits.[36]

35. Marland K. Strasser, James E. Aaron, Ralph C. Bohn, and John R. Eales, *Fundamentals of Safety Education* (New York: Macmillan Co., 1964), p. 233.
36. Lee O. Garber, "Legal Outlook: More 1968 Clashes Over Student Rights," *Nation's Schools* 81 (1968): 74, 78.

The laws concerning the liability of public school officials and personnel vary from state to state. In a few states the state and local governments and school districts can be sued; however, in most states restitution can be collected for a school-related accident only by bringing a lawsuit against a teacher, administrator, or school official.

Liability insurance is a must for all school officials and personnel. In some states, by law the school district cannot procure liability insurance for its employees. Even though other states allow for school districts to purchase liability insurance, usually with an upper limit of $10,000, it is wise for all teachers to procure an insurance policy of their own. A liability insurance policy can easily be obtained through most home or automobile insurance firms for a nominal rate.

Courtroom terminology is difficult to grasp. However, some understanding of the following terms can provide insight into how a teacher's actions, or lack of action, when an accident occurs are viewed by a court of law.[37]

TERMS IN SCHOOL LIABILITY

Negligence—the failure to act as a reasonably prudent person would act under a specific set of circumstances.

Tort—an improper act of commission or omission, without right, contributing to the injury of another in person, property, or reputation. An act of omission occurs when without intent an individual failed to foresee or perform an action that would have prevented an injury to another. An act of commission occurs when there was an intent to cause an injury to another.

Attractive nuisance—any type of structure, apparatus, or excavation that is left unguarded, thereby inviting a child to play on or in it. A common example of an attractive nuisance is a backyard swimming pool.

In loco parentis ("in place of the parent")—a phrase which states that because school attendance is required by law the teacher or school assumes the parents' responsibility for the child while he is at school.

Foreseeability—awareness of the consequences of a certain act or situation and avoidance of this act or situation. Ignorance is not a defense. If one assumes the responsibility of supervising or directing an activity, it is his or an administrator's responsibility to be qualified and skilled in directing the activity.

Last clear chance—the final opportunity to take action in preventing an injury.

Malfeasance—usually, performance of an illegal act by a school official.

Misfeasance—performance of a legal act such as giving first aid in an improper manner by a school official.

Nonfeasance—failure of a school official to perform his legal duty or responsibility such as giving first aid.

Proprietary function—the responsibility of a school for the safety of those attending school functions. In the eyes of the court this responsibility is increased when fees are charged for admission to a school function.

TERMS FOR THE DEFENSE IN A LAWSUIT

Assumption of risk—an adult's voluntary participation in an activity with full knowledge of the possible risks involved. This defense can almost never

37. Howard C. Leibee, *Tort Liability for Injuries to Pupils* (Ann Arbor, Mich.: Campus Publishers, 1965).

be used when the victim of a tort is of elementary school age. It is assumed that even though the student has an understanding of the risks involved in the activity he is not capable of making the proper judgment of whether or not to participate.

Comparative negligence—assigning to an adult victim of an injury a percentage of the responsibility for an accident. The concept is similar to that of assumption of risk. Again, this is rarely or never used as a defense when the victim of an accident is a minor.

Contributory negligence—negligence of an adult victim of an injury in failing to act prudently in preventing the injury to himself.

Stare decisis ("stand by settled matters")—the customary action of a court to follow the precedent set by previous court decisions.

Vis major—an accident or injury that could not have been avoided, for example, an earthquake.

If a qualified educator carefully protects the safety of students, the probability of a lawsuit is very low. In summary, a reasonably prudent teacher will take the following precautions:

1. Plan for safety.
2. Know the health status of the pupils.
3. Never use defective equipment.
4. Inspect the facility on a regular basis.
5. Carefully consider the readiness of the student for the activity.
6. Always conduct activities in a safe area.
7. Be professionally prepared to teach proper techniques and be aware of how injuries might occur.
8. Carefully train all students to perform the activity properly.
9. Perform first aid in a proper manner when an injury does occur.
10. Keep an accurate record of all accidents and always complete accident reports in detail as soon after the accident as possible.
11. Do not transport students in a private vehicle.
12. Do not leave students unsupervised.
13. Obtain parental permission slips for activities which are different from normal classroom activity.
14. Be alert for and correct those student actions which might lead to an injury.
15. If litigation does occur, seek a highly qualified attorney.[38]
16. Control the action of students under supervision.

SUMMARY
Healthful school living has two major components: (1) healthful school environment and (2) safe school environment. A commonality of each of these major components is the interaction of personal, social, economic, cultural, and other ecological factors. Providing for the health and safety of school children is the responsibility of both school and community.

Many factors within the school can influence the health and safety of students. These factors can include scheduling, sanitation, heating, ventilation, maintenance of facilities, working conditions, teacher-student rapport,

38. Raymond G. Kuntz, "How to Help Your Attorney Win Your Case When Your School District Is Sued," *American School Board Journal* 160 (1973): 35–37.

discipline codes, and other factors. A healthful school environment is a critical blend of adequate community support, qualified personnel, attitude, cooperation, and motivation.

School officials and personnel have both moral and legal obligations to provide a safe school environment. Students must be protected from injury and if injured must be provided with adequate emergency care. The protection of students from injury involves careful planning, adequate and well-maintained facilities, and safety instruction. Having teachers and students grasp the concepts that safety measures can provide for more fulfilling experiences and for the protection of others will aid in the prevention of accidents.

Safe school living can be developed within the concept of a program of emergency controls. This program combines safety education with fire prevention, first-aid organization, careful record keeping, cooperative safety programs with community agencies, and civil defense and disaster plans. Even though careful attention has been paid to preventing accidents, active student involvement in modern teaching strategies will create situations in which students can be injured. With this in mind, the modern educator needs a clear understanding of liability and the information necessary for making prudent decisions for the protection of the health and safety of students.

Discussion Questions

1. Why should there be an ecological approach to the school health environment?
2. List five major within-school factors that influence the health of students. Rank these factors in order of importance. Defend your ranking.
3. Conduct a survey to determine how different members of your community view rising school costs, the teaching profession, teachers' salaries, and modern teaching strategies.
4. How can the planning of school facilities influence the health of students and school personnel?
5. Discuss with teachers their view on who is responsible for a healthful school environment.
6. How can each of the following factors influence the health of students? (a) scheduling, (b) play and recreation, (c) teacher-student relations, (d) teacher-administrator relations
7. Describe the type of school facility in which you would like to teach.
8. What is your opinion on open schools, self-contained classrooms, and team teaching?
9. What are the pros-and-cons of tracking students? What is your opinion?
10. List all the implications of overcrowding in a school.
11. Why is the federally supported school lunch program in jeopardy?
12. Should teachers have to supervise lunchrooms, study halls, recesses, playgrounds, and bus loading and unloading? Defend your answer.
13. Since accident rates are very high for playground equipment, discuss the pros-and-cons of eliminating this equipment.
14. Suggest a series of rules for ensuring the comfort of students in terms of temperature and humidity control.
15. Where and under what circumstances are accidents likely to occur in schools?

16. Defend the concept of living safety in schools. Discuss ways of implementing this concept.
17. Observe safety patrols in action. How are they supervised? What are the opinions of the students involved of these activities?
18. Develop a plan for: (a) evacuation of your room in case of fire, (b) emergency procedures in case of a natural disaster, and (c) what to do in case an accident or sudden illness occurs.
19. Consider the school-related accidents you have witnessed or been involved in. How could these accidents have been avoided? What did the supervisor do after the accident occurred as well as before the incident? Could the teacher have been open to a lawsuit? How do you feel the court would have ruled on the case?
20. Describe a "reasonably prudent" elementary teacher.

References

Accident Facts. Chicago: National Safety Council, 1974.

Agran, Phyllis. "The National School Lunch Program." *Journal of School Health* 39 (1969): 440–442.

Babigan, George R., and Licht, Kenneth. "What Are Accidents Costing Your District?" *American School Board Journal* 157 (1970): 27–28.

Baron, Robert A. *The Tyranny of Noise.* New York: St Martin's Press, 1970.

Bedell, Robert K. "Heating Systems Provide Spark for School Environment." *Nation's Schools* 86 (1970): 58–59.

Benenson, Abram S., ed. *Control of Communicable Diseases in Man.* Washington, D.C.: American Public Health Association, 1970.

Berland, Theodore. "The Medical Consequences of Noise Pollution." Mimeographed. Springfield, Ill.: Environmental Protection Agency, 1970.

Florio, A. E., and Stafford, George T. *Safety Education.* New York: McGraw-Hill Book Co. ,1969.

Garber, Lee O. "Legal Outlook: More 1968 Clashes Over Student Rights." *Nation's Schools* 81 (1968): 74, 78.

Haag, Jessie, H. *School Health Program.* Philadelphia: Lea & Febiger, 1972.

Hansen, Burdette P. "A Study of the Effects of Room Temperature on Learning." *Research in Education* 2 (1966): 11.

"How Today's Noise Hurts Body and Mind." *Medical World News* 10 (1969): 42–47.

"If You Don't Want To Get Injured, Don't Get Near a School." *American School Board Journal* 158 (1971): 31–33.

Joint Committee on Health Problems in Education of the National Education Association and the American Medical Association, *Healthful School Environment.* Washington, D.C.: National Education Association, 1969.

Knirk, Frederick G. "Acoustical and Visual Environments Effect Learning." *Audiovisual Instruction* 15 (1970): 34–35.

Kuntz, Raymond G. "How to Help Your Attorney Win Your Case When Your School District Is Sued." *American School Board Journal* 160 (1973): 35–37.

Leibee, Howard C. *Tort Liability for Injuries to Pupils.* Ann Arbor, Mich.: Campus Publishers, 1965.

National Commission on Safety Education. *Policies and Practices for School Safety Patrols*. Washington, D.C.: National Education Association, 1966.

National Education Association. Research Division. "Teacher Lunch Periods: An Item of Negotiation." *National Education Association, Research Bulletin* 50 (1972): 38–40.

Rittelmann, Phillip R. "How Schools Contribute to the Energy Crisis." *American School Board Journal* 160 (1973): 49–52.

Smally, David E. "New Cleaning Techniques Free Floors From Dirt." *American School Board Journal* 148 (1964): 38, 42, 44.

Smolensky, Jack, and Bonvechio, Richard L. *Principles of School Health*. Boston: D. C. Heath & Co., 1966.

Stack, Herbert J., ed. *Safety for Greater Adventure: The Contributions of Albert W. Whitney*. New York: New York University Center for Safety Education, 1953.

Strasser, Marland K., Aaron, James E., Bohn, Ralph C., and Eales, John R. *Fundamentals of Safety Education*. New York: Macmillan Co., 1964.

Student Accident Reporting Guidebook. Chicago: National Safety Council, 1966.

Sugden, John H. "How Effective Are Open Plan Elementary Schools?" *American Schools and Universities* 45 (1973): 18–20.

"Twenty Steps to Programmed Washroom Maintenance." *Nation's Schools* 84 (1969): 106–107.

U.S. Department of Agriculture. Consumer Marketing Services. *The Type A Lunch Pattern*. Washington, D.C.: Department of Agriculture, 1969.

Chapter 10

THE
HEALTH
INSTRUCTION
PROGRAM

What is meant by the cognitive, affective, and behavioral components of a belief?

Why is insight into pupils' health attitudes important to the classroom teacher?

How can behavior change be facilitated in the classroom?

How does one determine the content of health instruction in the elementary and middle grades?

Discussions in chapter 8 and 9 deal with health services and healthful school living, two constituents of the school health program with which classroom teachers should be intimately familiar. The present chapter focuses on health instruction, the final, but by no means least important, element of the health program triad.

THE AIMS OF HEALTH EDUCATION

The term *instruction* has a didactic connotation, for it suggests a somewhat methodical, highly structured, teacher-centered process concerned essentially with the transmission of factual information or the development of specific skills. However, health instruction as described in this book encompasses a broader range of activities including formal classroom teaching, planned learning experiences outside the classroom, and incidental teaching, provided for individuals or groups.

Though the impartation of knowledge is basic to all instruction, where health is concerned, knowing is not enough. Virtually all cigarette smokers, for example, know that their habit is detrimental to health since a warning to that effect is clearly stated in bold print on each cigarette package. Of what value is this knowledge to them? Teaching children to wash their hands prior to eating serves little purpose unless the behavior is internalized and practiced regularly. Curiously enough, some schools teach children that this practice is desirable, but do not allow children the time to wash their hands before lunch. Health knowledge per se is practically useless unless it is accepted by the individual, incorporated into his attitude structure, and manifested as positive health behavior. The ultimate aim of health education, therefore, is to enable one to achieve and maintain positive well-being

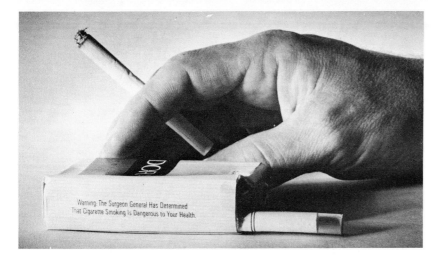

Fig. 10–1. Warnings are sometimes not enough!

through the application of basic health principles to life situations. Progress toward this end depends largely on how well teachers of health succeed in developing health-educated persons, rather than merely health-informed persons.

At the end of the first day on the job, an exhausted, yet enthusiastic beginning teacher described the class as having twenty-five odd children. This ambiguous reference was to the relative size of the class, rather than to pupil peculiarities observed during the first day on the job. Little did the teacher realize that as a neophyte her class and all other classes are indeed odd. The simple fact is that while children on a given grade level have much in common no two classmates match up like socks in a pair or bananas in a bunch. Apart from their obvious physical, emotional, and social dissimilarities, children enter classrooms with ideas, attitudes, knowledge, and behaviors that are characteristically their own. Insight into these differences is as vital to effective health instruction as is the teacher's command of subject matter and pedagogical expertise.

According to Rokeach, "an attitude is a relatively enduring organization of beliefs around an object or situation predisposing one to respond in some preferential manner."[1] In other words, an individual's attitudes are persistent, or relatively so, are a function of his beliefs, and are basic causes of behavior. Each belief that underlies an attitude has three characteristics, identified by Rokeach as cognitive, affective, and behavioral. A belief is cognitive to the extent that it represents a child's knowledge, however accurate or inaccurate, of what is good or bad, right or wrong, desirable or undesirable. The child who "knows" that dentists hurt people has formulated the evaluative judgment that characterizes the cognitive aspect of a belief. If and when this belief arouses feelings related to the object of the belief (dentists), the affective component comes into play. Children with a negative evaluation (belief) of dentists would have their affect (feelings) awakened if during health instruction the importance of regular dental

THE NATURE OF ATTITUDES

1. M. Rokeach, *Beliefs, Attitudes, and Values* (San Francisco: Jossey-Bass, Inc., 1968), p. 112.

checkups was stressed. Under these circumstances it would be important for instructional purposes that children express their feelings regarding dentists. The probability of this self-expression occurring increases in a relaxed classroom atmosphere where the verbalization of feelings is welcomed and encouraged, and fear of ridicule and reprisal is nonexistent. Only then does the teacher have an opportunity to provide immediate reinforcement of positive health beliefs and to identify and respond to belief systems that impede sound health attitudes and behaviors.

Occasionally, the behavioral component of a belief remains inactive until circumstances trigger its expression. In our example of the child with the negative evaluation of dentists, the prospect of actually visiting a dentist for even a routine examination could arouse avoidance behavior consistent with the affective and cognitive dimensions of his belief. Rosenberg's work supports the common observation that each of us strives for consistency among the affective, cognitive, and behavioral elements of a belief and the belief organization of which an attitude consists.[2] Failure to achieve this consistency or consonance creates a dissonant condition that is stressful to the individual. Therefore, since attitudes seem to provide a measure of uniformity to one's behavior, insight into the health attitudes of children makes it possible to more readily predict their health behavior.

FACTS ALONE ARE NOT ENOUGH

Man is considered a rational being, though at times his behavior is strangely irrational. During his rational moments, man is guided by the facts as he knows them, but at other times, old habits, emotions, and other conscious and unconscious forces motivate behavior that is contradictory to knowledge and reason. Without question, health education would be a cakewalk if everybody acted solely on the basis of health information substantiated by valid evidence.

Too many classroom teachers and other persons involved in the health education enterprise approach their task seemingly believing that *to know is to do.* While some educators clearly do not know any better, others recognize the serious limitations of emphasizing facts only, but choose to take the easy way out. Consequently, the emphasis that should be placed on attitude formation and behavioral change is largely omitted from their teaching.

Instructional objectives that stress the importance of memory and factual recall actually demand little from most teachers in terms of preparation and presentation, and are the easiest to measure objectively. Teachers who face restrictions imposed by insufficient preparation time, inadequate teaching resources, and limited or outmoded professional preparation frequently find themselves seeking the haven of a curriculum that is basically fact-oriented. One gains a sense of security when dealing with the relatively stable body of basic knowledge in the health sciences. Nowhere is this more evident than in those classrooms where instruction in human anatomy and physiology is misrepresented as health education. The organs of digestion, their functions, and their relative position in the alimentary canal have been known for decades, and with few exceptions, this knowledge will continue to be accepted and unchallenged for years to come. In all probability, more

2. M. J. Rosenberg, "An Analysis of Affective-Cognitive Consistency," in *Attitude Organization and Change,* eds. M. J. Rosenberg et al. (New Haven: Yale University Press, 1960).

teachers have studied a course (e.g., freshman biology) having this type of content than have been exposed to courses placing greater emphasis on health attitude and behavior change. Little wonder, therefore, that so much of today's health instruction emphasizes anatomy and physiology and essentially ignores recent health science developments and issues that are relevant to today's health problems and their possible solutions.

An obvious peril one faces in dwelling upon factual information that one either knows best or feels most comfortable in teaching, regardless of pupil needs or interests, is that children will become bored. Unless the instruction concerns topics that are of concern to the class and taught in an engaging manner, pupil attention and learning will suffer. Psychologists refer to "selective pereception" as the conscious or unconscious process by which each of us selects only those visual, auditory, and other sensory stimuli that have special meaning to us. Irrelevant, uninteresting, and meaningless messages are selectively screened out. Using pupil needs and concerns as the basis for health instruction is, therefore, of critical importance. This is much easier said than accomplished, though, because the health instruction needed by youngsters does not always correspond with their interests. An astute and effective teacher refuses to allow pupil apathy and disinterest to serve as barriers to the teaching of essential health concepts. Instead, one employs sound professional judgment in identifying that content that needs to be taught and uses ingenuity in relating the topic to the lives of pupils.

Children begin to acquire health knowledge long before they attain the age of school entry. Much of this is the result of direct teaching by parents, other adults, and siblings. Television including commercial advertisements also contributes substantially to the fund of health knowledge possessed by children. Neither the source nor the accuracy of this information is necessarily reliable. In fact, much of what elementary school children understand about health is incomplete, misleading, or incorrect.

We have seen that attitudes can be reduced to belief systems and individual beliefs, which in turn, reflect one's knowledge, however accurate or inaccurate. Therefore, the importance of correct health information is crucial to the development of positive health attitudes.

The teacher's role in presenting accurate and current factual information to correct pupils' misinformation and to fill informational voids is of critical importance. In doing so, however, educators must keep in mind that health knowledge is not an end in itself. Teaching factual information is justified to the extent that it expands the child's potential for further learning, promotes constructive health behavior, and contributes to the individual's appreciation of life itself.

LEARNING OF HEALTH CONCEPTS

Man's ability to conceptualize is a learned process that places him above other animals in terms of intellectual ability. Though concepts are learned in relation to words or other symbols that describe objects, events, or qualities of sensory stimuli, concepts are *not* words. Simply stated, a concept is an idea. Woodruff describes a concept as "a relatively complete and meaningful idea in the mind of a person. It is an understanding of something. It is his own subjective product of his way of making meaning of things he has seen or otherwise perceived by his experience."[3] A very simple example

3. A. D. Woodruff, "The Use of Concepts in Teaching and Learning," *Journal of Teacher Education* 20 (1964): 81–99.

that is well within the capacity of primary grade children is the concept of *food*. Admittedly, this concept will not arouse the same idea in all children. While all have eaten food, many have consumed food products foreign to their classmates. Some have grown food, shopped for food, or been involved in its preparation for eating. In short, how a child conceptualizes food or any other concept object is determined by his previous learnings and experiences. Johnson and Medinnus claim:

> . . . concept formation requires an organism to develop an understanding, which can be measured by the organism's behavior, that certain objects, events, or characteristics of a stimulus have a common element. On the basis of this element the organism then classifies the phenomena. The actual source of the concept lies in respondent or operant learning. It is the transfer—or generalization—of what is learned to other situations sharing common elements that constitutes the formation of a concept.[4]

With development, the child's ability to conceptualize becomes more complex and abstract. Few kindergartners have an accurate conceptualization of *nutrition*, for instance, despite its kinship with *food*, a concept they have developed. Obviously the idea of the body processing foods to meet its defensive, growth, and repair requirements represents a more sophisticated and abstract idea. By the age of school entry, many of the concepts that children have developed are poorly formed and rather loosely bound. Providing learning experiences that will add the relevant and eliminate the irrelevant qualities of conceptual systems is a major function of education.

THE IMPORTANCE OF CONCEPTUAL ABILITY

Since concepts enable one to generalize about all objects in a concept category, even in the absence of perceptual experiences (sensory stimuli), they are extremely important to learning. As the child's ability to conceptualize is augmented and his concept repertoire expands, so does his knowledge of his ecosystem and the world around him. The human experience and the stimuli that bear upon it are exceedingly complex today, and might easily overwhelm us, were we incapable of organizing events or objects into convenient categories.

Concepts are of added value especially in the classroom because a simple verbalization permits each child to develop essentially the same mental image of the concept object as those of his classmates. How useful it is to be able to mention a concept object such as *elephant* and feel confident that every member of a class is able to conceptualize it without actually displaying the beast in class. A third grade teacher requesting pupils to observe ways that the school playground could be made safer would have confidence that most of the children are able to conceptualize the task. If an example of the kind of suggestion pupils are expected to make is described, more of them would clarify the concept and understand what their assignment involves. Words, therefore, serve to arouse concepts that simplify teaching and facilitate learning.

4. R. C. Johnson, and G. R. Medinnus, *Child Psychology Behavior and Development,* 2nd ed. (New York: John Wiley & Son, 1969), p. 121.

The teaching of concepts requires that children think, observe, question, make decisions, and become active participants in the learning process. Health instruction approached in this manner, focusing on the children's questions, needs, and concerns, is likely to influence health attitudes and behavior. Moreover, a conceptual approach to health instruction enables pupils to assume increasing responsibility for their health decisions.

HEALTH BEHAVIOR AND MOTIVATION

Health behavior consists of habits and practices which have a direct influence on one's health behavior. The feature that distinguishes between habits and practices is the individual's awareness of the reasons for his behavior. By way of example, handwashing before meals would be considered a health practice if the behavior was engaged in primarily for health and disease prevention purposes. Habits, on the other hand, are simple, psychoneurological behaviors so deeply ingrained by repetition that the child is essentially unaware of the reason for his behavior. From an outcome standpoint, both positive health habits and practices are desirable, but practices should ultimately receive greater instructional emphasis, for they are based upon rational throught processes. And as the elementary grade child grows and develops, so does his appetite for understanding the reasons why some health behaviors are desirable and others are not.

Learning depends in no small way on the process of motivation. To motivate is to arouse and stimulate in such a way as to enhance the effort an individual is willing to put forth. Much of what is written in educational psychology textbooks concerning the arousal process deals with the learner, but the outcomes of a given learning experience are as much a function of teacher motivation as they are of learner arousal. When subject matter becomes old hat for the teacher, or is concerned with simple learnings, as it frequently is at the lower grade levels, teacher disinterest will invariably spread to pupils. Teacher interest and excitement are often revived by employing new approaches to old learnings and by using innovative means of involving children in the learning. One point is abundantly clear: that an apathetic teacher can just as effectively put the damper on a topic as can a poorly motivated class.

In general, traditional textbook learning with emphasis on memorization, recall, and recitation of factual information will not sustain a satisfactory level of motivation for elementary school children. *How* one teaches appears to be more critical from a motivational standpoint than *what* one teaches. An otherwise bland health topic can suddenly spring to life for youngsters if the techniques of teaching are appealing to them. In general, their interest is aroused when they are able to identify with what is being taught and are permitted active involvement in the learning process.

While observing an eighth grade student teacher attempting to acquaint a class with the process of community water treatment, I was not altogether surprised with the teacher's lack of success in arousing student interest in the subject. In spite of the teacher's clever chalkboard diagram and informative discourse on sedimentation, filtration, chlorination, and aeration, students were obviously unimpressed and disinterested. Several members of the class were talking quietly among themselves about other matters, while some were diligently working on assignments for other classes.

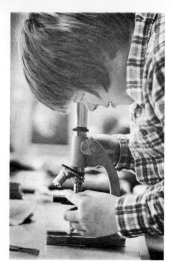

Fig. 10–2. By participating in a class laboratory project this student is actively involved in the learning process. The student is viewing a drop of water to determine the effectiveness of the class's water treatment process.

A brief conference was held at the close of school between the student teacher and supervisor for the purpose of discussing the successes and shortcomings of the lesson. The student teacher was very much concerned over the ineffectiveness of the lesson. By mutual agreement, the teacher decided to approach the subject differently by actively involving students in the learning.

Working together, students and teacher decided to arrange a field trip to the municipal water treatment plant. Two class members whose hobbies were photography volunteered to take pictures of various steps in the water treatment process. So resounding a success was the field trip that it generated several additional student-centered learning activities. A bulletin board was completed using photographs taken during the field trip and drawings completed in class. An article describing class activities was prepared for the school newspaper. Several students decided to create their own system of water treatment based upon the process used in their city. After gathering muddy water, they used a microscope to observe plant and animal life in the contaminated water. After the water was allowed to settle, it was filtered several times through gravel and sand. Chlorine tablets were then added to the clear solution to kill microorganisms. Upon macroscopic and microscopic examination, the water was found to be free of suspended particles with no sign of plant and animal life. Needless to say, the class was elated that they had succeeded in producing high-quality water by using the same basic procedures as those used to treat the water supply in their community.

Fig. 10–2 indicates how subject matter that tends to be unexciting and drab when taught by traditional classroom techniques can spark the interest of learners if special efforts are made to more actively involve them in the learning.

THE PROCESS OF BEHAVIOR CHANGE

An exploration of current theories of behavior change is not within the scope of this text. Nonetheless, the development of positive health behavior is so vital to health instruction that its complete omission would be a serious shortcoming of this discussion.

All learning involves behavior change since it modifies to some extent one's affect, cognition, or overt responses to stimuli. Kimble and Garmezy define learning as "a relatively permanent change in a behavioral tendency and is the result of reinforced practice."[5] This view is shared by McCandless, who adds that "Child and adult lives are full of such learnings: to *do* things and *not* to do things; to *approach* or master, and to *avoid*. Learning, then, refers to the acquisition of new skills, meanings, and orientations, including avoidances and simply *not doing* what one has once done."[6]

It was noted earlier that children possess an impressive array of health information by the age of school entry. Some of this information is basically sound, but much is erroneous, misleading, or partially understood. Ordinarily, health facts are loosely organized in the young mind, and some are in direct conflict with other facts learned. There is a real risk that as new pieces of information are added to the child's storehouse of knowledge,

5. G. A. Kimble, and N. Garmezy, *Principles of General Psychology,* 2nd ed. (New York: Ronald Press, 1963), p. 133.
6. B. R. McCandless, *Children: Behavior and Development,* 2nd ed. (New York: Holt, Rinehart & Winston, 1967), p. 178.

more confusion and contradiction will result. Instead of clarifying matters for the child, new learnings may further muddy the waters of understanding. Avoidance of this situation depends upon the teacher's willingness to concentrate on the *application* of new learnings. Time devoted to these activities will pay huge dividends since it promotes the adoption of positive health attitudes and practices and leads to the extinction of less desirable behavior.

When conflicting health information is held by children or adults, they are able to call forth beliefs that justify either positive or negative health behaviors, depending upon a whim of the moment. For example, adults who are aware of the health hazards of cigarette smoking might rationalize their smoking behavior since they have also learned that those who cease smoking often experience weight gain, which is also detrimental to health. Thus, poorly learned or seemingly conflicting health beliefs provide an ambiguous and convenient informational base that encourages intellectual copouts. Misuse of health information for the purpose of explaining or justifying unwise health behavior can be minimized if the application of health information, rather than facts, is given instructional emphasis.

Figure 10–3 illustrates a simple and effective model for changing health behavior. The elements of this model are isolated solely for discussion purposes, but overlap in actual practice. Initially, the child must recognize (perception) that a potential health problem exists. Since children (and many adults) have extreme difficulty conceptualizing that which cannot be seen, some health topics pose special perceptual difficulties for the learner. A second grade unit of instruction dealing with communicable disease is a case in point. This entire body of knowledge rests on the belief that organisms too small to be viewed by unaided vision cause considerable illness and death each year.

By actually demonstrating the presence of microorganisms on children's hands, the teacher permits the children to observe, probably for the first time in their lives, that living objects known as germs are present on unwashed or unclean hands. This experience is valuable especially if the importance of washing hands before meals is a learning objective. A relatively simple procedure, requiring nutrient agar, petri dishes, and an incubator, vividly demonstrates the presence of germs. Elementary science coordinators and secondary grade science teachers usually are able to provide the hardware and expertise required for this activity. Learning experiences of this type contribute to the child's perception that not only does a potential problem indeed exist, but also that it is a problem shared by all people.

Examples of skin, respiratory, and other diseases caused by germs and transmitted by contaminated hands help to modify the belief system. Pupil interaction is especially important in the *belief* phase, for this permits them to verbalize or otherwise express their existing understandings of germs, of communicable diseases, and of the importance of clean hands. Illustrations (e.g., a surgeon scrubbing before an operation) are essential at this point to further convince the class of the importance of clean hands. Several concrete examples may be necessary, for a child's mistaken ideas may be deeply ingrained and resistant to change.

Success in the third phase (importance) of the behavior change model depends largely upon motivation. Once children recognize a potential health problem and believe that it poses a threat, the next step is to relate

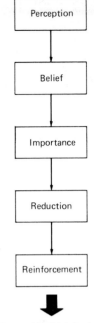

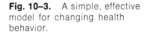

Changed health behavior

Fig. 10–3. A simple, effective model for changing health behavior.

the problem to their lives. Once this is accomplished, the belief is internalized and becomes a viable element in their attitude structure. Success in this process depends heavily upon the teacher's understanding of those interests, concerns, and learning activities that turn on pupils to learning.

Recognition of the steps or measures one can take to reduce the health risks is also essential to behavior change. That is, risk-reduction techniques must be included in the learning process. Regardless of the health problem under discussion, recommended risk-reduction procedures must be kept simple and well within the grasp of the age group. When teachers suggest health-promoting behaviors that are complex, time-consuming, or otherwise unrealistic to children, they are likely to become discouraged.

Finally, *reinforcement* of desirable health behaviors is necessary if children are to adopt them and incorporate them in their behavioral response patterns. Reinforcement of appropriate handwashing, therefore, is essential in the school setting. Soap, warm water, and towels are required, and time must be available to allow children to wash their hands before lunch and at other appropriate times. Reinforcement in the form of praise or recognition is very encouraging to youngsters and is recommended as a means of promoting behavior change.

Behaviors that are reinforced in the classroom may pass unnoticed in the home. Consistent support of positive health behavior in school and at home will evoke more persistent changes in behavior than will haphazard or intermittent reinforcement. Teachers must, therefore, be concerned with the kinds of responses children receive in the home as they practice behaviors learned in schools. Some educators insist that parent-teacher conferences are useful in informing parents of instructional goals and how these can be supported in the home. Realistically, though, such conferences are not often a solution to the problem, for the parents in greatest need of understanding what schools are attempting to accomplish are frequently those who, for myriad reasons, never seem to arrange conferences with teachers or attend the school's open house. Other possibilities exist for involving family members in their child's learnings. It is sometimes useful to plan classroom activities that have carry-over potential into the home. In the case of the handwashing behavior used as an example in this discussion glazed ceramic soap dishes, constructed by the children as an art activity, can be used as family presents. Those who know children realize how dearly they regard their own creations and given the opportunity how they will insist that the objects be put to use in the home. Thus, what appears to be a creative art object produced by the child serves also as a useful reminder in the home that handwashing is desirable health behavior.

CHILD INTERESTS: A KEY TO LEARNING

That pupil interests provide a strong motivation to learn is universally acknowledged by educators. Activities geared to their interests and concerns are not only more enjoyable for young learners, but they also encourage greater expenditures of pupil effort than do activities generating lesser amounts of interest. Teaching that disregards or falls short of capturing pupils' interests often fails to tap their learning capacity and thus results in lower levels of achievement than one might otherwise expect.

Knowledge of child development is invaluable in understanding grade level interests, for many concerns of the young parallel physical and mental development. For instance, the first permanent teeth usually appear during the first grade, and this event stimulates much interest in baby teeth and newly erupted six-year molars. Such curiosity provides a teachable moment not only to respond to pupil questions, but also to explore in a planned manner other basic dental health understandings at the primary level. Opportunities for health instruction emanating from growth and development patterns of children present themselves throughout the elementary school years. During the late intermediate grade experience, for instance, children exhibit ". . . high interest in the body, its growth, development and function, and in body differences in the sexes. They want to know all about it, no holds barred. They have intense interest in menstruation, the interest reaching an almost feverish pitch in grade six, where all children—boys and girls alike—are conscious of the imminence of puberty."[7] Just prior to puberty, many schools capitalize on these heightened interests and introduce studies of the physical, social, emotional, and physiological changes that mark the puberal and early adolescent phases of human development.

Too frequently pupil interests in important health topics do not appear spontaneously, nor are essential areas of health instruction clearly related to existing interests. We have discussed that curiosity about one's body and bodily functions does exist and is certainly a plus as far as health teaching is concerned. This is not to suggest that the only topics worthy of inclusion in the elementary grade health curriculum are those that children *want* to learn about. Instruction devoted only to the satisfaction of children's curiosity may fall short of responding to their health needs. Basic concepts regarding the importance of adequate sleep, exercise, and nutrition to one's health should be stressed in elementary grades, even though these topics are not generally of great interest to youngsters. This in no way diminishes the importance of instruction in these areas. The supreme test of teaching effectiveness is to arouse interest in what children perceive as comparatively unexciting topics.

WHAT CHILDREN WANT TO KNOW
The Connecticut Board of Education recently conducted an interest survey of over 5,000 students in grades kindergarten through twelve. Identified as the Student Health Concerns Project, this research attempted to identify the health interests, concerns, and problems of boys and girls living in four diverse regions of Connecticut. Recognizing the possible influence of geographic, socioeconomic, and cultural variables on the survey findings, members of the study team sampled children from inner city, suburban, rural, and high socioeconomic areas. Surprisingly, findings revealed that "The wide variance in geographic and sociological towns selected apparently mattered very little as far as health interests of Connecticut boys and girls were concerned."[8]

Children of elementary school age show considerable interest in their body, its functions, and its deviations from normality. In spite of this curiosity, they are not especially interested in positive health as a dynamic

7. R. Byler, G. Lewis, and R. Totman, *Teach Us What We Want to Know* (New York: Mental Health Materials Center, Inc., 1969), p. 47.
8. Byler et al., *Teach Us*, p. 166.

quality of life. As might be anticipated, primary grade children's interests encompass a wide range of topics, are easily aroused, but usually persist for only a short time. These tendencies usually change as children mature and progress through the fifth and sixth grades. At the junior and senior high school levels, student motivation is in many ways a more difficult task, but as a rule, once interest is aroused, involvement in learning activities is more intense and persistent than in the elementary grades.

Kindergarten children, first graders, and second graders in the Connecticut study encountered great difficulty when asked to define the meaning of health. According to the survey team, "Even at this early age, these boys and girls (K-2) show much interest in a wide variety of health problems—at their own level of curiosity and comprehension of course . . . Their primary health concern is *not to be sick,* rather than *to be healthy* so they can run and play and be very active. As with all children of this age group, they ask myriads of questions, many of which are directly related to their health, growth and development and offer excellent opportunities for functional health teaching."[9]

Third and fourth graders in the Connecticut study also expressed interest in the human body, although on a more sophisticated level than their younger schoolmates. In addition, third grade boys and girls indicated high interest in babies including where they come from, how they are born, and how they develop. Diseases and their causes, cures, and effects were of interest to children at this grade level. The interests of fourth graders, while strikingly similar to those of their third grade counterparts, included such topics as drugs of abuse and the health effects of smoking.

In addition to their intense interest in the body and its growth and its functions and in physical differences in the sexes, fifth and sixth graders expressed interest in the following:

> —understanding themselves: their personalities, reactions, behaviors, moods, and fears
> —understanding their peers and families: sixth graders reach out to know more about mentally retarded children, and about human differences and their causes. They also wish to alleviate the circumstances of unfortunate people.
> —knowing about babies: where they come from, how they are born, infant abnormalities. Their interests embrace little of pre- and post-natal care.
> —learning the causes of many diseases, and progress toward curing them
> —understanding the drug and smoking problems with greater precision.[10]

Results of the Connecticut survey of health interests provide clues to child responsiveness, rather than guidelines for curriculum development. What was done on a massive scale by the Connecticut Board of Education can be accomplished by teachers within their own classrooms.

9. Byler et al., *Teach Us,* p. 16.
10. Byler et al., *Teach Us,* pp. 47–48.

IDENTIFYING THE HEALTH INTERESTS OF CHILDREN

Careful observation of youngsters as they work independently or interact in groups provides considerable information about their concerns and interests. By listening instead of merely hearing and by observing rather than simply seeing, classroom teachers are able to identify those topics and methodologies likely to engage young minds and bodies. Kerlinger claims that "Basically, there are only two modes of observation: we can watch people do and say things and we can ask people about their own actions and the behavior of others."[11]

Both of these methods are used extensively by teachers as they assess the health behavior of children. Though observation appears at first glance to be a relatively simple means of collecting information, it involves a hazard that must be avoided. Observers face the risk of making incorrect inferences from their observations. The teacher who infers that a child does not like his classmates because of his observed aggression toward them may actually be observing a child who is basically nonaggressive but who knows of no other way to gain the attention of other children. Overt behavior becomes truly significant only when one is aware of the underlying reasons for the behavior.

Several techniques including small group discussion, teacher observation, free anonymous writing, incomplete story, dramatization, and role playing were employed to elicit student health concerns in the Connecticut survey. Some of these methods were judged most successful at certain grade levels and quite unsatisfactory at others.

In kindergarten through second grade, teacher observation, life situations, and group discussions proved most effective in revealing pupils' health interests. Life situations are actual events observed in the home (the birth of a baby) or other happenings experienced by class members. Teacher observation of children engaged in free, unstructured work and play activities was most productive in identifying interests. Techniques such as sentence completion and anonymous writing are of limited value with children of these ages due to their limited ability to express themselves in written forms.

From third grade on, group discussion, free and anonymous writing, and secret questions, in addition to teacher observation, were judged effective for interest-identifying purposes. According to the researchers, "Other methods, such as the unfinished story, role playing, structured quizzes, assigned composition topics, and the like, each of which has a worthy place in teaching and learning, did *not* prove helpful in this study for the reason they failed to reveal what students want to know."[12]

Classroom experiences are but one dimension of the child's involvement in the total school program. Learning also takes place in the library, cafeteria, hallways, and gymnasium; on the school bus; and in various school locations. Health and safety needs and interests not readily apparent to the classroom teacher emerge when children are being supervised by other

CONTRIBUTIONS OF OTHER SCHOOL PERSONNEL

11. F. N. Kerlinger, *Foundations of Behavioral Research* (New York: Holt, Rinehart & Winston, 1966), p. 504.
12. Byler et al., *Teach Us,* p. 167.

school personnel. Virtually all school employees including custodians, bus drivers, cafeteria workers, and school-crossing guards have opportunities to observe children in settings less structured than classrooms.

Personnel in the lunchroom, for instance, are aware of the nutritional quality of the bag lunches children bring from home. In schools having a hot lunch program, they are aware of children's food choices, the foods they consistently throw in the trash, and other matters related to nutrition that might easily be incorporated in classroom instruction. School nurses have a wealth of useful information since they maintain cumulative health records for each child enrolled in their schools. Their awareness of health problems affecting children and their families is of inestimable value to teachers. For this reason, the importance of close working relationships between teachers, school nurses, and other members of the health service team should not be overlooked.

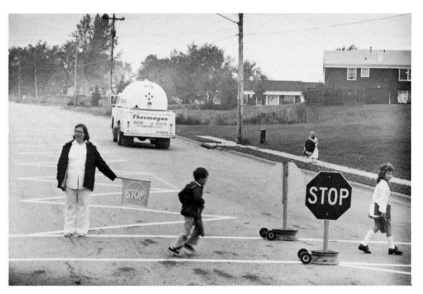

Fig. 10–4. This school-crossing guard is illustrative of one situation in which a school employee has the opportunity to observe the behavior of students in an unstructured setting.

SUMMARY

Health education is based on the firm conviction that behavior change is the single most important outcome of instruction. The acquisition of accurate health information and the development of positive health attitudes are basic ingredients of any effort to facilitate changes in health behavior. The entire process is complex and may well be the most difficult educational undertaking of the classroom teacher.

Health attitudes of children are as different as the individuals who hold them, and they consist of beliefs, each having cognitive, affective, and behavioral components. An understanding of health attitudes and their underlying belief systems is essential for the teacher who is attempting to discourage undesirable and encourage desirable attitudes and behaviors.

Instruction that relies heavily on factual information and is teacher centered does not lend itself to the discovery of existing beliefs, attitudes, and behaviors. Neither do these instructional approaches encourage the development of health practices that will enhance the health status of children. Experience has demonstrated that instruction with a strong motivational appeal that emphasizes learner involvement enhances the probability of behavior modification. Furthermore, when students recognize a health need or problem, believe in the need to find its solution, and recognize its importance to them, they more readily internalize attitudes and practice health behaviors that will help them avoid the problem. Consistent reinforcement, both in and out of school, is likely to bring about more or less permanent behavior change.

Interests of learners are another important consideration in teaching. Attention to learning tasks increases in direct proportion to the level of learner interest. Though these health concerns and interests must be taken into account when planning and implementing health education experiences, the content of health instruction should not be based solely upon interests. Successful teachers are those who are aware of child health needs, even those that children do not find interesting, and who plan experiences that create student interest in these needs.

Discussion Questions

1. What are the advantages and disadvantages of encouraging children to express their ideas and feelings concerning health?
2. Discuss the relationship between a child's socioeconomic experience and concept formation at the age of school entry.
3. Comment on the practice of some teachers to "answer any health questions their pupils may ask."
4. Support or refute the following claim: *How* one teaches is more critical from a motivational standpoint than *what* one teaches.
5. Using the behavioral change model outlined in this chapter, briefly describe how you would teach children to "respect the rights of others."
6. Under what circumstances should the health interests of children cease to serve as the primary criterion for instructional content?

References

Byler, R., Lewis, G., and Totman, R. *Teach Us What We Want To Know.* New York: Mental Health Materials Center, Inc., 1969.

Johnson, R. C., and Medinnus, G. R. *Child Psychology Behavior and Development.* 2nd ed. New York: John Wiley & Sons, 1969.

Kerlinger, F. N. *Foundations of Behavioral Research.* New York: Holt, Rinehart & Winston, 1966.

Kimble, G. A., and Garmezy, N. *Principles of General Psychology.* 2nd ed. New York: Ronald Press, 1963.

McCandless, B. R. *Children: Behavior and Development.* 2nd ed. New York: Holt, Rinehart & Winston, 1967.

Rokeach, H. *Beliefs, Attitudes, and Values.* San Francisco: Jossey-Bass, Inc., 1968.

Rosenberg, M. J. "An Analysis of Affective-Cognitive Consistency." In *Attitude Organization and Change,* eds. M. J. Rosenberg et al. New Haven: Yale University Press, 1960.

Woodruff, A. D. "The Use of Concepts in Teaching and Learning." *Journal of Teacher Education* 20 (1964): 81–99.

SECTION THREE

EFFECTIVE HEALTH INSTRUCTION

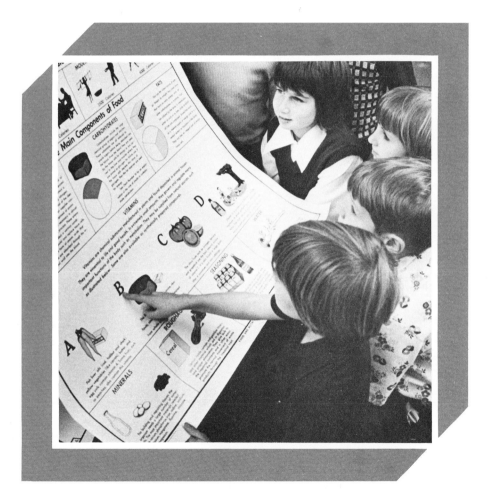

Chapter 11
TEACHING AND LEARNING: THEORETICAL FOUNDATIONS

What is the value of theory in education?

How would one distinguish between association and cognitive learning theories?

What roles do reinforcement, extinction, reward, and punishment play in learning?

What is meant by "information processing"?

What procedures or operations are involved in the problem-solving approach to learning?

How does the social climate of the classroom influence teaching and learning?

Teaching has been described as an art and psychology as a science. Both have upon occasion been criticized—teaching for being less than artful and psychology for lacking the precision of the natural sciences. While criticism of these two disciplines is to some extent justifiable, both have made substantial contributions to our understanding of the learning process. This chapter is concerned essentially with the interface between learning and psychology, commony recognized as educational psychology. As a behavioral discipline, "educational psychology is concerned with identifying and describing principles of learning and related conditions and procedures for improving educational practices."[1] An in-depth discussion of educational psychology is not within the scope of this text, and has been generously left to those who represent that discipline. Many of its principles, however, have application in health education and are included in the following discussion.

LEARNING THEORIES

Educational psychologists may be broadly classified into one of two categories, association theorists and cognitive (or field) theorists. This division may be more a matter of convenience than of anything else, for distinctions between the two schools of thought are not always clear.

1. H. J. Klausmeier, and R. E. Ripple, *Learning and Human Abilities,* 3rd ed. (New York: Harper & Row, 1971), pp. 30–31.

Associationists tend to view learning as an associative process that relates a given stimulus (S) to a response (R). They stress the significance of the learner's response to stimuli arising from outside the learner and pay particular attention to changes that occur within the learner as a result of S–R. Pavlov's early conditioning experiments with dogs are a classic example of association theory. Other learning models representative of the associationist school include E. L. Thorndike's Connectionism, Guthrie's Contiguous Conditioning, and Hull's theory of behavior.

Cognitive Theory, formerly referred to as Field Theory, is evident in the work of Tolman (Sign-Significate Theory) and Lewin (Topology Theory). Piaget's work with cognitive development and Bruner's views on conceptual development are more recent applications of cognitive theory. Representatives of this group believe that learning is largely a process of discovering and understanding relationships and of arranging and deriving significance from sensory experiences. Cognitive Theory infers that concepts, perceptual images, and feelings are involved in the learning process. While cognitive theorists tend to view learning as the acquisition of cognitive structures, association theorists see learning largely as habit formation. Moreover, those with a cognitive orientation stress the importance of insight in problem solving, while their association counterparts consider trial and error a principal mode of learning.

Both theoretical positions agree that the basic requirements for learning are a learner, one or more stimuli, and behavioral responses to the stimuli. Moreover, educational psychologists, regardless of their theoretical position, are generally agreed that learning is a process or operation inferred from more or less permanent behavior changes resulting from practice. How these changes occur and what precipitates them are questions that remain essentially unresolved. In terms of the application of present educational theory, Klausmeier claims that "learning theories in themselves do not present an adequate basis for understanding or managing the many variables associated with learning in school settings."[2]

A well-developed, widely applicable, and universally accepted theory of learning will not appear on the American educational scene in the next several years. In fact, it is conceivable that such a model may never be developed. Some educational leaders are not convinced that a single theory is possible, or even desirable. Theory is not necessarily synonymous with truth, though many theoreticians may appear to believe otherwise. Theory is simply a logical method of explaining phenomena. Some theories survive scientific inquiry and the passage of time, while others fail to stand up under scrutiny and are rejected.

TEACHING AND LEARNING: SELECTED PRAGMATIC PROPOSITIONS

School learning desperately needs an operational base, even if this framework fails to qualify as a theory. Without it, teaching and learning are little more than aimless activities the outcomes of which are in serious doubt. Educational psychology, perhaps to a greater extent than any other single discipline, adds purpose and meaning to the teacher's instructional efforts. Commenting on this shortly after the turn of the century, E. L. Thorndike suggested the following:

2. Klausmeier and Ripple, *Learning*, p. 9.

Anyone of good sense can farm fairly well without science, and anyone of good sense can teach fairly well without knowing and applying psychology. Still, as the farmer with the knowledge of the application of botany and chemistry to farming is, other things being equal, more successful than the farmer without it, so the teacher will, other things being equal, be the more successful who can apply psychology, the science of human nature, to the problems of the school.[3]

Many classroom teachers, consciously or unconsciously, frequently employ basic learning precepts, principles, or propositions derived from both associative and cognitive approaches to learning. Admittedly, these classroom applications must be described as eclectic because they typically consist of elements of different theories. The important consideration is not the theoretical genesis of a given principle but, rather, how effectively its application contributes to children's learning.

ASSOCIATIVE PRINCIPLES: CLASSROOM IMPLICATIONS

Associationism, sometimes referred to as Early Behaviorism, dominated American educational theory for nearly a half-century. Edward L. Thorndike's book *Animal Intelligence* (1911) proposed that learning was based upon the association (bond, connection) between sensory stimuli and learner responses. In recent years, some of Thorndike's hypotheses have become obsolete, while others have been modified. Nonetheless, the influence of Thorndike is still present in contemporary behavior theory and continues to be felt in the classroom.

Reinforcement   Environmental events that occur in conjunction with learner responses and influence the probability that the responses will be exhibited in the future are referred to as reinforcers. *Reinforcement* is the process by which reinforcers contribute to learning. Positive reinforcers strengthen the bond or connection between a stimulus and response, thus increasing the likelihood that the response will occur in the future. When a child responds properly to a question, correctly pronounces a word, or otherwise responds in a desirable manner to any stimulus, reinforcement should be provided. This is a key point, for evidence suggests that responses strengthened through reinforcement may be weakened through nonreinforcement. With children of elementary school age, reinforcers often consist of teacher verbalizations such as "good boy," "you surely have your thinking cap on," and similar comments that support or reinforce the child's response.

There is little doubt that positive reinforcement plays a key role in learning and that it is manifest in many ways and for a variety of reasons in the classroom. Let us consider the case of a quiet, retiring fifth grader whose lack of self-confidence precludes his participating in class discussions and answering questions raised by his teacher. Any effort by this child to emerge from his shell and become a more active class participant would certainly

3. E. L. Thorndike, "The Principles of Teaching," in *Learning: Theory and Practice,* ed. P. E. Johnson (New York: Thomas Y. Crowell Co., 1971), p. 17.

be worthy of reinforcement because such behavior would represent a giant step forward for him. According to association theorists, positive reinforcement from peers or teacher would encourage the boy's future involvement.

In a situation such as the one described, it is possible for the teacher to employ negative reinforcers which would tend to discourage the child's effort to become actively involved in classroom affairs. In other words, the stimulus-response bond would be weakened as a consequence of negative reinforcement. Assume that the learner mustered all of his courage and intellect, only to offer an incorrect answer to a question asked by the teacher. An insensitive teacher, oblivious to the process of reinforcement, might respond by saying, "That's wrong," or as one practice teacher I observed once said, "You *never* know the right answer!" Such a response is the supreme put-down for a child such as we have described. In fact, reinforcement of this nature has a negative effect upon most children. The salient point is that the child's participatory behavior should have been positively reinforced, for it was much more important to his development as an individual and to his future school performance than was his answer to a specific question, however incorrect it might have been.

Notwithstanding the fact that the reinforcement phenomenon is universally acknowledged as a contributor to learning, researchers do not agree on the precise mechanism by which reinforcement takes place. Bugelski claims that learners apparently derive reinforcement from success.[4] The notion that it serves a drive-reducing or anxiety-reducing function has been proposed by several researchers. Others explain it in terms of ego-satisfaction or self-enhancement. Regardless of the physical, psychological, or emotional dynamics inherent to reinforcement, one point is clear to those who work with children: when a child's responses are perceived by him as worthy or successful, his behaviors are positively reinforced and are likely to be repeated.

Extinction Earlier in this discussion the point was mentioned in passing that specific learner responses discontinue as a result of nonreinforcement. This behavioral principle, known as *extinction,* was formulated following years of research with laboratory animals. While it may appear to the casual observer to be a rather simple process, extinction is exceedingly complex and is the source of much disagreement among learning theorists. Does the extinction process represent unlearning or relearning? To what extent does the strength of reinforcers play in extinction? How important is the frequency of reinforcement in the process? In spite of these and other essentially unsolved questions surrounding the matter of extinction, it continues to be relied upon in educational settings. Children whose obnoxious behavior is designed to elicit a response from their teacher (reinforcement) will often refrain from the behavior if it is ignored. However, unless their positive behaviors are adequately reinforced, children may resort to other undesirable behaviors in an effort to achieve the reinforcement they seek.

Reward and punishment Reinforcement is inextricably interwoven with other forces operating in the learning environment which, for lack of a better term, may be called learning incentives. *Incentives* are objects or

4. B. R. Bugelski, *The Psychology of Learning* (New York: Henry Holt Co., 1956), p. 477.

situations occurring outside the learner which influence learning. They are not to be confused with motives, which are intrinsic learner qualities. Reward and punishment, two learning incentives having their roots in early behavioral theory, are used quite extensively in classrooms.

When used judiciously, reward generally operates as a positive reinforcer. Many teachers object to the use of gold stars, special privileges, and similar forms of reward because of their conviction that these incentives are hedonistic in nature and may teach children to expect, if not demand, rewards for their efforts. Reward can take the form of praise which if dispensed carefully is a much more satisfactory incentive and one that teachers are not averse to using.

Greene and Lepper tested the hypothesis that "a person's intrinsic interest in an activity may be decreased by inducing him to engage in that activity as an explicit means to some extrinsic goal."[5] Working with nursery school children and using objective rewards as the extrinsic goal, the researchers showed in each of three studies that if children enjoy an activity, the practice of giving rewards will often lead to decreased interest in the activity. As a result of their findings, the researchers recommended that extrinsic rewards should be employed only when necessary and never to the extent that they undermine children's intrinsic motivations.

Clearly, the improper use of rewards can backfire for the uninitiated teacher. However, as the following example illustrates, the apparent hazards of extrinsic rewards can be an ace up the teacher's sleeve:

> He lived alone on a street where boys played noisily every afternoon. One day the din became too much, and he called the boys into his house. He told them he liked to listen to them play, but his hearing was failing and he could no longer hear their games. He asked them to come around each day and play noisily in front of his house. If they did, he would give them each a quarter. The youngsters raced back the following day, and made a tremendous racket in front of the house. The old man paid them, and asked them to return the next day. Again they made the noise, and again the old man paid them for it. But this time he gave each boy only twenty cents, explaining he was running out of money. On the following day, they got only fifteen cents each. Furthermore, the old man told them, he would have to reduce the fee to five cents on the fourth day. The boys became angry, and told the old man they would not be back. It was not worth the effort, they said, to make noise for only five cents a day.[6]

When punishment follows a human response, it generally serves an aversive purpose. That is, when a child has learned from experience that certain of his actions are punished, either verbally or physically, he avoids those behaviors that promise unpleasant results. Occasionally, an individual may so highly value the other consequences of his act that he will persist with

5. D. Greene, and M. R. Lepper, "How to Turn Work Into Play," *Psychology Today,* September 1974, p. 50.

6. M. Casady, "The Tricky Business of Giving Rewards," *Psychology Today,* September 1974, p. 52.

the behavior, convinced that its satisfactions will outweigh the punishment he knows will follow. This is sometimes the case with children whose chronic misbehavior fails to yield to severe ridicule and punishment from their teacher. Perhaps the peer recognition they receive as a result of their behavior is more important to them than the expectation of punishment.

Parents and teachers should constantly remind themselves that punishment tells a child what *not* to do, rather than what to do. I am reminded of a kindergarten teacher who warned her pupils never to run in the halls in their school. To be caught doing so, she threatened, would result in a severe reprimand and a trip to the principal's office for disciplinary action. For most of the children in class the threat of punishment was sufficient to discourage them from running in the halls. Two of her boys, after making certain that no one was watching, raced down the hall, one of them colliding with a classroom door that suddenly swung open into the hall. Fortunately the most serious injury sustained was a badly bruised leg. Had the teacher taken time to explain and demonstrate that the doors in the school opened outward instead of inward, the children would have recognized the real hazard. As it was, all that the boys had worried about was the punishment and not the dangers posed by improperly hung doors.

Punishment as a technique for behavior modification appears to be unwise, according to Clarizio and Yelon, for the following reasons:

1. Punishment does not eliminate the response; it merely slows down the rate at which troublesome behaviors are emitted.
2. This technique serves notice to stop certain negative behaviors; it does not indicate what behaviors are appropriate in the situation.
3. Aggressive behaviors on the teacher's part may provide an undesirable model for the pupil.
4. The emotional side effects of punishment such as fear, tenseness and withdrawal are maladaptive.
5. Punishment serves as a source of frustration which is apt to elicit additional maladaptive behaviors.[7]

In spite of these well-recognized hazards of punishment, the authors acknowledge that "Teachers, whatever their motivations, use verbal reprimands and other forms of correction in their approach to classroom management, and the judicious use of punishment as an intervention technique is most likely necessary in that it is impossible to guide behavior effectively with positive reinforcement and extinction alone."[8]

EMERGENT LEARNING APPROACHES

Much of the current research on learning indicates that a shift in thinking is occurring as investigators are increasingly looking beyond the S-R theoretical base which explains learning in terms of connections (bonds) between stimuli and responses. This is not to suggest that association theory has been altogether abandoned, for it is generally accepted that S-R associations are involved in the young preschooler's acquisition of basic skills and simple

---

7. H. F. Clarizio, and S. L. Yelon, "Learning Theory Approaches to Classroom Management: Rationale and Intervention Techniques," in *Designing Instructional Strategies for Young Children*, eds., B. Mills and R. Mills (Dubuque, Iowa: Wm. C. Brown Co. Publishers, 1972), p. 231.
8. Clarizio and Yelon, "Learning Theory Approaches," p. 231.

learnings. As children grow older, the complexity of their learning intensifies as the influence of individual motives and experiential factors are brought to bear on the learning process. Most recent learning research, especially that having direct classroom implications, regards learning as an information-processing operation dependent upon such things as the learner's developmental level, perceptual ability, conceptual ability, and problem-solving capabilities.

A DIRECTED APPROACH TO CLASSROOM LEARNING

An approach to learning that represents a synthesis of educational principles, derived mainly from cognitive theory, can be easily and effectively used by teachers of the elementary and middle grades. The following suggested sequence of events includes both teacher and learner involvements.

**A Directed Approach
to Classroom Learning**

Teacher Actions	*Learner Actions*
1. Manages teaching materials and learning activities so as to generate and maintain learner interest and attention.	1. Responds to situation by attending to learning task.
2. Helps learner formulate specific goals based upon instructional objectives.	2. Establishes goal or alternative goals; initiates preliminary goal-directed behavior.
3. Provides instructional resources including reference books, diagrams, models, and other materials; encourages learner's use of appropriate resources.	3. Initiates goal-directed trials requiring productive thinking in connection with activities in the cognitive and affective domains.
4. Assesses learner abilities, learning rate and style, and degree of motivation, while providing direction to learner study, practice, and other activities.	4. Gains proficiency and progresses toward goal through practice; continues development of cognitive and psychomotor abilities.
5. Evaluates learner progress and shares this assessment with learner; counsels with student, corrects errors, provides positive reinforcements.	5. Assesses own behaviors.
6. Works with learner in making a summative evaluation of extent to which goal has been achieved.	6. Achieves goal.
7. Establishes situations that permit learner to apply recently acquired skills, knowledge, and abilities; encourages the application of these learnings to more complex situations.	7. Experiences a sense of accomplishment and satisfaction; applies new learnings in other situations.

Perhaps the most effective means of familiarizing the reader with the application of this learning sequence in health education is through the use of an example. For purposes of illustration, let us briefly consider the involvement of a third grade class in a study of foods and nutrition.

Directed Learning Sequence	*Learner Activities*
1. Attends to learning.	1. Pupil interest generated by television documentary on world hunger. Spontaneous discussion of illness and death caused by the lack of food in underdeveloped nations.

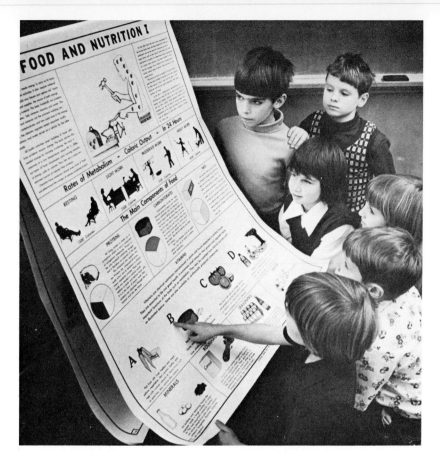

Teacher suggests that poor nutrition exists and causes health problems in the United States.

2. Sets goals.

2. Class decides that it would be interesting and important to learn more about foods and health.

With teacher guidance, two basic goals set: (1) to learn why foods help to make you strong and healthy, and (2) to be able to select those foods that make for a good diet.

3. Makes preliminary trials involving the following:

3. Field trip to local supermarket. During art period, pupils construct papier-mâché models of foods they learned about while on their field trip.

Film shown emphasizing nutrients and their importance to growth and health; Basic Four Food Groups also emphasized.

Educational game played in which each child is blindfolded and then "fishes" a papier-mâché food model from a carton; must identify the food and indicate the Basic Food Group it represents.

4. Practices to gain proficiency, etc.

4. Each pupil draws pictures to represent foods in nutritious breakfast, lunch, and dinner.

	Children keep a record of all foods and snacks eaten for one day.
	During math period, some children calculate daily caloric intake; others learn how to use household scales and weigh food portions.
5. Evaluates own behavior.	5. Teacher works independently with pupils, assessing each individual's dietary recall sheet and reviewing pictures of nutritious meals drawn by each child. Teacher stresses the positive aspects of the child's diet and encourages children on the basis of what has been learned to suggest dietary improvements.
6. Reaches goal.	6. Class divided into three groups (breakfast, lunch, and dinner groups).
	Using magazine pictures of food, each group prepares bulletin board to illustrate a nutritious example of the meal they are responsible for.
	Several children work on meal display (using papier-mâché models) for display case in hall.
	Others develop and practice a short play about food and health.
	Remaining food models used to construct mobiles to be hung in classroom.
7. Experiences satisfactions, etc.	7. Children suggest and conduct a school-wide collection of canned foods for needy families in their community.
	Dramatization of the importance of food to health presented in class.
	Other third grade classes invited to attend the play and to observe bulletin boards, hall display, mobiles.
	New learnings used in social studies unit as children study "foods from other lands" and reasons for malnutrition and illness in underdeveloped countries.

This illustration includes both learner and teacher involvements in the Learner Activity column. A host of alternative experiences may be substituted for those suggested, depending upon the amount of time available, concomitant curriculum concerns, pupil interests and abilities, class's readiness to work in groups, and myriad factors existing in the classroom. In any case, the directed learning sequence offers a logical, systematic, and effective means of approaching health instruction.

LEARNING AS INFORMATION PROCESSING

Some types of learning tasks lend themselves to teaching strategies collectively identified as information-processing (IP) techniques. Included among these approaches are inquiry, discovery, problem solving, and exploratory learning. Information processing as a general approach to learning is based upon the premise that the learner's intellectual performances, which are dependent upon such rational processes as perception, memory, information gathering and collating, decision making, and generalizing, enable him to draw conclusions, apply them to other situations, and thereby better comprehend events in his environment. Since these capabilities are not inherent human qualities, they must be learned if IP is to bear fruit as a teaching-learning approach. Some pupils achieve this by the time they reach third grade, even though their information processing is conducted at a relatively simple level.

The pupil-centered nature of the IP process does not in any way diminish teacher involvement as a facilitator of learning. If anything, successful outcomes demand greater efforts, more sophisticated skills, and extra measures of patience from teachers than do the more traditional, teacher-centered, expository teaching techniques.

> Student-identified involvement in the content of any subject can best be accomplished when the teacher can create an atmosphere in which students and the teacher mutually identify the most relevant issues and proceed cooperatively to plan how best to investigate the topic. A student-centered approach to learning, as such, should not lead to a laissez-faire attitude on the part of the teacher, for the success of this approach relies heavily on carefully guided student participation in the learning situation. If we agree that man is interactive, not just reactive, the teacher must actively lead, guide, or facilitate structuring of the learning; however, the student's interests within the structure of the course, as well as those of the teacher, become the center of the class. Thus, when the classroom environment allows students to inquire into their perplexities and when students have a significant part to play in the selection and planning of learning experiences, conditions present should allow more meaningful learning to take place.[9]

Closer study of one specific IP strategy will better acquaint the reader with the process and to what extent its success is dependent upon the mutual involvement of teacher and learner.

Problem solving A problem exists when a learner encounters a situation, must respond to it, but momentarily does not possess the information, labeling vocabulary, concepts, principles, or strategies necessary to solve the problem. Many educators are convinced that by developing flexibility, resourcefulness, originality, and problem sensitivity, individuals can apply problem-solving processes in many learning experiences at the elementary grade level. Needless to say, the application of problem-solving techniques in no way guarantees that a given problem will be solved.

No single teaching-learning approach including problem solving should be used exclusively in the classroom. Ausubel claims that information-processing techniques involve inordinate amounts of time and therefore are often unfeasible.[10] In his view, it makes better sense, especially when large bodies of subject matter are to be learned, to rely on approaches other than those involving IP. While he is supportive of problem solving and similar discovery methods, Ausubel makes the following claims:

9. R. L. Wendel, "Developing Climates for Learning," *Journal of Secondary Education* 45 (1970): 330.

10. D. P. Ausubel, "Reception Learning and the Acquisition of Concepts," in *Analysis of Concept Learning,* eds. H. J. Klausmeier and C. Harris (New York: Academic Press, 1966).

. . . . discovery learning, on developmental grounds, is pedagogically sound for the meaningful acquisition of subject matter only in the case of more difficult and unfamiliar material, and more frequently during the elementary school than in subsequent periods.[11]

In spite of minor differences, usually involving terminology or operational emphasis, educators agree that problem solving involves the following procedures:

1. Perceiving a need, difficulty, or problem
2. Assessing or defining the problem
3. Gathering and processing information
4. Formulating and testing hypotheses
5. Selecting a suitable solution

Perceiving a need, difficulty, or problem—Pupils from Miss Wally's sixth grade class returned from their lunch period day after day, complaining of the dirty eating utensils in the school cafeteria. Obviously concerned, the children claimed that the forks and spoons were "never clean," and they were determined to see what could be done to correct the situation.

Assessing or defining the problem—At their teacher's suggestion, a committee of four students was chosen to determine if students in other classes shared their concern. Since the class was anxious that Miss Wally realize that their complaints were justified, one member of the class volunteered to bring several forks and spoons to class for her examination.

As it turned out, several pupils from other classes shared the concern of Miss Wally's group, but had more or less accepted the situation. The uten-

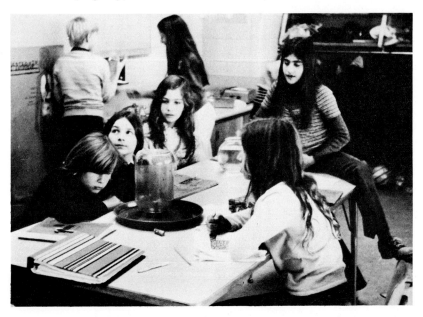

Fig. 11–2. These students are involved in a problem-solving activity dealing with oxidation. (Photograph by L. K. Olsen.)

11. Ausubel, "Reception Learning," p. 162.

sils provided as evidence were indeed soiled, with many of the forks containing encrusted food between the tines. Having previously learned that *Salmonella* and other disease organisms can be transmitted via unclean eating utensils, the class was convinced that the problem posed a health hazard.

Gathering and processing information—Upon closer scrutiny, it was learned that the knives and spoons merely appeared soiled because of water spots and mineral deposits. Food residue was clearly evident on several forks.

A restaurant inspector from the health department was invited to visit Miss Wally's class to discuss his job and local ordinances that applied to sanitation practices in eating establishments. At no time was the class's concern over the school cafeteria mentioned to the health department representaive.

Interested in discovering more about food-borne illnesses, a small group of students researched the topic, prepared a brief report, and shared it with their classmates.

Formulating and testing hypotheses—Several alternative courses of action were suggested by the pupils. These included boycott the school cafeteria, report the situation to the school superintendent, and notify the health department of their findings. One enterprising youth suggested that they prepare an exposé to be submitted to a local newspaper. Ultimately, under the leadership of Miss Wally, reason prevailed, and the class decided to pursue an internal course of action that appeared promising. Perhaps the situation could be attributed to inefficient dishwashing operations that could easily be remedied.

After much deliberation, the following hypotheses were formulated by members of the class:

—Not enough detergent was used to wash the dishes.

—The dishwashing detergent was of poor quality.

—Dishes were merely rinsed, rather than washed and rinsed.

—Water in the dishwasher was not hot enough.

—Some of the younger children in school were placing dirty utensils in trays reserved for clean silverware.

—The dishwasher was not working properly.

Selecting a suitable solution—One by one, each tentative hypothesis, except one, was rejected by the class. After meeting with the cafeteria supervisor, they learned that the dishwasher was not operating efficiently. The supervisor had been aware of the situation and demonstrated the source of the problem to the students. A rinse nozzle, designed to forcefully remove food from eating utensils, was defective. In fact, a replacement part ordered at the beginning of the school year had never been received.

Follow-up by a committee of students revealed that the requisition for the replacement part had never left the desk of the district's business manager. Once the situation was discussed and the business manager became aware of student concern over the potential health hazard, the requisition was quickly processed. Within three weeks the replacement part arrived at the school and was installed, and to the delight of Miss Wally's class, the problem they had identified was solved.

Obviously, children derive considerable satisfaction and confidence when their problem-solving efforts succeed. In those instances where problems are not resolved or issues are left hanging, the child also benefits. Involvement in the process of problem solving is itself a learning experience, as is the realization that in spite of one's best efforts some questions remain unanswered. No classroom experience surpasses this learning approach in encouraging children to think critically, do research, and approach an issue systematically and logically.

No discussion of problem solving would be complete without emphasizing the fact that the skills and abilities required of this activity do not come easily. Kingsley and Garry point out that successful problem-solving techniques require considerable expertise from the teacher.[12] Frequently she must set the stage for a problem. This may be accomplished either by posing a question or by structuring a learning task that will create pupil awareness of and interest in a problem. For elementary grade children, problems must be relatively simple, deal with concrete situations, and require investigative materials and techniques with which they are familiar.

Once a problem surfaces, young children frequently have difficulty in defining or clearly comprehending it. Without concise clarification, a problem may confuse children and confound the entire problem-solving process. Teachers must frequently remind children of dimensions of the problem they may have overlooked, thus enabling them to appreciate and address themselves to the total issue.

Teachers should be prepared to lend assistance to their pupils if superficial thinking, faulty assumptions, and erroneous conclusions are to be

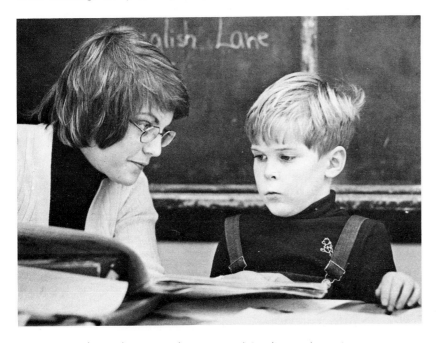

Fig. 11–3. Young children often need help in understanding how to use a book effectively.

12. H. L. Kingsley, and R. Garry, *The Nature and Conditions of Learning,* 2nd ed. (Englewood Cliffs, N.J.: Prentice-Hall, 1957), pp. 429–434.

avoided. In general, this leadership consists of teaching children which materials are useful in learning more about a problem, where these sources of information are available, and how they may be used. With younger children this help may involve an understanding of how to use a table of contents, a glossary, and an index in reference materials. However, most children at the intermediate level need advanced experiences such as understanding and utilizing the card catalog, reference books, and classifying system in the school library.

Experience in dealing with problem solving is the teacher's best teacher, for it quickly provides insight into the IP capabilities of children on a given grade level. For those who lack this experience it is helpful to remember the following advice:

> Young children solve problematic situations mainly by overt trial-and-error exploration and manipulation. The ability to solve problems by thinking develops gradually with growth in experience and understanding. Children are inferior to adults in problem thinking principally because of their smaller range of experience. They are less sensitive to problems, have fewer concepts to work with, lack critical judgment, are less capable of sustained attention, and are less able to take an objective attitude toward their problems.[13]

HUMAN DEVELOPMENT AND CONCEPT FORMATION

Jean Piaget, a Swiss psychologist, has probably contributed more to our understanding of cognitive development than any other single individual. A biologist by training, Piaget has devoted most of his career to the study of children, their thought processes, and how they interpret environmental stimuli. Largely as a result of his basic work, educators now recognize that conceptual structures develop quantitatively and qualitatively as the child develops.

During the preschool years, children begin to acquire expressive language, an ability that enables them to learn concrete, and eventually abstract, concepts. Words are essential if the child is to succeed in labeling events and objects in his environment. Kagan believes that certain analytic concepts also emerge during this period and that these include among others the concepts of big—small, adult—child, good—bad, and male—female.[14]

According to Piaget, during the first two years of life the child progresses from a reflex organism in a world that is totally undifferentiated to him to an individual who gains remarkable sensorimotor control and begins to systematically organize his near environment. This is referred to by Piaget as the *sensorimotor period* of cognitive development.

Roughly between the ages of two and seven years, children enter a transitional era of cognitive development known as the *preoperational period*. Many object concepts ordinarily of a simple nature are formed, and an awareness of object sameness develops. This is concept formation at its most primitive level. Nonetheless, this phase must necessarily precede the more complex conceptual operations that follow during future developmen-

13. Kingsley and Garry, *Nature and Conditions,* p. 435.
14. J. Kagan, "A Development Approach to Conceptual Growth," in *Analysis of Concept Learning,* eds. H. J. Klausmeier and C. Harris (New York: Academic Press, 1966), pp. 97–115.

tal periods. Relational concepts (e.g., smaller, shorter, more) usually are evident during the preoperational period, but frequently are loosely organized. It is not uncommon for one between the ages of two and seven years to be inconsistent when making relational choices, for he continues to operate largely from perceptual experiences, instead of relying upon critical thinking.

Between the ages of seven or eight years and eleven or twelve years, children experience what Piaget describes as the *concrete operations period* of cognitive development. Ordinarily, children of these ages are able to deal with single concepts and to interpret relationships. Their mental operations, while more sophisticated than those of younger children, typically relate only to the child's world of reality. For this reason, health teaching during the primary grades should avoid learning experiences that require abstract reasoning. Classroom activities that produce the greatest return in terms of learning must, therefore, be related to the child's life and ecological experience. In classrooms consisting of pupils from different social and economic circumstances, this is an important point. Even though, as we have previously noted, health interests of children reared in rural, suburban, and inner city areas may not differ markedly, their ability to comprehend and deal with concepts foreign to their life experience is limited.

Ordinarily during the fifth and sixth grades, youngsters enter the *formal operations period* of cognitive development. The process of reasoning is awakened, and according to Piaget, this marks the first time children can be taught logical reasoning. During this, the most advanced, stage of cognitive development, children and adolescents are capable of dealing with fore than concrete or real-life situations. For the first time a consideration of the *possible* as well as of the *real* becomes a reality. According to Stott:

> The child's ability to think then grows directly out of his varied direct contacts and sensory experiences with his world outside. He develops the ability to represent mentally these experiences in the absence of actual objects of sensory experience and to manipulate, reorganize, and transform them. His cognitive structure is augmented. He can now *conceptualize*.[15]

Inferential operations, scientific reasoning, and insight into causal relationships are evident at this point and greatly influence the child's problem-solving ability.

SOCIAL CONDITIONS FOR LEARNING

Much of the discussion to this point has dealt with theoretical formulations and strategies relating to teaching and learning. Not all of these will prove useful to every elementary school teacher, but each has obvious implications for educational programs at early grade levels. Regardless of the approach or combination of strategies one employs while working with the young, it is essential that at least one other condition in the learning environment be given careful attention. Those who ignore or largely overlook the social climate of the classroom may find their teaching efforts falling short of expectations. On the other hand, teachers who are cognizant of the importance of a positive learning environment and who strive to maintain it find that their efforts are more than compensated by high levels of pupil enthusiasm and achievement.

15. L. H. Stott, *Child Development: An Individual Longitudinal Approach* (New York: Holt, Rinehart & Winston, 1967), p. 285.

In a very real sense, the school is a microcosm of society, and for children who live, work, and play in this setting, the school is the most important element of their social world. There is no longer any doubt that how a child responds to the social milieu of his classroom will, in large measure, determine the outcomes of his school experience.

Of all the social elements to be considered, none deserves more attention than the "success atmosphere" of the classroom. By this is meant that each child regardless of intellectual capacity or past performance can experience success in school. More important, the child must himself *believe* that success is a realistic expectation of his efforts and activities. Educators recognize that many learning disabilities and much of the negativism that some children manifest toward school are results of repeated failure that serves a self-fulfilling prophesy. This is not to suggest that failure should or can be entirely eliminatetd from the classroom. Just as every individual experiences some successes in life, each will have his share of failures. There is no better time for this realization to be grasped than in the lower grades. The value of failure notwithstanding, it is important to learning in the elementary grades that the child's successes far outstrip his failures. Whether or not this occurs is dependent upon the teacher's understanding of individual differences among pupils and her ability to take these into account as she strives to create a "can do" atmosphere in her classroom.

Socialization of the child begins in the preschool years and by the age of school entry has advanced to the point that the youngster has learned to depend upon others. Most kindergarten teachers are well aware of this dependence and what it demands in terms of tying shoes, zipping jackets, providing direction, making decisions, and otherwise responding to young children's need to depend on others. However, a primary function of schools is to augment the socialization process. This means that children must develop the self-determination and independence that characterize the socialized individual, but at the same time preserve a level of dependence that also typifies a socialized person in American society. In short, the child must learn to think and act for himself as well as to accept assistance from others.

Self-assertion often becomes evident shortly after the child is thrust into the school milieu. In a sense, it is a matter of either asserting oneself or being overwhelmed by other personalities and forces in the school. The development of independence is a gradual process, but one which teachers influence a great deal.

Child behavior that is independent and desirable should be reinforced so as to increase the likelihood that it will become a recurring element in the child's behavior pattern. Also in keeping with the formulations of association learning theory, dependent behavior should be ignored or unreinforced so as to discourage its reappearance. Under no circumstances should a dependent child be scolded or severely reprimanded for his behavior, for as we have learned this may serve a reinforcing function. The secret in dealing with these children is to make certain that even their most feeble attempts to function independently are commended by the teacher.

Classrooms that tend to be teacher-centered and rigidly structured fail to allow for pupil initiative and self-determination and thus nurture the dependence that the child should be striving to overcome. The complexity of the educator's task is readily apparent, for she must, on the one hand, establish a classroom social atmosphere that encourages independence and, on the other hand, involve children in experiences that help them to derive value and satisfaction from group activities and interpersonal relationships.

Elementary children who are heavily dependent on their teachers and classmates can be expected to encounter serious difficulty when faced with problem-solving or other information-processing situations that require independent thought, research, and choice making. More important, perhaps, is the fact that as the child grows and develops, so must his ability to make sound and independent health decisions based upon his personal values, knowledge, and conscience. Realizing this, many classroom teachers choose to approach some aspects of health instruction in a manner that develops the pupil's ability to think and act independently.

So complex are the factors that determine the social climate in any classroom that it is impossible to even mention them in this discussion. The following statement, however, successfully touches upon several characteristics of a setting that is conducive to learning:

> Learners do not function well in a sterile or unrealistic setting, nor in a classroom which reflects tensions and pressures. The teacher should strive toward achieving a classroom atmosphere free of fear, threat, punishment, suspicion, distrust, and uncertainty. Although the learning process may consist of placing learners out of equilibrium, for efficient results such procedures must be attempted in a classroom environment in which learners experience security, consistency, and sincerity. In this kind of setting pupils can become involved in the learning.[16]

SUMMARY

While this chapter makes no attempt to provide an in-depth discussion of learning theory, distinctions are made between Association and Cognitive theories. Neither of these two major schools of thought adequately explains all of the complexities of learning, yet each contributes to what is presently accepted as sound learning theory.

Associationism dominated educational thought for several decades, beginning in the early 1900s. Principles of Association Theory such as reinforcement, extinction, and reward and punishment continue to have impact on contemporary education.

Cognitive learning emphasizes problem solving, information processing, and similar learning strategies that place high value on the student's concepts, perceptions, and feelings.

In our synthesis of learning principles we suggest a Directed Approach to learning which has many applications in elementary and middle grade health teaching. Problem solving, another useful learning technique, is discussed, and a realistic example of how one class identified a problem and proceeded to solve it is provided. Success in these and other essentially cognitive approaches to learning depend largely upon the child's ability to deal with relatively complex concepts and to work with some degree of independence.

Regardless of the theoretical principles one decides to employ, social climate within the classroom has a pronounced effect upon the outcomes

16. J. W. Renner, G. D. Shepherd, and R. F. Bibens, *Guiding Learning in the Elementary School* (New York: Harper & Row, 1973), p. 192.

of learning. Children need an atmosphere in which the possibility of success is an omnipresent force. Environments that encourage student initiative and enable one to become increasingly responsible for individual decisions are particularly conducive to learning.

Discussion Questions

1. Compare and contrast the basic elements of association and cognitive approaches to learning.
2. Discuss how reinforcement can contribute to a positive classroom social environment.
3. How can reinforcement undermine the social climate of a classroom?
4. Make a case for or against the use of objective rewards as a means of reinforcing desirable classroom behavior.
5. Select an area of study in health (e.g., family life, safety, dental health, nutrition) and develop a learning experience based on the Directed Learning sequence.
6. To what extent does a child's success with problem-solving activities depend upon his level of cognitive development?

References

Ausubel, D. P. "Reception Learning and the Acquisition of Concepts." In *Analysis of Concept Learning,* eds H. J. Klausmier and C. Harris. New York: Academic Press, 1966.

Bugelski, B. R. *The Psychology of Learning.* New York: Henry Holt Co., 1956.

Casady, M. "The Tricky Business of Giving Rewards." *Psychology Today,* September 1974.

Clarizio, H. F., and Yelon, S. L. "Learning Theory Approaches to Classroom Management: Rationale and Intervention Techniques." In *Designing Instructional Strategies for Young Children,* eds. B. Mills and R. Mills. Dubuque, Iowa: Wm. C. Brown Co. Publishers, 1972.

Greene, D., and Lepper, M. R. "How to Turn Work Into Play." *Psychology Today,* September 1974.

Kagan, J. "A Developmental Approach to Conceptual Growth." In *Analysis of Concept Learning,* eds. H. J. Klausmeier and Harris. New York: Academic Press, 1966.

Kingsley, H. L., and Garry, R. *The Nature and Conditions of Learning.* 2nd ed. Englewood Cliffs, N.J.: Prentice-Hall, 1957.

Klausmeier, H. J., and Ripple, R. E. *Learning and Human Abilities.* 3rd ed. New York: Harper & Row, 1971.

Renner, J. W., Shepherd, G. D., and Bibens, R. F. *Guiding Learning in the Elementary School.* New York: Harper & Row, 1973.

Stott, L. H. *Child Development: An Individual Longitudinal Approach.* New York: Holt, Rinehart, & Winston, 1967.

Thorndike, E. L. "The Principles of Teaching." In *Learning: Theory and Practice,* ed. P. E. Johnson. New York: Thomas Y. Crowell Co., 1971.

Wendel, R. L. "Developing Climates for Learning." *Journal of Secondary Education* 45 (1970): 330.

Chapter 12
TOWARD A PHILOSOPHY OF HEALTH TEACHING

Why does the health educator need a philosophy of teaching?

What are the advantages and the disadvantages of being a health information giver and of being a health initiator?

What is functional health teaching?

What is the role of values growth in health education?

Should certain health topics be integrated with other subject areas or should other subjects be integrated with certain health topics?

Who should teach elementary school health education?

The aim of health education has been described as "personal fitness for survival, fulfillment, and meaning in life."[1] To achieve this aim the health educator attempts to develop attitudes, influence the development of healthful life styles, sway opinion, develop habits, sell ideas, and promote valuing activities for many of today's most controversial issues. The controversial issues in health education include many sensitive personal, moral, and legal issues such as population growth, sex roles, drug laws, medical payment alternatives, and interpersonal relations. In order to be effective, a health educator needs to have personal value judgments concerning each health issue and a philosophical base from which to teach these controversial topics.

An effective health teacher has a philosophy of education and health education.[2] This philosophy should include clear, personal convictions concerning the following factors:

THE NEED FOR A TEACHING PHILOSOPHY

1. The role of education in a democracy
2. The role of the modern health educator

1. Howard S. Hoyman, "New Frontiers in Health Education," *Journal of School Health* 7 (1973): 423–430.
2. Earle F. Ziegler, "The Health Teacher Needs a Philosophy," *New Directions in Health Education,* ed. Donald A. Reed (New York: Macmillan Co., 1971), pp. 65–92.

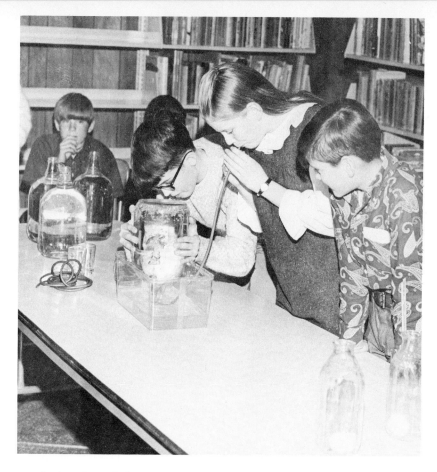

3. A system of classroom management
4. A procedure for teaching controversial issues
5. The role of valuing and decision-making activities in health education
6. A system of keeping up with the rapidly changing information in the field of health education.

A teacher should not operate in a vacuum. Teachers must come to grips with a wide range of issues which do not have clear-cut right or wrong answers. Listed below are several examples of issues an effective educator needs to take a stand on:

1. What is your personal stand on each controversial health issue?
2. Should a health educator be an information giver or a health initiator?
3. What is your view of the current criticisms of our nation's schools?
4. What are the moral implications of perpetuating our society through our public school systems?
5. What are the implications of taking a stand on an issue that opposes the stand of the majority of your community members?
6. When, if ever, should a teacher take a stand on a sensitive issue?

7. Is an educator an innovator for changes in society or a perpetuator of the status quo?
8. Is health education a panacea or a tool for the prevention of disease?
9. Should public schools teach morality?
10. How does a teacher reach students?
11. How involved should a teacher become in counseling a student?
12. What should be done about students who are unmotivated, under-achievers, or both?
13. What do young people really want to know?
14. How do students really view teachers?
15. Would you report a student who confides in you that he is on drugs?
16. What is your stand on corporal punishment?
17. What is your approach to teaching each of the major health topics?
18. Why should there be student involvement in your classes?
19. What is your philosophy about grading? How would you explain your grading system?
20. Does health education merit being a "major" subject area in elementary education?
21. What teaching strategies do students prefer?
22. Why should reinforcement be used as a motivating device?
23. Do students need authority?

Traditionally, health teaching has involved heavy emphasis on information giving. The philosophy behind the emphasis on the cognitive domain reflected an underlying trust that a child provided with enough of the right facts will make a correct health decision. Unfortunately, knowledge of facts may not influence behavior in the face of pressure from peers, situation ethics, or imperious urge. For example, even though most young people are aware of the health hazards of smoking, the incidence of teenage smoking is rising. In this regard, health educators are advised to utilize decision-making and valuing activities. In decision making, students participate in reaching their own conclusions and course of action for health through the study of both sides of issues. In valuing activities, students are asked to reach conclusions about what health factors are important to them and why they are important. Logically, the practice of decision making on health topics under adult guidance with support of class members will provide a basis for rational health behavior. Again, health education facilitates healthful behavior, may prevent occurrence of health problems, and can assist individuals in making correct decisions when disease occurs, but cannot act as a panacea for the prevention of all drug abuse, all premarital pregnancies, all cases of venereal disease, and all other attitude-behavior health problems.[3, 4]

Most health educators can be placed on a continuum somewhere between being information givers and being health initiators. The identifying characteristics of this philosophical dichotomy are found in figure 12–2.

HEALTH INFORMATION GIVING VERSUS HEALTH INITIATING

3. Godfrey M. Hochbaum, "How Can We Teach Adolescents About Smoking, Drinking, and Drug Abuse" Journal of Health, Physical Education and Recreation 4 (1968): 36.
4. Blum, Richard, "Schools Are Not Effective in Drug Education," Drugs and Drug Abuse Education Newsletter 3 (1972): 2.

Fig. 12–2. Are you a health information giver or a health initiator?

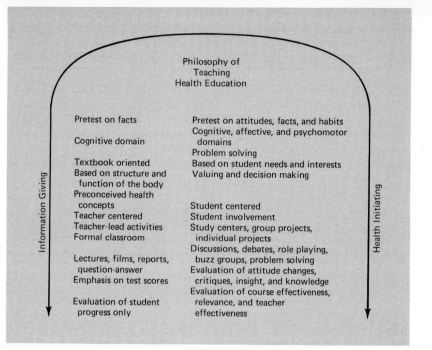

Philosophy of Teaching Health Education

Information Giving | Health Initiating

Pretest on facts

Cognitive domain

Textbook oriented
Based on structure and function of the body
Preconceived health concepts
Teacher centered
Teacher-lead activities
Formal classroom

Lectures, films, reports, question-answer
Emphasis on test scores

Evaluation of student progress only

Pretest on attitudes, facts, and habits
Cognitive, affective, and psychomotor domains
Problem solving
Based on student needs and interests
Valuing and decision making

Student centered
Student involvement
Study centers, group projects, individual projects
Discussions, debates, role playing, buzz groups, problem solving
Evaluation of attitude changes, critiques, insight, and knowledge
Evaluation of course effectiveness, relevance, and teacher effectiveness

FUNCTIONAL HEALTH TEACHING

Hoyman coined the term *functional health teaching* to denote that health educators should use valuing and decision-making activities as integral parts of health instruction.[5] Functional health teaching involves the development of health instruction based upon student needs and interests, teacher-student planning, and emphasis on personalized, student-centered activities. The practice of decision making in functional health teaching utilizes the development of the facts on all sides of all controversial issues, formation of value judgments, establishment of criteria for evaluation, and careful critique of all sources of information. In addition, evaluation in functional health teaching not only involves measuring student knowledge, but also places emphasis on evaluating course content, course organization, instructor effectiveness, relevance of information, implications of decisions made, and student attitude and behavioral change.

THE TEACHER'S ROLE IN CONTROVERSIAL ISSUES

The teacher's role in any controversial issue is to serve in guiding, motivating, clarifying, and resource-gathering capacities. The teacher should remain unbiased. More specifically, the teacher's role encompasses the following services:

1. To sell the importance of the topic
2. To aid students in defining the problems to be investigated
3. To aid in the development of essential evaluative criteria
4. To ensure the reliability of all resources
5. To evaluate student progress
6. To aid in analyzing data

5. Howard S. Hoyman, *Functional Health Teaching* (Goshen, Ind.: Mc-Connell School Map Co., 1949), pp. 33–34.

7. To guide students through the problem-solving process
8. To ensure that decisions are reached and follow-up activities pursued
9. To take a stand on a controversial issue if it is appropriate to do so

Values have been defined as concepts or constructs on which decisions are based and, in a broader context, on how a value is developed. Dalis and Strasser suggest that "a value is a characteristic or attribute of some general realm of human experience which is considered desirable by an individual or group."[6] Whatever the definition adopted, values remain subject to change and are often incompatible with behavior.

It is generally accepted that value activities in health education may contribute to the development of positive health attitudes and behavior through practice in personal and group decision making. Since facts, needs, and attitudes change throughout one's life, careful attention to the process by which students can arrive at value judgments and personal decisions may be the most important contribution of the value activities approach.

Today's generation might be described as a race of brilliant giants. Certainly, this generation is the best prepared to meet life's challenges. Why, then, do health problems such as venereal disease, drug abuse, and quackery persist? It has become apparent that the cognitive aspects of a given health problem, no matter how convincingly presented by an authority, do not necessarily bring about positive health attitudes or behavior. Carefully memorized facts for an examination may not be viewed within a value framework of existing motivation, peer pressure, personal need, relevance, and emotion.

While students in general seem to benefit from a values approach, value activities are pointed at those individuals who have yet to make their decision about a health problem or have made their decision without critical insight or the right information or because "others were doing it." The intent of value activities is to have students utilize factual information for personal decision making. These decision-making activities involve the gathering of reliable information concerning both sides of an issue. Students are expected to take part in judging, ranking, voting, and discussing the information. Finally, they should participate in developing measurable criteria for evaluating the information and in assessing both the short-range and long-range effects of their decisions.[7] These decision-making and value activities may fulfill the following objectives:

1. To have students rate particular value objects
2. To help students make rational, defensible judgments on controversial issues
3. To have students become aware of and utilize the various procedures needed for making rational, defensible health judgments and decisions
4. To have students participate in individual decision-making activities

6. Gus T. Dalis, and Ben B. Strasser, "The Starting Point in Values Education," *School Health Review* 5 (1974): 2–5.
7. Sidney B. Simon, Leland Howe, and Howard Kirschenbaum, *Values-Clarification: A Handbook of Practical Strategies for Teachers and Students* (New York: Hart Publishing Co.), 1972.

and to practice the skill needed for operating within a group in attempting to develop common value judgments and decisions.[8]

WHO SHOULD TEACH ELEMENTARY AND MIDDLE SCHOOL HEALTH EDUCATION?

Elementary school health education should be taught by the regular classroom teacher, rather than by a health specialist who visits different classes in one or more schools each day. On a day-to-day basis, the regular classroom teacher is in a position to counsel, remind, teach, and meet the immediate and long-range health problems of the students. In addition, the regular classroom teacher can continuously observe and evaluate the health of students and discuss current health problems and topics. The health specialist who visits a number of classes each day is not in a comparable position to meet the health needs of students.

Health education is very effective when a skilled classroom teacher integrates health topics with other subject areas. For example, concepts of nutrition might be reinforced while the class studies the culture of other countries. Also, two of the major components of health are human relations and mental health. The classroom teacher can develop formal instruction in these topics and follow through by guiding students in these important health factors on a day-to-day basis.

Recently, many states have begun to mandate that health education be taught in grades kindergarten through twelve. Such state laws often call for upgrading the quality of teacher preparation in elementary school health education. The American Association for Health, Physical Education, and Recreation has offered the following endorsement for certification programs in health education:

1. Each state department of education establish health education as an academic subject area.
2. All states develop health education certification standards requiring separate subject area preparation for health education teachers.
3. Health education certification requirements include preparation in: the physical, biological, and behavioral sciences; methodology; use of educational materials; communication skills; in-depth knowledge of a variety of health content areas as they relate to the individual, the family unit, and community groups; and the successful completion of a student or intern teaching experience in health education.
4. School systems move toward the development and implementation of comprehensive health education programs, the designation of health coordinators, and the employment of full-time health education teachers.[9]

The elementary school health educator needs competency in the following areas:

1. Understanding of the total school health program: (a) health services, (b) healthful school living, (c) health instruction, and (d) community interaction

8. Jerrold R. Coombs, "Objectives of Value Analysis," in *Values Education,* ed. Lawrence E. Metcalf (Washington, D.C.: National Council for the Social Studies, 1971), p. 4.
9. "Separate Certification for Health Education Teachers," *School Health Review* 5 (1974): 3.

2. Understanding of the health needs of school children
3. Knowledge of the total scope of health education and skill in the planning of health education
4. Special preparation in the teaching strategies best suited to health education
5. Skill in health counseling
6. In-depth knowledge of at least five of the following health components:
    a. Human growth and development
    b. Ecology and health
    c. Community health
    d. Chronic and communicable disease control
    e. Human sexuality and family life
    f. Nutrition
    g. Consumer health
    h. Safety education
    i. Drug education
    j. Mental health
    k. Care of the body senses
    l. Epidemiology

BASIC TEACHING APPROACHES IN HEALTH EDUCATION

Several different teaching approaches are available for most major areas in education. At the present time, health education seems to have four major teaching approaches: direct, integrated, correlated, and incidental health teaching.

DIRECT HEALTH TEACHING

Direct teaching of health indicates sequential kindergarten through sixth grade curriculum plans that include all major health topic areas. When approached in this manner, health education requires as much time as all other major elementary school subject areas. Along these same lines, most health educators agree that this would amount to approximately twenty minutes of health instruction per day. Equivalent plans utilizing larger blocks of time are encouraged.

The term *direct teaching* has also been referred to as a teacher-led, lecture-type approach to teaching. Direct teaching also refers to health instruction utilizing all modern teaching strategies within the context of a carefully planned, sequential kindergarten through sixth grade health education curriculum.

INTEGRATED HEALTH TEACHING

Integrated health teaching is a highly recommended approach to elementary school health curriculum construction and implementation. In integrated teaching traditionally separate subject matter areas are combined in a multidisciplinary approach. For example, a language arts project could integrate history, communication, art, drama, and music within a broad area such as the American Frontier 1824–1850.

Fortunately, many of the major health topics involve problems, issues, and concepts that are multidisciplinary in nature. For example, a study of pollution includes historical, legal, biological, economic, and cultural topics. In order to understand the importance of this major health topic, an integrated multidisciplinary approach is necessary.

In the past, health topics such as pollution were integrated into other subject areas. Because of the importance of many present-day health problems, it seems logical that "other" subjects might best be integrated into the study of certain health problems. Planning for integrated teaching can be more complex than planning in the traditional, separate discipline approach. The rewards, however, in terms of relevant topics, value activities, student involvement, and teaching strategies that relate to the needs and interests of students are well worth the extra effort.

CORRELATED HEALTH TEACHING

Correlated health teaching is an approach to health education in which health topics are scattered among other subject matter areas. Unfortunately, correlated health curriculum plans have long been used as a ruse by school districts for meeting state guidelines in health education without really teaching health or having health materials, sequential curricula, separate health courses at the secondary level, or qualified personnel. In the past, extensive efforts have been made to develop endless lists of health topics that could be covered in mathematics, science, language arts, physical education, and social science. The logic behind such efforts includes the following: (1) health topics can be tied in with other subjects, (2) careful planning will limit overlap of subject areas, and (3) savings in materials, personnel, space, and curriculum time are achieved.

The negative aspects of the correlated health teaching approach seem to outweigh possible advantages. The negative aspects of a program relying heavily on correlated health teaching include the following:

1. Health topics are generally given little emphasis in the classroom or not covered at all.
2. Teachers do not make the health topics meaningful to students.
3. Because of rapid changes in curricula and in personnel, health education is not taught in a logical, sequential manner.
4. Health materials and teaching strategies are not fully developed.
5. Because the various aspects of a major health problem are covered on a hit-or-miss basis, students are not prepared for facing present-day health problems.

To ensure that health be taught in the most effective manner, the profession might best be served by abandoning the correlated teaching approach. It is important, however, that health topics be brought up at appropriate times while other subjects are being taught. This will reinforce the concept that solving health problems requires a multidisciplinary approach.

INCIDENTAL HEALTH TEACHING

The type of health teaching that incorporates health topics into the teaching of other subjects is called *incidental health teaching*. Such an approach has merit, provided that it does not deteriorate into "accidental teaching." In this approach, health topics are incorporated as they logically occur during lessons on other subjects and as health and safety incidents occur during the school day. A new medical breakthrough, a provocative newspaper item, or an injury on the playground are best discussed when they occur, rather than wait for coverage later during a planned lesson or unit. An experienced teacher makes use of such teachable moments. Why, for example, should a political science teacher dwell on the impeachment of Andrew Johnson when the impeachment of a modern government official is imminent?

SUMMARY

Elementary school teachers need a philosophy of health education. As educators they need to take a personal stand on the role of education in society, on the role of health education, on good classroom management, on how to teach specific health areas, on controversial issues of health education, and on how to keep up with the rapidly changing information in the health field. Included in this philosophy is the personal decision on whether to be a health information giver or a health initiator.

Modern health educators are concerned with their role in guiding students through decision-making and value-judgment processes. Finally, because of an already crowded elementary curriculum, the modern elementary teacher needs to decide whether health will continue to be taught on an incidental basis or whether modern health problems are important enough to become major topics in elementary education.

Discussion Questions

1. Why should health education be taught in the elementary school?
2. What is your philosophy of education?
3. What is your philosophy of health education?
4. Define the role of the modern health educator.
5. Why do children need authority?
6. What is your philosophy of classroom management?
7. List what in your opinion are the ten best means of motivating students.
8. When are you a health information giver? a health initiator?
9. Would you take a stand on a controversial issue opposite that of most of the people in your community? Under what circumstances?
10. Should a health educator remain unbiased on all controversial issues? Discuss your position.
11. What is your detailed philosophy of evaluation?
12. What is your concept of functional health teaching?
13. Why should there be valuing activities in health education?
14. List your qualifications, strengths, and weaknesses for teaching health education.
15. Which approaches to teaching health do you prefer: direct? integrated? correlated? incidental?
16. Should health education be a *major* subject in elementary school? Defend your answer.

References

Blum, Richard. "Schools Are Not Effective in Drug Education." *Drugs and Drug Abuse Education Newsletter* 3 (1972): 2.

Coombs, Jerrold R. "Objectives of Value Analysis." In *Values Education*, ed. Lawrence E. Metcalf. Washington, D.C.: National Council for the Social Studies, 1971 .

Dalis, Gus T., and Strasser, Ben B. "The Starting Point in Values Education," *School Health Review* 5 (1974): 2–5.

Hochbaum, Godfrey M. "How Can We Teach Adolescents About Smoking, Drinking, and Drug Abuse?" *Journal of Health, Physical Education and Recreation* 4 (1968): 36.

Hoyman, Howard S. *Functional Health Teaching.* Goshen, Ind.: McConnell School Map Co., 1949.

Hoyman, Howard S. "New Frontiers in Health Education." *Journal of School Health* 7 (1973): 423–430.

"Separate Certification for Health Education Teachers." *School Health Review* 5 (1974): 3.

Simon, Sidney B., Howe, Leland, and Kirschenbaum, Howard. *Values-Clarification: A Handbook of Practical Strategies for Teachers and Students.* New York: Hart Publishing Co., 1972.

Ziegler, Earle F. "The Health Teacher Needs a Philosophy." In *New Directions in Health Education,* ed. Donald A. Reed. New York: Macmillan Co., 1971.

Chapter 13
INSTRUCTIONAL MEDIA

How should one describe the process of communication?

What are some of the barriers to effective classroom communication?

How does the use of instructional media contribute to learning?

What specific instructional methods involve still projection techniques?

How can one determine the strengths and weaknesses of an educational film?

Why are some educators critical of textbook teaching?

In what sense is the community a learning resource?

Health teaching and instruction have as their primary goal the facilitation of learning which in its broadest sense involves the acquisition of knowledge, the formation of attitudes, and the development of behaviors that serve health-promoting purposes. Effective learning reflects the teacher's awareness of rapidly expanding knowledge in the health sciences and current issues and trends having health implications, as well as the ability to translate these developments into experiences that have meaning, value, and relevance to pupils. What is taught must be scientifically accurate, well communicated, and stimulating to the members of the class. This is no small task, but experience has demonstrated that the effective selection and utilization of instructional media can substantially enhance the quality of teaching and enrich classroom learning.

Basically, the communication process consists of a sender, a signal, and a receiver. Successful classroom learning depends upon the clarity and understanding with which communication is conducted between the sender and the receiver of messages. While this fundamental process appears quite simple, it is more complex than our description implies.

As is shown in figure 13–1, a message is originated by a source (e.g., teacher) and is then converted into transmittable form (encoded). Upon transmission, messages stimulate one or more sense organs and are de-

THE COMMUNICATION PROCESS

Fig. 13–1. Transmission and reception of a message during the process of communication.

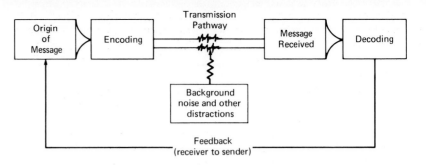

coded by the central nervous system of the receiver (destination). The model also includes the process of *feedback* which in Kemp's view is essential for the following reason:

> .... effective communication depends upon the receiver being active. He reacts by answering, questioning, or performing, physically or mentally. There is then a return or response loop of this cycle, from receiver to sender. It is termed *feedback*. Feedback may enable the originator to correct omissions and errors in the transmitted message, or to improve the encoding and transmission process, or even to assist the recipient in decoding the message.[1]

Unfortunately, intended communications in the classroom are frequently impeded by extraneous background noise, lack of attentiveness on the part of the receiver, communications medium that is of poor quality, discomforting environmental conditions, and hosts of factors that disrupt transmissions. Kinder suggests that these intrusions include poor physical reception, inaccurate interpretation of feedback, dissimilar background experiences, jargon, and differences in conceptions of time and space.[2]

BARRIERS TO CLASSROOM COMMUNICATION

Accurate physical reception of auditory and visual communications is dependent upon the undistorted transmission of messages. The spoken word must be enunciated with sufficient clarity and volume that the receiver can hear precisely what is said. Material written on the chalkboard or experience chart must be written in heavy print and large enough that students can easily read it. Glare, too much or too little light, poor color contrast of visual materials, and annoying teacher mannerisms are among the classroom forces that can impede the sending and receiving of messages.

When feedback is incorrectly interpreted, the success of communication is seriously jeopardized. Pupils often show some evidence (e.g., facial expressions) that they have or have not received an intended message. A blank stare on the face of a child is good reason to repeat directions or any other communication, perhaps using a different communications channel. However, even when receiver reactions suggest that the message has

1. J. E. Kemp, *Planning and Producing Audiovisual Materials,* 2nd ed. (San Francisco: Chandler Publishing Co., 1968), p. 11.
2. J. S. Kinder, *Using Instructional Media* (New York: D. Von Nostrand Co., 1973), pp. 45–48.

indeed been received, one can never be certain from this feedback that the receivers *understand* it or are able to relate it to previous learnings. Further evidence of understanding is desirable. A technique such as asking children to repeat a communication in their own words is a useful way of accomplishing this. The risk of inaccurately assessing pupil feedback is something that teachers must constantly be conscious of, especially in non-face-to-face teaching such as that involving television, programmed learning, and other independent learning techniques.

In all classrooms vast differences exist between the background and experiences of the teacher and of children in the class. While this is hardly a profound statement, it is something that one can easily lose sight of. Naturally, the experiential gap between teacher and child is widest at the earliest grade levels. One common mistake is to assume that words, ideas, and relationships that seem simple to the teacher are fully grasped by the very young. For instance, concepts such as health, fitness, and preventive medicine are virtually meaningless to youngsters in kindergarten and first grade. Processes such as digestion and circulation, which involve several discrete as well as overlapping functions, must be explained carefully and deliberately through the use of multiple media. A good rule of thumb to follow when working with children is to *take nothing for granted and never assume that anything is "common sense."* To believe and act otherwise is to invite communications breakdowns.

Every group of professionals employs jargon to facilitate communication among themselves, and educators are no exception. There is nothing inherently wrong with this practice, but it can obscure or confound the meaning of a message, particularly when one is communicating with others who are unfamiliar with the jargon. To "evaluate pupil progress" means little to children of elementary age, but "giving a test" leaves little doubt as to their teacher's intent. Children also use terms, phrases, and gestures whose meanings are perfectly clear to their peers, but are poorly understood by their teacher. A sixth grader reported by her classmates to be "going with someone" could mean that she received a phone call from a boy or walked home from school with him. In any case it has a different connotation than that with which the teacher may be familiar. A child's use of the term *queer* to describe a classmate may be an indication of disapproval of the other person, rather than a reflection upon his sexuality. Instead of interpreting what children mean by a communication that is unclear to the teacher, it is a wise practice to have children themselves explain what they mean. A child once approached me in tears complaining that while on the school playground one of her classmates gave her the "one-finger salute." Naturally, my initial reaction was to consider the gesture a vulgarity and to reprimand the guilty party. In a rare moment of self-restraint, however, I decided to discuss with the lad what he meant by the gesture. Surprisingly, the child explained that it did not mean anything except that he did not like the girl. Needless to say, this was not the interpretation most adults would be inclined to ascribe to the behavior. When we impose our own interpretations on what children say or do, messages become muddled and their true meaning is lost.

Differences in the time orientations of receivers and originators of messages also are responsible for ineffective communication. Elementary teachers who refer to heart transplants and kidney dialysis as recent medical innovations are in terms of their personal time orientation quite correct. To children, however, who were born since both of these medical procedures were introduced heart transplantations and dialysis are old hat. To successfully avoid the time orientation barrier to communication, one must first recognize that time differentials exist between teachers and pupils and attempt to compensate for them. One effective way to accomplish this is through the use of a variety of teaching aids.

SCOPE, FUNCTION, AND VALUE OF EDUCATIONAL MEDIA

Educational (or instructional) media is a relatively new term officially recognized in 1963 by the Association for Educational Communication and Technology of the National Education Association and is described by that group as follows:

> Educational media are defined here as those things which are manipulated, seen, heard, read or talked about, plus the instruments which facilitate such activity. Educational media are both tools for teaching and avenues for learning. . . .[3]

Educational media are not in themselves teaching methods, though they are necessary adjuncts to effective instruction. A filmstrip concerned with school safety is an example of a teaching aid. It becomes an essential step in teaching methodology when it serves as a springboard to other related learning experiences. A class discussion of the filmstrip, the development of a safety bulletin board theme, and a school safety survey based upon the filmstrip are examples of useful follow-up activities. Under these circumstances, the filmstrip is considered an integral part of teaching methodology. The distinction between educational media as teaching aids or as teaching methodologies is subtle, but nonetheless important. When teaching aids are used as ends in themselves without being integrated into a series of learning activities, their educational value is seriously limited. On the other hand, planned and systematic use of media and other learning activities contributes greatly to successful classroom experiences.

ADVANTAGES OF EDUCATIONAL MEDIA

There was a time in the not too distant past when teachers had to rely upon single sets of textbooks (often greatly outdated) and limited additional materials for instruction. Today the situation has changed dramatically, largely as a result of improvements in educational technology and the realization that media play an important role in educational processes. Yet, some classroom teachers appear to be unaware of the media opportunities that exist. Lack of awareness is not the only reason why a variety of media approaches are not used in some classrooms. A major factor is that these resources are not easily available to some teachers; another is that teachers are not willing to take the time required for the effective use of these resources.

In general, health education instructional aids are classified under three major groupings. Some are used mainly to develop and refine basic learning

3. B. Morris, ed., "The Function of Media in Public Schools," *Audiovisual Instruction* 8 (1963): 1.

skills such as reading, writing, and information gathering. Textbooks, work sheets, and study guides are representative of this category of instructional materials.

Other resource aids are intended to provide *indirect* learning experiences that would otherwise be difficult or impossible to arrange. A film describing the operation of a municipal water treatment plant and its role in protecting the public's health is one example of instructional aids that serve this purpose. Use of a model of the human torso to help pupils in the identification of anatomical landmarks also qualifies for this category.

Provision of *direct* experiences is the function of the third category of instructional resources. Field trips, work with animal organs (e.g., beef heart), and similar firsthand opportunities fall into this third category.

Collectively, all instructional media contribute to elementary school health instruction in one or more of the following ways:

1. *Provide multiple sensory experiences*

   Different types of learning are dependent upon the stimulation of various senses. For instance, when color is essential to the learning of a concept, it should be provided to enhance the child's learning. The same generalization applies to sound, shape, texture, and any other quality upon which conceptualizations depend. Instructional media are able to provide these stimuli.

2. *Offer common learning opportunities*

   Due to the wide experiential differences evident in the classroom, it is extremely difficult to identify experiences shared by all pupils. Through the use of appropriate health teaching aids which provide common experiences for the class, background dissimilarities can be lessened.

3. *Stimulate interest and involvement*

   Instruction that relies heavily upon verbalism, one-way communication, or any other single medium channel can be exceedingly dull. Perhaps the reader's own experience in college courses attests to this. Children in the elementary grades face essentially the same dilemma when their teachers use textbooks day in and day out, or constantly "talk to" their pupils. Boredom and apathy give way to excitement and enthusiasm when children are told that a field trip, film, or other "special event" has been planned. This heightened interest improves their receptivity to learning and also encourages them to become involved in subsequent activities related to the special event. Teaching strategy should include on a fairly regular basis a variety of educational media to help maintain a more or less constant climate of excitement and enthusiasm in the classroom.

4. *Make the abstract more concrete*

   Earlier discussion focused on the difficulties faced by most children when they are required to deal with concepts or abstractions that are not a part of their concrete life experiences. Instructional media by converting abstractions to real life objects and experiences add much to classroom learning.

5. *Provide enrichment experiences*

Only through the use of instructional aids are some educational experiences possible. For schools in the inner city, it may be all but impossible to arrange a field trip to a dairy farm to observe livestock and milk production and processing. However, a film on this subject is a perfectly acceptable alternative for children who may never have a firsthand opportunity to observe where milk comes from and how it is made safe for human consumption. Rural youngsters who may never have seen the mantle of polluted air that shrouds our metropolitan areas can do so via instructional media. Experts, multiple resources, and similar enrichment possibilities are presently available to teachers and pupils if only they will utilize media opportunities.

GUIDELINES FOR USING EDUCATIONAL MEDIA

Like the tools of a master mechanic, educational media must be wisely selected and skillfully employed if they are to accomplish the task that is expected of them. Unfortunately, no definite set of principles has been developed that will guide classroom teachers in their use of media under all circumstances. The following guidelines have proved very useful in helping educators improve their use of resources, regardless of the learning task required:

Guideline 1: Choose instructional media which fit specific objectives of the instruction. By listing your objectives first, then selecting materials that best further the attainment of those objectives, you avoid using materials merely for the sake of using materials.

Guideline 2: Prepare yourself in advance. Once you have selected the media you will use for your lesson, thoroughly familiarize yourself with them (for example, preview the slide, filmstrip, or film you have chosen) and consult study guides and manuals. Further, integrate the materials you have chosen into your lesson plan, considering sequence, timing, and proper coordination of all learning materials used.

Guideline 3: Prepare the class in advance. Student readiness ensures an 'atmosphere' for association and assimilation. Discuss with the class in advance the materials to be used, by name, type, source, and other pertinent information. Make the students aware of the reasons for using those particular materials, things to look for, associations to be made or considered, and new or unusual words, phrases, or symbols. Explain beforehand, too, any negative features of the material.

Guideline 4: Prepare physical facilities in advance. Although students are a captive audience, they are entitled to the use of all learning materials under optimum conditions. All equipment and media should be ready before the class assembles and should be in good working order. Alternative materials should be available in case of breakdown. Schedule student operators, if used, and be sure that you and/or the student operator know how to operate the equipment easily. Attend to seating arrangements, speaker's location, screen placement, light control, volume of sound equipment, and similar factors.

Guideline 5: Ensure student participation either before, during, or after presentation. The actual degree of student participation will depend on the type of materials used, their purpose, and the students' age or grade levels. Audio material does not necessarily eliminate student discussion during preparation, for example.

Guideline 6: Follow up use of instructional materials with related activities and an evaluation of the materials by the class. Facilitate the students' forming of associations and conclusions which have resulted from the use of the instructional materials, encouraging them to summarize the content imparted by the materials, set forth generalizations based on that content, or discuss the materials in the light of the purposes for which they were used. You might test the students on the lesson or repeat use of the media. Follow-up projects which involve individual students, committees, the entire school, or even the community may result from the use of the materials. If time permits, such projects may involve extended research and a challenge to creativity.

Guideline 7: Evaluate the materials you have used. Judge how well the materials did the job for which they were intended, also considering whether or not the students responded positively to them. You might then ask yourself what other materials, if any, might do a better job.[4]

Allen studied the relationships between instructional media and learning objectives.[5] His judgments of media effectiveness in relation to broad instructional objectives are shown in Table 13–1. Though his findings are not based on exhaustive research, they do provide a basis for determining which instructional media one should select to satisfy a specific learning objective.

Table 13–1. Relationships Between Instructional Media and Learning Objectives

Instructional Media Type	Learning Factual Information	Learning Visual Identifications	Learning Principles, Concepts, and Rules	Learning Procedures	Performing Skilled Perceptual-Motor Acts	Developing Desirable Attitudes, Opinions, and Motivations
Still pictures	medium	high	medium	medium	low	low
Motion pictures	medium	high	high	high	medium	medium
Television	medium	medium	high	medium	low	medium
Three-D objects	low	high	low	low	low	low
Audio recordings	medium	low	low	medium	low	medium
Programed instruction	medium	medium	medium	high	low	medium
Demonstration	low	medium	low	high	medium	medium
Printed textbooks	medium	low	medium	medium	low	medium
Oral presentation	medium	low	medium	medium	low	medium

Source: Allen, "Media Stimulus and Types of Learning," *Audiovisual Instruction* 12, no. 1 (1967):27–31.

4. J. S. Kinder, *Using Instructional Media* (New York: D. Van Nostrand), pp. 29–30. © 1973 by Litton Educational Publishing, Inc.

5. W. H. Allen, "Media Stimulus and Types of Learning," *Audiovisual Instruction* 12, no. 1 (1967): 27–31.

Media technology has kept pace with technological advances in other fields in recent years. Some of the hardware presently available (videotape equipment, computerized learning devices, audio-cued learning systems) are not commonly found in most schools, and for this reason will not be discussed in this section. Only those instructional media to which most elementary grade teachers have access are included in the following discussion.

STILL PROJECTION TECHNIQUES

When nonmoving images are projected on a surface, the process is known as *still projection*. All forms of this technique except one involve the passing of light through a transparent material (e.g., film) containing images. The image is then transmitted to a screen or other projection surface. Opaque projection is the single exception to this process since it is made possible by shining a powerful light on an opaque surface (e.g., magazine picture). The image of the opaque object is then *reflected* to a screen or wall. Filmstrips, transparencies, and two-by-two-inch slides are other forms of still projection that have gained wide popularity in schools.

Two-by-two-inch slides   Color slides are very popular as teaching aids at all grade levels. Many commercial slide sets dealing with a broad range of health topics are presently available for use in the elementary grades. Ordinarily these are relatively inexpensive and of good quality, but it is unwise to purchase such slides until you have had an opportunity to view them and determine how well they will satisfy your purposes.

Since 35 mm. cameras and color film are widely available at low cost, many teachers take their own pictures and create their own slides. When the film is returned from the processor, each slide is finished in a cardboard mount ready for use. Pictures of class projects, field trips, and other activities prepared as slides are very useful to teachers and of great interest to their classes.

The primary advantages of two-by-two-inch slides are their low cost, convenience, and ease of storage. If their color quality is good, this adds an important advantage to learning because of the realistic quality of the projection. Individual mountings enable the teacher to select slides at random for showing or to arrange slides in a special sequence. The fact that slides sometimes get out of order may be considered a disadvantage, but with minimal effort this can be avoided.

Projection requires either a special slide projector such as the carousel device illustrated or a filmstrip projector having a slide adapter. The former, since it is automatic and accommodates several slides at one time, is far superior for most purposes to the manually operated slide adapter.

Filmstrips   The popular filmstrip consists of a fixed sequence of still pictures on a strip of 35 mm. film. Commercially prepared filmstrips ordinarily contain about twenty to fifty frames and can be rolled up for easy storage in a small canister. Unlike the individually mounted two-by-two-inch slides which can get out of order, the sequence of frames in a filmstrip cannot be changed.

Filmstrips are available at low cost on a variety of health subjects and

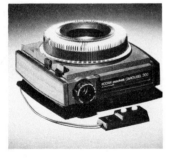

Fig. 13–2.   Carousel projector. (Courtesy of Eastman Kodak Co.)

are simple to use, and projectors for their use are available in most schools. Occasionally the strip of film becomes jammed in the projector and is damaged. Children who operate these pieces of equipment must be trained to insert the filmstrip properly and operate the equipment efficiently. With reasonable care filmstrips will last for years.

Some filmstrips have written captions on all or most of the frames, while others do not. In either case, the projectionist can pause on any frame for purposes of clarification or discussion. This is an advantage that all still projection techniques have over moving projections. Many filmstrips are available with accompanying record disks synchronized with the picture frames. When this audio aid is used, one cannot hesitate on a given frame or return to a previous frame without getting out of phase with the recording. All considered, filmstrips are very useful media devices and for certain teaching objectives are unsurpassed in ease of use and effectiveness.

Transparencies Transparencies are ten-by-ten-inch sheets of clear acetate material which are used with overhead projectors (see fig. 13–3). Special felt-point marking pens are used for writing on the transparency sheet, either prior to projection or while the transparency is situated on the overhead projector. By means of a moistened tissue, one can easily remove marks made on the acetate sheets.

This media technique became popular in schools during the early 1960s, and since then its versatility and effectiveness have made it a favorite of teachers. The projector is operated from the front of the room and requires very little darkening to be used with a high degree of effectiveness. This is a distinct advantage, for if viewers are required to be involved in reading, writing, or other seat work while the projector is in use, there is sufficient light to do so. Another advantage is that the teacher faces the class and can maintain eye contact with students as the image is projected on a screen behind her. One unique characteristic of transparencies is that they accommodate overlays (multiple acetate sheets) to illustrate a sequence of events or progressive phases of development.

Opaque projection As was previously noted, the principle of opaque projection differs from that underlying other methods of still projection. By contrast, this technique uses reflected light to project an image from nontransparent materials. Images of flat pictures, sample work sheets, newspaper articles or photographs, diagrams, and similar opaque objects can be projected on a wall or screen. By adjustment of the distance from the projector to the projection surface and refocus of the lens, images are enlarged or made smaller and can be traced or transferred to other surfaces. Many teachers use this process to produce object outlines for bulletin boards, to construct models, and for other instructional purposes.

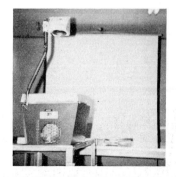

Fig. 13–3. Overhead projector.

Opaque projectors are very easy to operate but are somewhat bulky and difficult to store. Their effective use requires that the projection room be well darkened. In classrooms that are not equipped with effective light-screening window shades, this resource technique will not be satisfactory. In spite of these major disadvantages, opaque projection has a unique capability with which all teachers should be familiar.

MOTION PICTURES

Learning from motion pictures has proved so successful in schools that these instructional aids are now considered essential for some teachings and highly desirable for others. Research findings indicate that "Where motion is a defining attribute of a concept, it is better to present that concept using motion picture film than by nonmotion media."[6] Without question, motion pictures represent the most accurate means yet devised of capturing human events and environmental phenomena that would otherwise go unrecorded.

In the production of films, four basic techniques are employed. These are direct photography, changed-speed photography, photomicrography, and animation, each of which is used extensively in health-science motion pictures.

Direct photography   This process is used when the camera photographs an event as it actually occurs. A film showing gaseous and particulate emissions spewing from an industrial smokestack and the effects of wind currents in scattering these emissions is an example of direct photography. Naturally, not all events lend themselves to this photographic technique. When it is used effectively, it provides a documented, indirect experience for children.

Changed-speed photography   Some of the topics studied by elementary school children occur either too rapidly or too slowly to be perceived visually. Photography that either speeds up or slows down action is known as changed-speed photography. Time-lapse pictures showing the sequence of events in embryonic development can illustrate in a few seconds human development that actually takes place over a period of several months. The value of safety belts in protecting victims of automobile accidents is another example of the value of changed-speed photography in illustrating something that is, at best, difficult to show using any other media technique.

Photomicrography   Also known as microphotography, this method of filming permits the learner to experience visually objects and processes that are too small to be seen by unaided vision. Accomplished with the help of a microscope, it is possible to take pictures of blood passing through a capillary network or view microorganisms in water samples. Since children have considerable difficulty conceptualizing that which they cannot see, photomicrography lends itself to many health education films. Occasionally this technique is used in conjunction with changed-speed photography to show a microscopic series of events.

Animation   That which is theoretical, hypothetical, or otherwise inaccessible to the senses can be effectively illustrated by photographing a sequence of carefully drawn visualizations that suggest movement. The end product is an animation. This technique has much to offer children who are having difficulty understanding verbal or other explanations of phenomena they are unable to sense directly. For instance, the health concept *disease immunity* poses learning problems for many children primarily because it repre-

6. R. L. Houser, E. J. Houser, and A. R. Van Mondfrans, "Learning a Motion and Nonmotion Concept by Motion Pictures versus Slide Presentation," *AV Communication Review* 18, no. 4 (1970): 425.

sents difficult abstractions. When animated, as it is in many health films, the immune process becomes "real," and its basic features can be readily understood by youngsters. One must be careful when using animated films that content and technical accuracy of the film are not sacrificed for the sake of entertainment.

Film types Beginning in the mid-1920s, 16 mm. motion pictures have been used extensively for educational purposes. These movies were in themselves a tremendous innovation, but during 1929 and 1930 when sound tracks were added to films, their application in education was greatly broadened. "The interest that is produced when two of man's primary sensing mechanisms are simultaneously challenged and activated creates a sense of involvement and response which fulfills most of the conditions necessary for learning to take place."[7]

For years, 16 mm. films dominated the educational scene, with 8 mm. films used much less frequently. Super 8 mm. film was introduced by Eastman Kodak in 1966, and since that time has become very popular in schools. Being smaller than 16 mm. films, those of 8 mm. size require different equipment and are projected on a small screen. Their image is highly visual and better defined than that of 16 mm. films. Super 8 produces even better motion pictures than standard 8 mm. film.

One clear-cut advantage of Super 8 is that it is available in continuous-loop cartridges that can be easily used by children engaged in independent study. Silent 8 mm. films are usually from three to four minutes long, and the increasingly available 8 mm. sound films are from ten to twenty minutes in length.

Selecting films for classroom use Earlier it was noted that films and other educational media should be selected on the basis of how effectively they can assist the teacher in meeting established learning objectives. Mayshark and Foster have suggested that teachers ask themselves the following questions when considering a film for classroom showing:

1. Is it interesting and appropriate to the age and grade level?
2. Does it convey the desired facts and concepts, and is it likely to contribute to the formation of desirable attitudes?
3. Is it accurate and up-to-date?
4. Can it be correlated with and integrated into the course of study at the particular grade level?
5. Is the language well suited to the intended audience?
6. Is it likely to be understood by students?
7. Does it meet reasonable standards of technical excellence in terms of good-quality pictures, satisfactory sound, and natural acting?
8. Is the film of suitable length?
9. Are there commercial overtones that are distasteful and detract from the educational message?[8]

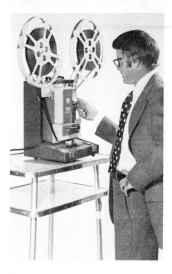

Fig. 13–4. Sixteen mm. projector. (Courtesy of Eastman Kodak Co.)

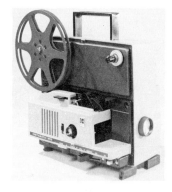

Fig. 13–5. Super 8 movie projector. (Courtesy of Eastman Kodak Co.)

7. W. A. Wittich, and C. F. Schuller, *Instructional Technology: Its Nature and Uses,* 5th ed. (New York: Harper & Row, 1973), p. 468.

8. C. M. Mayshark, and R. A. Foster, *Health Education in Secondary Schools,* 3rd ed. (St. Louis: C. V. Mosby Co., 1972), pp. 268–269.

Film Preview Information   (front)

Title _____ Date of Prev. _____

16 mm ____ 8 mm ____ So. ____ Silent _____ Color ____ B/W _____

Produced by _____ Date _____

Length of film _____ Free _____ Rental _____

Target audience, age group _____

Purpose of film _____

_____

_____

Techniques used (animation, changed-speed, etc.)

_____

_____

_____

                                                        (back)

Strengths of film: _____

_____

_____

Weaknesses of film: _____

_____

_____

Rating: _____ _____ _____ _____
                Excellent   Good   Fair   Poor

Additional comments _____

_____

_____

_____

_____

Without exception, all films should be previewed prior to their use in the classroom. One efficient and timesaving practice is to maintain a card file on all films reviewed for class use. Both sides of the cards can be mimeographed, as shown in figure 13–6.

MODELS

Models are three-dimensional likenesses of objects that add realism to instruction when an actual specimen is either not available for use or does not lend itself to instruction. Models are commonly used to acquaint children with the structure and function of body parts, although their use is not limited to these purposes. A model of a fire extinguisher showing the internal mechanism might be useful in explaining how this device operates. Similarly, a model of a sewage disposal plant showing the various steps of treatment could be used to good advantage in preparing children for an actual visit to their municipal sewage treatment facility.

The depth or thickness quality that is unique to models contributes substantially to their realism. If this third dimension is not necessary for students' appreciation of the structure and organization of an organ, object, or process, a flat picture, chart, or other two-dimensional representation will serve just as well and should be used.

When the actual size of the object being depicted (e.g., human heart) is large enough to be easily observed, life-size models are appropriate for classroom use. However, other models (e.g., tooth) must be considerably larger than the objects they represent if their component parts are to be easily discernible. In the case of models representing massive structures such as the sewage plant mentioned earlier, care must be taken not to distort relationships between parts when the scaled-down version is constructed. This assumes, of course, that models of this type will be constructed by children, rather than by companies specializing in instructional resources.

Color contributes to the attractiveness and lifelike qualities of a model and assists in the identification of its parts. Color is sometimes misused on models when attractiveness or color balance, rather than technical accuracy, is the manufacturer's primary concern. Use of these models should be discouraged because of the possibility of conveying faulty impressions and misinformation.

Elementary grade children enjoy working with models, especially those that provide interior views by means of cutaway construction and removable parts. Pupils' senses of sight and touch are stimulated when they explore models that can be disassembled and reassembled. Multiple sensory stimulation is more effective from a learning standpoint than is the stimulation of a single sense.

In summary, size, color, construction, and technical qualities determine the usefulness of instructional models. However, even those that satisfactorily meet these requirements do not necessarily contribute to learning. As is true of all instructional media, models must be used effectively by the teacher in conjunction with her other teaching strategies.

INSTRUCTIONAL TELEVISION (ITV)

As recently as a generation ago television was a novel and essentially untested communications medium accessible to relatively few Americans. Few, if any, people in those early years of the television industry could have imagined that by 1969 an estimated two billion worldwide viewers would witness via live television transmission man's first moon landing. That event and the technical sophistication it demanded indicate how rapidly television has progressed in a relatively short time. Educational institutions have benefited from the technological advancements in television. Technical developments plus improved production techniques have made educational television an important and exciting aid to classroom teaching.

The success of television as a communications medium was largely responsible for the establishment of public education broadcasting networks in this country. Among these are the Public Broadcasting Service (PBS) and National Educational Television (NET), both of which operate separately from commercial television networks and are dedicated to public education.

"Sesame Street," a popular program for young children, was first aired by PBS in 1969 and is without a doubt one of the most widely researched of all instructional television programs.[9] In general, research on ITV shows that television can be used effectively in teaching any subject where one-way communication facilitates learning.

> The advantages to the learner of carefully produced and wisely used television thus include its high visual impact as it presents lifelike and realistic experiences. When television is available to teachers, it has the effect of enlarging instructional experiences, expanding curriculum learning opportunities, and stimulating both pupils and teachers. The obvious reason for this is that it is far beyond the energies or capacities of any one or a few teachers to match the literally hundreds of hours of planning and production and other professional work necessary for *good* television.[10]

Health topics are being presented with increasing frequency on ITV, and when they are utilized for instruction, they should be closely related to classroom health education experiences. Additionally, pupils must be prepared for the telecast, viewing conditions should be of high quality, and appropriate follow-up activities must be planned. Clearly, the successful use of ITV requires considerable teacher skill, planning, and effort.

TEXTBOOKS

Considering all of the health instructional materials employed in elementary (and secondary) schools, textbooks are probably the most widely used and misused. One must bear in mind that textbooks, like all other teaching materials, are aids to learning, nothing more and nothing less. Properly used they are a most effective teaching and learning tool. Yet, more youngsters have been turned off from health education because of improper use of textbooks than as a result of any other single cause.

Critics maintain that textbook teaching restricts both teachers and pupils, stifles interest and creativity, and leads to a highly structured and formalized learning environment. Without question, those teachers who rely heavily if not exclusively on textbooks are deserving of this criticism. It is clear to me that many teachers who utilize textbooks in conjunction with other learning aids are doing a superb job of health teaching. Therefore, criticism should not be leveled at textbooks, but instead at the unwise manner in which they are used by some teachers.

To categorically denounce textbook use in the elementary grades is to deny pupils and their teachers an important learning aid. Educators recognize that well-written and up-to-date textbooks provide accurate and important health information organized in an orderly and understandable style. They are usually written by authorities and provide a common core of reliable health information for pupils. Moreover, textbooks and their accompanying manuals for teachers include a compilation of pertinent illustrations, graphs, diagrams, questions, resource suggestions, and other important aids.

9. G. A. Bogatz, and S. Ball, *The Second Year of Sesame Street: A Continuing Evaluation* (Princeton, N.J.: Educational Testing Service, 1971).
10. Wittich and Schuller, *Instructional Technology*, p. 514.

These features are of value to all teachers, but are especially useful to those with limited background in the health sciences.

Kilander believes that the likely causes of unwise textbook teaching include the following:

1. those traceable to the want of suitable teaching materials, for example, an inadequate library, a lack of proper classroom references, or a dearth of such teaching aids as films, records, maps and specimens and,
2. those resulting from such deficiencies on the part of the teacher himself as lack of competence in health education, insufficient training in educational method, imperfect understanding of children and the principles of learning, or meager teaching experience.[11]

Kilander's statement implies, and correctly, that textbooks should not be substituted for other teaching aids or media that can better satisfy a given teaching purpose. Textbooks should be used to provide background information and to stimulate pupils' thinking, but only in conjunction with other learning activities that encourage creativity, initiative, and exploration. The printed word merely verbalizes concepts and understandings, whereas other media can provide movement, animation, color, sound, texture, and other stimuli that are more effective than textbooks in generating interest and assisting in concept learning.

Textbook selection   When beginning teachers assume their first teaching position, they usually must use the textbooks currently available for the grade level they are assigned to teach. Eventually they will be in a position to recommend the ordering of new editions of these publications or to request the adoption of new health textbooks from a different publisher. In either case, the selection process needs to be objective and systematic, perhaps in collaboration with grade level colleagues and the health coordinator. The checklist recommended by Kilander (page 248) serves as a useful guide in this appraisal process.[12]

Textbooks for the elementary and middle grades   Most current textbooks available for health instructional purposes in grades one through eight are a vast improvement over those written in previous years. Generally, they have been written by authorities in health and education. Selected examples of these instructional materials include these choices.

Textbook Series

1. Bobbs-Merrill Company, Inc., 4300 West 62nd Street, Indianapolis, Indiana 46268.
   Health for Young America Series, Wilson and Wilson, 1968.

Grade	Title
1	*Health at School*
2	*Health Day by Day*

11. H. F. Kilander, *School Health Education,* 2nd ed. (New York: Macmillan Co., 1968), pp. 345–346.
12. Kilander, *School Health,* p. 347.

Fig. 13–7. Checklist for appraising textbooks in health education. (From Kilander, *School Health Education*, Macmillan, 1968.)

TITLE OF BOOK OR SERIES —————————————————————
AUTHOR(S) ——————————————————————————————
PUBLISHER ——————————————————————————————

Book	1	2	3	4	5	6
Name of book if in a series						
Grade for which intended						
Length in pages						
Year published						
Cost						

A. PHYSICAL FEATURES (10 points)
   1. Appearance attractive   2
   2. Cover and binding strong   2
   3. Print of desirable size   2
   4. Lines of desirable length   2
   5. Book of handy size   1
   6. Paper of good quality   1
B. CONTENT (50 points)
   1. Scope and emphasis of topics adequate†   20
   2. Sequence of topics good   5
   3. Length of book appropriate   5
   4. Style satisfactory for age level   5
   5. Vocabulary satisfactory for age level   5
   6. Situations within pupil experience   5
   7. Attitudes, habits, and facts stressed   5
C. AIDS FOR USE OF TEXTBOOK (25 points)
   (When desirable for grade level)
   1. Index adequate   4
   2. Illustrations adequate and good   4
   3. Activities adequate and interesting   4
   4. Questions appropriate and challenging   4
   5. Table of contents adequate   3
   6. Glossary or word meaning adequate   3
   7. Bibliography and references adequate   3
D. MISCELLANEOUS (15 points)
   1. Authors qualified   5
   2. Text published recently enough   5
   3. Content accurate and sound   5
E. GRAND TOTAL FOR BOOK   100

*Direction: Give the number of points on each item that you think the book deserves. The numbers shown are the maximum points assigned to the respective items.
†For "scope and emphasis of topics adequate," examine to determine whether each of the health areas is covered to the extent desirable for the grade level represented by each textbook. The health areas include:

1. Personal health
2. Nutrition
3. Community and environmental health
4. Consumer health
5. Mental and emotional health
6. Stimulants and depressants
7. Family life—sex education
8. Safety education
9. First aid
10. Home nursing

  3   *Health and Fun*
  4   *Health and Growth*
  5   *Health and Living*
  6   *Health and Happiness*
  7   *Men, Science, and Health*
  8   *Health, Fitness, and Safety*

Teacher's editions and separate teacher's manuals are available for each grade level.

2. Laidlaw Brothers, Thatcher and Madison Streets, River Forest, Illinois 60305.

The Healthful Living Program, Fodor, Glass, Gmur, Moore, Neilson, Byrd, 1974.

Grade	Title
1	*Your Health*
2	*Being Healthy*
3	*Your Health and You*
4	*Keeping Healthy*
5	*Growing Up Healthy*
6	*Health for Living*
7	*A Healthier You*
8	*Your Health and Your Future*

Teacher's editions are available for each grade level, and tests with answer keys are available for grades 3 through 8.

3. Scott, Foresman and Company, 1900 East Lake Avenue, Glenview, Illinois 60025.

Health and Growth Program, Richmond, Pounds, Jenkins, Sussdorf, 1974.

Grade	Title
1	*Health and Growth, Book 1*
2	*Health and Growth, Book 2*
3	*Health and Growth, Book 3*
4	*Health and Growth, Book 4*
5	*Health and Growth, Book 5*
6	*Health and Growth, Book 6*
7	*Health and Growth, Book 7*
8	*Health and Growth, Book 8*

Teacher's editions are available for each grade level. Preprimary materials (pictures and songs) are available also.

Supplementary Textbooks

1. *Laidlaw Brothers*

Basic Concept Books, Needle, et al.

Basic Concepts of Alcohol
Basic Concepts of Drugs
Basic Concepts of Tobacco and Smoking
Basic Concepts of Human Life: Facts for Youth to Know

2. *Scott, Foresman and Company*

Health and Growth Enrichment Booklets (primary grades)

Drugs and Your Safety
Moving, Moving, Moving About
Primary Pollution Packet

Supplementary Materials, Grades 4 through 8

> *The Human Story: Facts on Birth, Growth, and Reproduction* (Spanish-language edition also)
> *V.D.: Facts You Should Know*
> *Drugs: Facts on Their Use and Abuse* (Spanish-language edition also)
> *About You and Smoking*

Paperback Health Booklets, Grades 7 and 8

> *Pollution and Health*
> *A Healthy Personality for You*
> *Sleep, Exercise, and Nutrition*
> *Consumer Health*
> *Safety for Teen-Agers*

INSTRUCTIONAL RESOURCES CENTER

Considering its most embryonic stage, the instructional resource center (IRC) is hardly a new idea in education, but it is a concept that has changed dramatically in recent years. Prior to the modern era of instructional resources, the IRC was little more than a collection of reading materials located in practically every classroom. As newer and more complex teaching media were developed, teachers found themselves unable to keep informed of media innovations and their implications for teaching and learning. Space required to store the increasing quantities of printed and nonprinted media and the equipment to use them was far more than that available in the individual classroom. Of necessity, our concept of the learning resources center experienced and continues to undergo an exciting metamorphosis.

Beggs has aptly described the purpose and scope of the modern IRC as it functions to improve the quality of teaching and learning.

> The instructional media center, when properly organized, is the heart of the school. Rather than being only a place where ideas and facts are stored in printed, recorded, and illustrated forms, the IMC is a beehive of activity. Both students and teachers use the IMC—students for learning and teachers for designing and developing learning experiences.
>
> The instructional media center is the place where the broadest possible range of information in multiple and diverse forms is stored and readily available for use by both partners in instruction, the student and the teacher. Students can go to the IMC to read, listen, write, view, and construct. The IMC houses a wide range of books in terms of subject and complexity, along with pamphlets, magazines, newspapers, and mimeographed materials. Records, electronic tapes, photographic slides, transparencies, maps, posters, charts, mock-ups, models, teaching machines, films, and filmstrips are included.[13]

Instructional resources centers vary considerably in their organization, location, and scope. In general, larger school districts are able to develop

13. D. W. Beggs, "Storehouse and Laboratory," in *Instructional Media Center*, ed. H. S. Davis (Bloomington, Ind.: Indiana University Press, 1971), pp. 2–3.

better equipped and more comprehensive facilities. Large school districts often employ professionals whose primary responsibilities include the operation and development of a centralized district IRC. In some locations, regional IRCs have been established, serving students and teachers in several adjoining school districts. On a much smaller scale, individual schools may have a decentralized resources center. This type of facility often takes on the appearance of a school library, but with expanded services. Learning resources centers range from those with minimal equipment, materials, personnel, and services to those which are well staffed and well equipped with the latest materials and most sophisticated equipment. Any teacher, new or otherwise, should acquaint herself with the IRC in her district and become fully aware of how this facility can assist her and her pupils in teaching and learning.

The community is an educational resource that is readily available to all teachers regardless of where they teach. Exciting opportunities for health education exist in this setting, but too frequently they are not taken advantage of. Sometimes they pass unnoticed by the teacher who is not aware of the educational potential of community activities. Other teachers, bound by the chains of tradition, by rigid classroom scheduling, and by the mistaken belief that all worthwhile school learning occurs in the classroom, restrict their teaching to that environment and ignore opportunities for learning in the community. In either case, stimulating real-life experiences which usually cannot be replicated by the teacher in her classroom remain untapped.

Community study can be an extremely effective means of expanding the school's learning resources. Enrichment results either by bringing useful community resources into the school or by arranging for students to go into the community. Both approaches to community study offer situations where children can learn firsthand about people, things, processes, and services upon which the health and welfare of their community depends.

USING COMMUNITY RESOURCE PEOPLE

In an earlier section we discussed a problem that developed in a school cafeteria and how one class decided to learn more about the situation by asking a public health sanitarian to speak to them. They were in need of technical information that their teacher was not able to provide. What better way to handle this situation than to invite an expert to class? Occasionally, physicians, nurses, pharmacists, veterinarians, firemen, representatives of official and voluntary health agencies, and other persons in the health or health-related occupations can add unique dimensions to classroom learning. Planning for this involvement needs to be careful and complete if the class is to realize maximum benefit from the experience. Not infrequently, casual and haphazard planning results in wasted time and effort for the teacher, pupils, and resource person.

Ideally, when a resource person is to make a class presentation, the decision to invite the person should be made jointly by pupils and teacher. This process is quite simple since children are always thrilled over the prospect of having a visitor come into their classroom. Actually, all a teacher has to do is to suggest that a given resource person might be helpful to pupils in their understanding of a subject. Almost without exception, class response is positive. In general, resource persons are less familiar than is the

UTILIZING COMMUNITY RESOURCES

grade level teacher with the educational process and the variables that influence its outcomes. With this generalization in mind, the teacher should take the initiative in apprising the resource person of the following factors prior to the class visit:

1. The time, duration, location, and subject of the presentation
2. What the teacher expects pupils to learn as a result of the presentation
3. What the children have learned previously about the subject
4. The general ability levels represented by pupils
5. The kinds of activities that generate most pupil interest

Additionally, it is a thoughtful gesture, as well as a wise pedagogical practice, to determine whether the teacher can be of any assistance by providing projection materials or other equipment required by the resource person.

Earlier, mention was made of the importance of involving pupils in the preliminary planning for community study. In this regard, the key consideration is to involve children in deciding what they hope to learn from their community experience. This may require nothing more than a loosely structured class discussion, but it is recommended that a limited number of questions be developed that teachers and pupils would hope to have answered by the resource person. One reason for having predetermined questions is that they provide direction for the resource person. A second and more important reason is that one can easily involve class members in evaluating the experience by having them express how well their questions were answered.

FIELD TRIPS

Planned learning situations in which pupils leave the confines of their classroom range from brief walking trips in the vicinity of the school to extensive tours that require more time and distance. Broadly speaking, this range of activities encompasses what are referred to as field trips. In the elementary grades, health field trips often include visits to a fire station, the health department, a hospital, the police department, water treatment facilities, and food processing operations.

Visits within the school should be the starting point for children in the earliest primary grade. After all, the school community is a strange and awesome world to children of this age. Trips to the kitchen, health office, and heating plant, as well as those that emphasize the locations of emergency exits and fire extinguishers and how a panic bolt operates, are certainly beneficial for kindergarteners. Children who have attended school for one or more years do not express as much enthusiasm over these awareness experiences as do children who are new to a school. Within-school trips provide an opportunity for children to learn about the basic community study process. Their experience in planning trips, asking questions, being observant, and evaluating involves skills upon which the success of extra-school field trips will depend.

As they proceed through the elementary grades, children are eager for and capable of active involvement in field experiences. For instance, they may choose to survey sources of noise pollution in their community and then arrange interviews or meetings with public officials to determine what can be done to control this problem. They may observe the bicycle-riding habits of their schoolmates, compile a list of common traffic violations, and discuss what can be done to make their school environment safer for pedestrians and bike riders.

Teachers considering the advisability of a specific field trip must ask themselves whether this type of activity is superior to discussion, lecture, textbooks, films, or other instructional media for realizing their teaching objectives. If other media will do as well or better, those alternatives should be used. This decision may appear simple, but in actual practice is not, especially for those new to teaching. Beginning teachers can more effectively plan community study experiences once they are aware of the field trip successes and failures of more experienced colleagues. In fact, many questions relating to the broad subject of instructional resources can be answered quickly and with authority if one is willing to ask questions of other teachers.

SUMMARY

Most classroom learning depends more upon clear communication than upon any other single consideration. Effective selection and utilization of instructional media not only provides diversity and clarity to communication between teacher and students, but it also enhances the learning of students who are working independently.

Basically, to communicate a message one needs nothing more than a transmission channel and a receiver of the message. However simple the process appears, communication is subject to many intrinsic and extrinsic conditions that impair its effectiveness. This is particularly true in a classroom filled with energetic, enthusiastic children who are subject to many distractions including noise, excessive light, and similar environmental conditions. Background differentials between teacher and pupils, inappropriate communications channels, use of jargon, and incorrect interpretation of feedback are among the factors that undermine communication.

Proper use of instructional media significantly reduces the probability of breakdown in the communicative process. Health instructional resources assist in the development of basic learning skills, provide *indirect* learning experiences, and enable students to have firsthand or *direct* experiences they might otherwise not have.

The effective use of media requires considerable teacher skill, effort, and knowledge of the advantages and shortcomings of various media techniques. Familiarity with both still and moving projection methods is extremely valuable, as is a knowledge of other resources including models, instructional television, and textbooks.

One readily available though often overlooked resource, the community, is discussed at some length. Local resource people are able to augment classroom instruction, and trips into the community when properly planned provide learning experiences impossible to replicate within the classroom.

Discussion Questions

1. Respond to the criticism that instructional resources are little more than educational frills.

2. What specific suggestions can you make for improving the use of instructional media in a course you are presently enrolled in?
3. Distinguish between educational media as teaching aids and as teaching methodologies.
4. As teachers plan their basic instructional program, why must they determine teaching objectives before deciding upon their educational resource needs?
5. Under what conditions can films facilitate learning?
6. Support or refute this book's claim that textbooks are important learning tools.
7. How can teachers successfully use their community as an effective resource for health instruction?

References

Allen, W. H. "Media Stimulus and Types of Learning." *Audiovisual Instruction* 12, no. 1 (1967): 27–31.

Beggs, D. W. "Storehouse and Laboratory." In *Instructional Media Center,* ed. H. S. Davis. Bloomington, Ind.: Indiana University Press, 1971.

Bogatz, G. A., and Ball, S. *The Second Year of Sesame Street: A Continuous Evaluation.* Princeton, N.J.: Educational Testing Service, 1971.

Houser, R. L., Houser, E. J., and Van Mondfrans, A. R. P. "Learning a Motion and Nonmotion Concept by Motion Pictures versus Slide Presentation." *AV Communication Review* 18, no. 4 (1970): 425.

Kemp, J. E. *Planning and Producing Audiovisual Materials.* 2nd ed. San Francisco: Chandler Publishing Co., 1968.

Kilander, H. F. *School Health Education.* 2nd ed. New York: Macmillan Co., 1968.

Kinder, J. S. *Using Instructional Media.* New York: D. Van Nostrand Co., 1973.

Mayshark, C. M., and Foster, R. A. *Health Education in Secondary Schools.* 3rd ed. St. Louis: C. V. Mosby Co., 1972.

Morris, B., ed. "The Function of Media in the Public Schools." *Audiovisual Instruction* 8 (1963): 1.

Wittich, W. A., and Schuller, C. F. *Instructional Technology: Its Nature and Uses.* 5th ed. New York: Harper & Row, 1973.

Chapter 14
TEACHING
STRATEGIES
IN
HEALTH
EDUCATION

What are some commonalities of all teaching strategies?

What are the available practical considerations for motivating students?

What are the more effective health teaching strategies?

What is the role of classroom organization in effective teaching?

How does the teacher implement decision-making and valuing activities?

Teaching strategies, or methods, are the tools an educator utilizes for the development of health attitudes, knowledge, and behavior. The term *teaching strategy* has been chosen over the term *method* in order to denote a broader concept of teaching tools. Teaching strategies can include motivational devices, classroom interpersonal relationships, specific classroom activities, and organization of classroom activities.

LESSON INTRODUCTION

A carefully developed introduction can be a major factor in the success of any teaching strategy. Students need to be informed of the why and how of a health lesson and, more important, what will be expected of them. As a rule, poorly given directions are a common cause of classroom confusion, disorder, and poor performance. An effectively delivered lesson introduction reflects the preparation of the teacher. Carefully prepared and explained handouts, concise directions, and a statement about the importance of the topic clearly illustrate the teacher's interest in the lesson.

ASSIGNMENTS

Poorly given assignments or directions can be a major cause of stress in the classroom. Confusion seems to breed doubt, panic, lack of trust, and frustration. A poorly thought-through assignment discourages motivated students and reinforces unmotivated ones. A bitter experience occurs when a motivated student has spent hours on an assignment only to find that his preparation is unnecessary or, worse, ignored. Students deserve and need

COMMONALITIES OF HEALTH TEACHING STRATEGIES

to know where they stand, what is expected of them, why they are involved in the activity, and what evaluative criteria are to be utilized.

MOTIVATION

Health teachers should consistently plan for classroom motivation. The following list of everyday practical reminders and suggestions should be useful in planning for motivation:

1. Reward, as discussed in chapter 11, is perhaps the most effective motivational device. Teachers can reward students by praise, interest, approval, trust, and recognition and by giving extrinsic awards ranging from stars to elaborate prizes. The key is to enhance a student's self-image and self-concept. Students need success. A kind word or conversation indicating that a teacher is interested in the student can be very effective.

2. It should be understood that motivation is contagious. The teacher must show enthusiasm and interest.

3. A clear understanding of the purposes of a lesson enhances motivation. People are goal orientated. They are more likely to push forward when they are aware of what lies ahead and how they are going to get to their destination. A carefully developed lesson introduction is an effective way of generating enthusiasm for the task at hand.

4. Self-imposed tasks tend to create more interest than teacher-imposed tasks. Have students share in the planning of health activities and setting personal goals.

5. Varied teaching strategies and procedures are necessary for maintaining interest.

6. Try to capitalize on existing interests. Teachable moments occur when student interest is high. This interest can be stifled by the ubiquitous comment "Let's wait and continue this discussion when we are in our _____ unit."

7. Be aware that each individual handles praise, success, criticism, and failure in a different manner.

8. Gear activities to the level of the students. Activities too difficult or too easy quickly inhibit interest.

9. Avoid fear as a motivational device. While the threat of important deadlines and possible failure can get us moving, we tend to ignore constant threat. Most students look for alternatives to high-anxiety situations. One particularly inviting alternative to constant pressure is to not bother.

10. The physical aspects of the classroom such as cheerful colors, attractive bulletin boards, comfortable heating, room size, and proper lighting and ventilation can seemingly shorten or lengthen a school day.

11. Stress health teaching strategies that are personalized and pointed at real student problems and involve student decision making. Promote problem solving.

12. Provide up-to-date materials and plan self-discovery activities around these materials.

STUDENT INVOLVEMENT

Having the students actively involved in the teaching activity should be a commonality in all health education lessons. Student involvement consists of more than having students work in study groups, participate in discussion, or complete special interest projects. Involvement in health education can include the following activities:

1. Topics that are personalized to the student's immediate needs and interests
2. Emphasis on student decision-making activities
3. Discussion activities that involve student-student dialogue rather than teacher-student dialogue or recitation
4. Emphasis on practical problem-solving activities in which the solutions can be directly applied to daily living
5. Students interacting among students and adults to determine their own course of action
6. Utilization of valuing activities in which students are forced to follow the personal decision-making process of fact-finding, critiquing of sources, and defending their own position on the issues
7. Student participation in the planning of health education and the evaluation of themselves, the teachers, and the program
8. Opportunities for special interest activities within the scope of any health topic
9. Unbiased exposure to all sides of controversial health issues

LESSON SUMMARY AND FOLLOW-UP ACTIVITIES

Teaching a few things well is a basic philosophy in the teaching of health. In order to implement this philosophy, teachers must avoid the traditional pattern of having students take copious lecture notes, do an outside reading assignment, and regurgitate the information on an examination. If the pattern of student involvement is followed, it is important that the key points in a health lesson be covered in such a manner that students will have a firm grasp of the subject matter and have completed the decision-making process by the end of the lesson. Lesson summaries and follow-up activities serve the purpose of immediate feedback as to whether the lesson teaching strategy was successful.

The approaches to a lesson summary include the following:

1. Teacher-led discussions on the key points
2. Students explaining what they received from the lesson
3. Student decision making and defense of their decisions
4. Surveys or votes on the controversial issues involved
5. Follow-up value activities utilizing the key points and issues developed in the lesson

The follow-up activity approach offers an alternative to a paper-and-pencil evaluation of student progress. This evaluation approach fits well with special interest activities and student-teacher contracts. It allows both slow and fast learners to be evaluated at their own pace.

CHOOSING TEACHING STRATEGIES

Choice of strategy is dependent upon the objectives of a lesson, the abilities of the students, the existing time limitations, the available facilities and resources, and the importance of the topic. Utilization of many strategies provides variety and increases student interest. Along these same lines, the use of differing strategies can reflect the quality of a teacher's ability, preparation, and motivation.

Readiness is a factor in the choice of an activity. While it is unlikely that a kindergarten or primary grade class can follow the complexities of a debate or that an upper grade class would look forward to show and tell, most teaching strategies with some modifications can be used at any level. The most effective approach is to involve the students in some type of decision-making process.

A health lesson should evolve from carefully stated objectives and directions clearly explaining what is expected of the student. Most activities should include decision making if possible. In following the philosophy of teaching a few things well, teachers should strive to have the learning take place during the lesson, not during some outside actvity such as studying for an examination. For most strategies this involves seeking out the information on both sides of an issue in an unbiased manner, utilizing the information in personal decision making, and reinforcing the learning that took place with some type of lesson summation.

Many strategies include group activities and discussions. At times the carefully developed lesson objectives may be of less importance than the concomitant communication and human relations skills employed in these activities. Teachers are encouraged to use their creative talents and try many different strategies. The extra preparation time and extra classroom time required for many of these activities are very worthwhile.

The choice of a clever, well-thought-through teaching strategy does not ensure that learning will take place. Teaching is not analogous to programming a computer. The skills and personality of the teacher determine the outcome of a lesson.

IMPLEMENTING HEALTH STRATEGIES

DISCUSSIONS

Classroom discussions are basic to functional health teaching. When effectively conducted, class discussion can develop student involvement, reinforce value judgments, generate further discussion, and make a positive contribution to a student's self-image.[1] While spontaneous discussion can be the highlight of a school day, the basic ingredients of successful classroom discussions are usually the following:

1. Careful planning
2. Controversial topics students are interested in
3. Communication among students and within a positive social environment
4. Skilled discussion leader

Planning for a discussion requires insight into the abilities, interests, and social interactions of the students. Very careful preparation needs to be made for these elements: (1) choosing a topic students are willing to discuss, have opinions on, and need to make decisions about; (2) introducing and selling the topic in order for students to grasp the purpose and direction of the discussion; (3) developing key questions that are capable of generating discussion; (4) providing structure to the discussion

---

1. Richard A. Schmuck, and Patricia A. Schmuck, *Group Process in the Classroom* (Dubuque, Iowa: Wm. C. Brown Co., 1973), pp. 2–14.

and ensuring its flow in a logical manner; (5) developing closure on a few topics rather than touching on many, and (6) having a plan for summarizing the lesson or developing follow-up activities for reinforcing the key points and decisions of the discussion. The leader must also plan for remaining unbiased and must ensure that all sides of an issue are covered. In addition, the leader needs to generate student opinions and decisions, not instill or force students to accept his or her view of the issues involved.

The social atmosphere of a classroom influences the effectiveness of a discussion. An autocratic teacher, a few students who distract or dominate a discussion, and a lack of cooperation and courtesy will stifle effective communication. In addition, students who are afraid to respond or have been embarrassed by peers or teachers for previous responses will also negatively effect a group process. Social and communicative skills are difficult to develop. Patience and guidance are prerequisites for the elementary school discussion leader.

Some important by-products of classroom discussions are the skills and self-confidence students can gain while communicating and cooperating with peers. In effect, the sharing of ideas, self-expressing, compromising, voting, listening, and debating in the spirit of a common goal provide a foundation of group process skills that are fundamental to a democratic way of life. The discovery that many other persons have the same thoughts, fears, and problems can also aid in the creation of a positive self-image. Groups guided by a skilled discussion leader have the opportunity to practice thinking through both sides of issues, choosing alternatives, and making decisions. Students experiencing this process should be better equipped to deal with their own personal and interpersonal problems.

Leading a discussion is a skill that requires considerable practice and planning. The ability to get all students into the discussion, to avoid answering your own key questions, to remain unbiased, to ask the right kinds of questions, to reach decisions, and to make sense out of a discussion is not easy to acquire. The following list includes suggestions for structuring and leading a discussion:

Structuring a discussion

1. Define and sell the problem or topic to be discussed.
2. Inform the group about the kinds of key questions that will be discussed or have students help plan the outline of key questions.
3. Use the blackboard or some other visual aid for listing the key questions and summarizing the key points developed from the discussion.
4. Summarize at appropriate times to bring the direction and key points more sharply into focus.
5. Strive for consensus among the students.
6. When appropriate, include follow-up valuing activities that utilize the information and concepts generated from the discussion.
7. Always summarize the discussion by reviewing the key questions, key points, and opinions on both sides of issues.
8. Have individuals or groups reach conclusions or decisions about the controversial issues discussed. Expect them to defend their decisions.

9. Hold students responsible for the key points on all sides of all issues.

Leading a discussion

1. Be thoroughly prepared on the topic to be discussed.
2. Prepare the class for a meaningful discussion through assignments and advance information concerning the key questions and what they will be responsible for.
3. Use visual aids for stimulating conversation.
4. Avoid the traditional seating arrangement in which the students are in rows, all facing the front of the room. This arrangement effectively stifles discussion. Try arrangements in which the students can face one another such as in circles or semicircles.
5. In order to keep the group on track, periodically summarize.
6. Be democratic rather than autocratic.
7. State key questions that call for opinions, reasons, and ideas, not for yes-or-no responses.
8. Strive for contributions from all members of the class.
9. Make sure that all understand what has been said. Use discussion for developing listening skills.
10. Discourage teacher-student conversation. Try to get the students to talk to one another and not always through you.
11. Strive for closure on an issue before moving on to the next key question.
12. Address the key questions to the class, not to individuals.
13. Through careful eye survey continually look for the individual who has that I-think-I-am-ready-to-say-something look.
14. Carefully make eye contact first with those students who have not been active in the discussion before calling on anyone.
15. Avoid the tension of frequently calling on someone who has not volunteered to respond.
16. Do not restate a student's comments. Force the class to listen.
17. If a student's statement is unclear, have that student repeat the statement.
18. Avoid the temptation of elaborating on every point yourself. This type of teacher domination defeats the purpose of the activity.
19. When writing a student's contribution on the board, use the student's own words. Do not rephrase the words the way you would like them to be.
20. Give some type of positive reinforcement to each contributor.
21. If a student is wrong, use a subtle statement such as: That is one way of looking at it. What other ideas might be involved?
22. Be alert to develop compromise solutions to issues.
23. Strive for a relaxed, cooperative exchange of ideas where humor is in evidence. In such an atmosphere ideas come under scrutiny or attack, never classmates.

PANEL DISCUSSIONS

A panel discussion is a discussion among a small group (panel) of experts who speak to a specific issue or issues. It is not a series of student reports or speeches.

Different organizational patterns can be effectively used for panel discussions. In one type, the panel members and moderator have been given the assignment well in advance so that each individual becomes a specialist in one area of the topic to be discussed. In another type of panel the members consist of students who are not experts, but who have been asked to discuss a controversial topic they can relate to: for example, parent-child relations for fifth graders. Students could also be asked to role play the position of experts. For example; one student could role play a conservative housewife; another, a flaming women's liberator; and so on. Although more difficult to arrange, a very effective panel can be made up of experts from the community such as a counselor, pastor, social worker, and parent.

In a panel discussion the emphasis is on the panel members discussing a series of key questions concerning a controversial area. The success of a panel discussion often depends upon the skill of the moderator. The moderator, either the teacher or a skilled student, asks each key question, strives for participation from all the panel members, keeps the discussion on track, periodically summarizes, and strives for a consensus. The moderator usually does not contribute his or her opinion.

The emphasis in a panel discussion is on meaningful dialogue between the panel members and on getting the audience involved. Audience participation can be accomplished by assigning the class members responsibility for the information discussed. Prior to each panel discussion the teacher should carefully explain the role of the audience. A handout of the key questions will help the students keep track of the discussion. In addition, the audience should be asked to participate in the discussion after the panel has reacted to each key question or after the panel has discussed all the key questions. It is very important that a carefully developed lesson summary occur.

DEBATES

The debate activity combines a game situation, detailed factual content, and communication skills. Since the nature of any debate is to present a detailed documented argument, this activity can present an almost overwhelming amount of factual information on both sides of a controversial issue in a very short period of time. Topics for a debate should be controversial, timely, and personally important to the students.

While several debate formats are available, the most common pattern is a modified interscholastic type of debate. Other patterns include a panel on which one-half the members are for or against an issue, a game type of activity in which members attempt to refute the statements made by the opposing team, and a more informal discussion in which students with different positions try to convince others to agree with them.

The modified interscholastic type of debate consists of two students on the affirmative side and two students on the negative side of an issue. A recommended pattern is to give all four students the assignment well in advance so that they can prepare documented information on both sides of the issue. Just prior to the debate, toss a coin to see which side each student will debate. This can eliminate the emotional involvement sometimes common in real health issues.

Because of time limitations and need for class participation, the following debate patterns seem to work well.

Pattern A	Time
Affirmative no. 1	3 minutes
Negative no. 1	3 minutes
Affirmative no. 1 rebuttal	2 minutes
Negative no. 2 rebuttal	2 minutes
Affirmative no. 1 summary	2 minutes
Negative no. 2 summary	2 minutes

Pattern B	Time
Affirmative no. 1	5 minutes
Negative no. 1	5 minutes
Affirmative no. 2 rebuttal and summary	2 minutes
Negative no. 2 rebuttal and summary	2 minutes

The teacher's role in this activity is to guide the debaters during their preparation and to ensure that accurate information is presented and quality resources used. The teacher introduces the lesson by explaining the rules for the debate and telling the class they will be held responsible for the key points of both sides of the issue. Once the debate has been completed, the class participates by asking questions of the debaters and continuing the discussion. Classmates can also determine which team won the debate and take a vote on the issue. Because of the large amount of detailed information covered in a very short period of time, a very careful summary and discussion of the key points on both sides of the issue are in order.

BUZZ GROUPS

In this very useful strategy the class is divided into small discussion groups. The groups should be small enough to facilitate discussion and large enough that in the course of the lesson all groups have time to report their findings to the rest of the class. In a class of twenty-five members three to four groups usually work best.

A successful buzz group activity depends upon the following important factors: careful choice of topics, careful planning by the teacher, and precise directions to the participants. In most classes, buzz groups work best

Fig. 14–1. A class divided into typical buzz groups. (Photo by L. K. Olsen.)

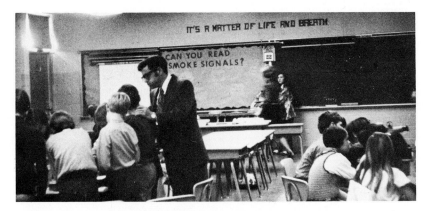

when the discussion topics involve human relations and problem solving. The technique also works well for planning sessions, for value activities, and for analysis of dramatization.

The teacher needs to plan for special seating arrangements, for proper movement of students, and for configuration of each buzz group. Discussion leaders and recorders must be appointed. Preliminary preparation such as handouts and assignments are often needed. The inexperienced teacher may be in for a difficult time if the directions for the activity are not well conceived or explained carefully. Since the groups will be working on their own, they need to understand clearly what each group is to do, how they will do it, what is expected of them, what the time limitations are, and what will happen once they complete their group assignment.

An important consideration is to have all groups report their findings before the end of the lesson. Knowing that responses will be used or compared with the efforts of others usually provides the motivation necessary for adequate performance. Careful consideration must be given to how the groups will report their findings. As in most lessons, the final teacher-guided discussion and summary are a major part of the learning process. The teacher must decide whether each group should simply read its report, write the report on the board, compare responses, discuss each point given by each group, or discuss the results after all groups have reported.

BRAINSTORMING

This technique has been adapted from industrial and governmental think tank approaches to solving problems. The rules for this lively and enjoyable activity are simple. In this teacher- or student-guided discussion, students are asked to come up with solutions to any health-related problem. The discussion leader records *all* answers and suggestion on the board, reminding the students that there are no wrong answers. Any idea or scheme is acceptable, no matter how farfetched. The answers should be given as rapidly as the recorder can write them down.

Once all the potential ideas or plans seem to have been offered, a discussion occurs in which each offering is accepted or rejected. Follow-up activities include reaching a consensus plan of action, taking a class vote or an opinion poll, or some other type of value activity. Brainstorming can be effectively pursued in small buzz groups where students might be less reluctant to express their wildest ideas.

ROLE PLAYING

Role playing is an enthusiasm-generating activity that may be the most effective way of exploring real-life human relations problems. The best topics for role playing seem to deal with such human relations problems as asking for something from mom or dad, receiving or giving criticism, accepting or rejecting help, starting a conversation with someone you have never met before, solving parent-child situations, and the like.

Suggestions for leading a role-playing strategy include the following:

1. Choose a topic that deals with mental health and everyday human relations problems.
2. Set the scene for both the role players and class.
3. Inform the class what to look for during the role play and mention

the key questions that will be asked after the activity has been completed.

4. Make a careful choice of role players. Normally it is best to use volunteers or individuals whom the teacher knows enjoy being in front of an audience or in drama activities. Teachers are often surprised to find that some rather quiet students seem to shed their inhibitions in a role-playing scene. The key is to protect those who might not benefit from the experience.

5. A role play is spontaneous, is without a script, and, once the scene is set, is completely up to the players. In this relaxed, humorous atmosphere teachers should expect most anything to happen.

6. Teachers need to be alert for when to end the drama, when to have another group perform, and when to reset the scene. Normally the psychodramas last less than five minutes.

Once the drama has been completed, students usually wish to discuss the more emotional aspects of the scene. For example: If someone said that to you, what would you do? What should she have done? and the like. The teacher should use this opportunity to promote discussion about the communication problems brought up in the drama. Once this has been accomplished, it is then appropriate to move on to the key questions and major objectives of the lesson. Role plays often serve as springboards for a number of student-suggested problems that can be investigated in future lessons.

PLAYS AND PUPPET SHOWS

These dramas serve the same purpose as role plays. However, instead of players "winging it" through a scene, the actors read from a carefully prepared script. Again, the topics of mental health and human relations work well in dramatizations.

A drama or play has the advantage of careful dialogue and structure. The teacher can plan key discussion questions and lesson objectives more easily than in a role play. Although several published dramas are available, many students have the interest and ability to author their own scenarios complete with script, costumes, staging, and moral overtones.

The teacher's role in the drama lesson is to inform the audience what is expected of them during the play, to lead the discussion after the play, and to carefully plan a lesson summary and follow-up activity.

ORAL QUIZZES

With a few simple modifications, this traditional classroom activity can become an interesting teaching strategy. Among the modifications is avoiding the pattern of having students recite carefully memorized facts or statements. Students should be asked to express opinions or give argumentative statements in which they defend their stand on a controversial issue. Oral quizzes can be used as lesson summaries, as games, as motivational devices, and as relaxed or high-pressure evaluation devices.

Suggestions for leading an oral quiz include the following:

1. Use questions that involve opinions and defense of a position.
2. Give questions either well in advance or at the time of the quiz.
3. Establish criteria for effective answers such as replying with clarity,

stating both sides of the issue, defending personal decisions or
stands, and answering in depth and with accuracy.
4. Give examples of a typical question and of a model response.
5. Determine whether the answers will be graded or ungraded.
6. Provide a summary of the key points and correct erroneous information.

CLASS SURVEYS

A survey can serve as a useful tool for promoting decision making and providing a solid basis for class discussion. Student-developed questionnaires
and opinionnaires offer the opportunity to seek information from parents,
teachers, and other students on a variety of interesting topics. In the process,
having to ask the right questions in the right manner is an efficient tool for
developing communication skills. Seeking adult opinions on such issues as
Why would a person smoke? can provide baseline data for student decision
making, inform members of the community about health problems, and
bring pressure on adults to help solve health problems.

A survey can be as simple as a show of hands concerning an issue or
as complex as a study using several questions and demographic variables,
comparing groups, defining trends, and the like. The key to discussing the
results of a survey is to present the results in an easily grasped, graphic
manner. The graphic presentation of the data should include the following
information: totals, trends, rank, and comparison of groups. As the questions for the questionnaire are being developed, careful consideration should
be given to how the results can be tabulated and presented to students.

GUEST SPEAKERS

Being a guest speaker before a group of elementary students can be a nerve-
shattering experience for many adults. A capable guest speaker may be able
to mesmerize a group of three hundred adults with a provocative or clever
talk, but may not be effective in the classroom. It is the teacher's responsibility to invite those speakers best suited for the elementary level. Several
community agencies have professionals who have presentations designed
for this age group. Invariably the presentations of these guest speakers include clever visual aids, demonstrations, stories, and skills that capture the
attention of students. The fire chief who brings along a special training film
or demonstrates life-saving equipment or a police officer with a trained dog
demonstrating safety with animals are the types of guest speakers who will
be the most effective.

Teachers should avoid using a guest speaker as a Friday afternoon fill-in.
The topic presented by the guest speaker should carefully fit in with the
objectives and structure of the health topic currently under investigation. In
addition, the students should be held responsible for the information
presented.

The teacher's role in this strategy is as follows:

1. To contact the guest speaker well in advance and carefully discuss
what will be covered during his visit.
2. To contact the speaker again as a reminder a few days before his
scheduled appearance and finalize details.
3. To inform the class a few days in advance what topic the speaker will

be discussing with them and to give assignments that will help them understand the information and ask appropriate questions.

4. To give the students a series of key questions and key points to look for in their guest's presentation and to also discuss their role during the presentation.
5. To introduce the speaker carefully.
6. To encourage the class to write thank you notes, a well-received courtesy.

Following the visit the teacher should review the key points of the guest speaker's presentation, summarize the presentation, and follow through with appropriate related activities.

LECTURES

The term *lecture* conjures up visions of sermons, college professors, political speeches, and reprimands for misdeeds. A straightforward lecture may be the most common and most ineffective teaching strategy. Verbalization without benefit of any visual aid or related illustration is very difficult for most people to comprehend.

The lecture method, however, is a tool that all teachers use and find effective when topics are complex, time is a factor, and efficiency is called for. Since verbalization is difficult for most students to comprehend, special effort must be made to enhance or embellish the key points of the lecture. A successful lecture involves these factors: (1) an introduction so that students can anticipate the direction of the verbalization, (2) the use of visual aids to slow the pace and elaborate on the key points, (3) the observance of appropriate stops and review, (4) the provision for periodic discussions and question-answer periods for clarification of key points, and (5) the presentation of a careful summary and review of the lecture objectives and goals.

The introduction, as in any strategy, serves the purpose of warning the students what to look for, what key questions will be answered, and what is to be the role of the students during the presentation. The audiovisual aids are the major parts of a successful lecture. Chalkboard, feltboards, charts, diagrams, transparencies, handouts, tapes, and illustrative anecdotes provide the structure of this strategy. These visual aids give a visual or mental picture of the key concepts and points of the lesson. In addition these aids slow the pace of the lecture, provide for questions, provide concrete points of reference, and allow for digressions that elaborate on the main points of the lecture.

Each lecture, whether it is a two-minute or an hour presentation, should allow for students to interject questions. In effect, most lectures might better be classified as lecture-discussions. Student involvement aids in clarifying and reinforcing the important points of the lesson. Other aspects of a meaningful lecture technique include showmanship, humor, and use of personal examples that relate to the students.

STUDENT REPORTS

Student reports, guest speakers, and lectures fall into the category of strategies in which the audience plays a passive role. The student report has an advantage in that the teacher can be reasonably certain that the student giving the report has learned something. This activity can act as a motivating device and also provide a valuable communication experience.

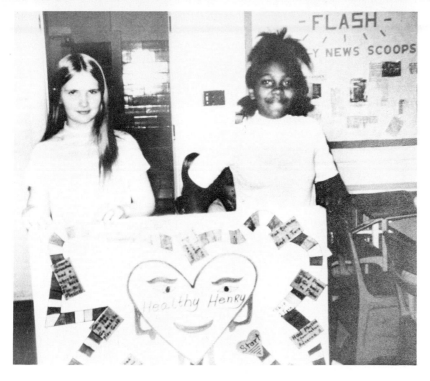

Fig. 14–2. Student reports.
(Photo by L. K. Olsen.)

The following suggestions have proved useful in utilizing student reports as a teaching strategy:

1. Have the report deal with a specific part of a unit or lesson.
2. Assign the report well in advance, preview the report, and tell the members of the class what to look for.
3. Hold the class responsible for the information presented in the report.
4. Encourage students to develop audiovisual aids for their reports.
5. Avoid having a series of student reports back to back.
6. Allow time for class discussion and to review the key points of each report.
7. Gear the reports to small topics or segments of topic areas so that students can explore a topic in depth rather than generalize.
8. Insist that quality sources be used in the development of each report.

In general, students enjoy this type of activity, particularly when reports are voluntary and the students are sure they are making a contribution. Rather than grade oral reports, try grading the written reports if you have to grade at all. Teachers must plan to give considerable assistance and individual attention in helping students select topics, gather resources, form outlines, and present their findings.

PROBLEM SOLVING

Problem solving is one of the basic tools in health education. Problem solving can involve developing a year's activities around a complex problem such as ecology and health or can simply be the strategy for a single lesson.

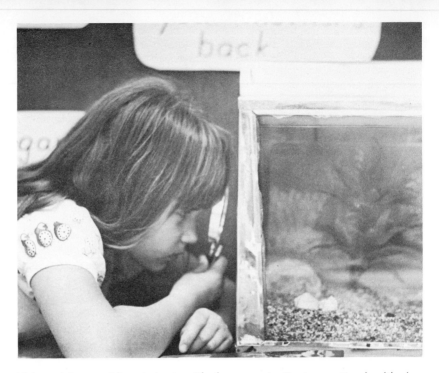

Fig. 14–3. Illustrated is a typical problem-solving activity. (Photo by L. K. Olsen.)

This activity provides students with the opportunity to practice health decision making. Problem solving works well as an individual, a class, or a small-group activity.

The purpose of problem solving in the health classroom is to give students the chance to plan, interpret, and utilize the information at their disposal for making rational health decisions. Also involved should be development of arguments for all sides of issues and development of alternative solutions. In all cases the students should be expected to defend their decisions.

The teacher's role in this activity includes developing resources, guiding the students in defining the problem, and aiding them in the development of criteria and plans for solving the problem. The teacher should remain unbiased, but insist that all sides of all issues be explored carefully. The teacher's role is as motivator and facilitator. The teacher does not dictate the solutions to be reached.

Health topics suitable for problem solving range from complex multidiscipline problems to everyday human relations problems. Problem solving is particularly effective in developing skills for handling the emotional-social problems all students have to some degree.

EXPERIMENTS

Experiments in health education can be undertaken in many topics including ecology, nutrition, human growth, personal health, and human relations. These activities provide excellent illustrations of key health concepts and some exciting avenues into scientific inquiry. Students are given the opportunity to define problems, set up an experimental situation, possibly form hypotheses, control variables, and test and record their findings.

Teachers have had success with experiments in the social science fields. For example: Students could try smiling at and striking-up a conversation with someone they do not know, stopping and assisting someone, or making a list of things they feel least capable of doing socially. They could try role playing a grouch, a genius, a teacher, and the like, for a part of one day and record and analyze what took place during and after the experiment. These experiments can provide an excellent basis for discussions concerning some everyday self-image and human relations problems.

DEMONSTRATIONS

A demonstration might best be described as a lecture with a clever visual aid. Unlike an experiment, students usually know what the outcome of a demonstration will be. Students are given the opportunity to view a process rather than to visualize something from verbalization.

The teacher has the option of having the demonstration performed by (1) a guest speaker, (2) a student expert, (3) a student beginner, or (4) the teacher. Each has certain advantages and some disadvantages as well. An outside guest expert offers the advantage of being specially prepared and thereby becoming a motivating factor. Disadvantages include the problems in scheduling, commitment time, equipment needed, and special preparation of the students. Using a student expert probably offers the most advantages. The teacher can control the subject matter, equipment, and time factors, and the demonstration can be easily scheduled into the sequence of a planned instructional unit. In addition, the positive recognition received by the demonstrator is a distinct advantage. Using a student beginner offers the opportunity for the class to observe a typical step-by-step learning process and the typical mistakes made in learning a new skill. If the beginner can achieve a new skill that all members of the class are expected to accomplish, the members of the class will progress very rapidly when it is their turn to participate. Care should be taken not to embarrass the pupil beginner. When the teacher gives the demonstration, pace, continuity, and key points are usually under control. The disadvantages of having the teacher demonstrate are that the teacher may be unskilled or unable to describe what is going on while performing the demonstration.

Care should be taken to inform the students what to look for during the demonstration. If a series of rules or procedures are needed, they should be written on the board or provided in handouts rather than verbalized. As in a lecture, allow for appropriate stops, student questions, clarifications, and class discussion. Demonstrations provide visual experiences that aid in the learning process; however, in most demonstrations the students are in a passive learning role. This passive role can be overcome by planning to have students perform the activity that has been demonstrated. In fact, teachers should normally give students the opportunity to perform the demonstrated activity or skill.

FIELD TRIPS

Field trips are looked forward to by students and are often remembered for a very long time. Unfortunately, unless they are carefully planned and supervised, teachers may think of field trips only as nerve-shattering experiences. In addition to the problems of scheduling, transportation, supervision, and meal arrangements, teachers have the problem of convincing students that a field trip is a learning experience rather than an amusement excursion. Ideally, the students should be able both to have fun and to learn.

A major concern on a field trip is the safety of the students. Particular care must be given to safe transportation and to proper supervision. Travel should be in school buses, never in private cars. Teacher aids, room mothers, or additional school personnel should be used to aid in the supervision of students. Correspond carefully with the hosts so that they understand the time of your arrival, the number of people involved, the length of your visit, and the age of your students. In most cases, facilities that do encourage visits from school children are well aware of and provide for the safety factors involved.

Field trips are effective learning experiences when they fit carefully into a unit plan or series of sequential lessons. As in a classroom experience, students should be given information concerning their role during the excursion and what will be expected of them, what things to look for on the trip, and what follow-up assignments to expect. As in all lessons, a summary should be done in which the key questions and key points of the learning experience are carefully reviewed.

GAMES

Games represent a favorite classroom learning experience at any level. Games that have been successfully used range from playing hangman to complex games that involve extensive rules and strategies. They are a welcome break from classroom routine and a useful technique for reviewing key points of information. The keys to successful classroom gamesmanship are clear-cut rules and maximum participation.

The following suggestions have proved helpful in the organization of classroom games:

1. Avoid spelldown types of games. Strive for maximum participation in which no individual or team can be eliminated from the contest.
2. Clearly state the rules and scoring. Have a short practice run to assure that the rules and scoring are understood.
3. Use questions that call for straightforward objective answers rather than for difficult-to-judge subjective statements.
4. Strive for evenly balanced teams.
5. Avoid games or rules in which decisions need to be reached to determine which side raised their hand or yelled first, and the like.
6. Feel free to try games that require strategy and teamwork.
7. Be fair, consistent, and unbiased. Students become very upset when rules are not followed or when someone gets more or less than he deserved.
8. Have a review system for missed questions.

AUDIOVISUAL AIDS

Films, filmstrips, tapes, television, and videotapes are available to most elementary schools. These aids when well produced offer information, perceptions, and demonstrations that are not accessible to classroom teachers. For example, visual aids can reproduce unique auditory stimuli and provide color

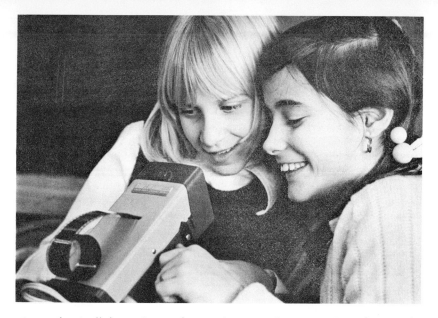

views of unicellular action under an electron microscope. In order to gain the most from audiovisual aids, the teacher should keep in mind a few simple factors:

1. Select aids suited to the age group in terms of complexity, accuracy, and taste.
2. Preview all audiovisual aids before using them in the classroom.
3. Be sure that the aids fit carefully into the lesson or unit under investigation.
4. Before presenting the aid, give the students key questions and key points to look for during the presentation and explain what will be expected of them following the presentation.
5. Stop the presentation when appropriate to discuss key points.
6. Following the presentation, carefully review and discuss the key points developed in the audiovisual aid.
7. If appropriate, present the audiovisual aid again.
8. Remember that audiovisual aids have been developed to help teachers, not to replace them.
9. Remember that in many cases learning takes place during the teacher-led activity following the presentation of an audiovisual aid.

Teachers need to become experts in the use of audiovisual equipment. This expertise should include being able to make simple repairs such as changing bulbs and splicing films. Faulty equipment or improperly set-up equipment can be a very frustrating experience for everyone. Most upper level elementary school students can learn to operate the equipment. Having student operators not only provides high-status tasks for students, but also frees teachers to perform other classroom duties.

The selection and ordering of films can be a perplexing task. Fortunately, most audiovisual aid retail and rental companies include descriptions of content and grade level recommendations. However, a more reliable source may be one's grade level teaching colleagues. Teachers should keep a log of the source, content, and value of each audiovisual aid. Each school or school district usually has established procedures for purchasing and renting teaching aids. It is the responsibility of new teachers to find out what the procedures for ordering are. Most procedures include requirements for ordering aids well in advance and for coordinating them for use in several classrooms.

Filmstrips and tape recordings have advantages over other audiovisual aids. They are less expensive and are easily stored, and the equipment is easier to operate. In addition the teacher can skip parts that are not relevant and can very easily stop the presentation to reinforce key points. Tape recorders and filmstrip projectors can be easily operated by students and can be used in teaching-learning stations, special interest projects, and individualized investigation.

STRATEGIES IN CLASSROOM ORGANIZATION

Most of the strategies discussed have been teacher-oriented group activities in which all class members participate at the same time. Health education has been classified as a self-discovery process in which the student is asked to utilize information for making personal health judgments and decisions. With emphasis on decision making, it follows that careful attention should be given to organizing the classroom to facilitate individual activities. Strategies in classroom organization include use of the following: (1) special interest activities, (2) health science fairs, (3) learning stations, (4) materials centers, (5) student contracts, (6) language arts activities, (7) programmed learning, and (8) displays and realia.

SPECIAL INTEREST ACTIVITIES

Health education represents such a widely based science that a large number of interesting topics must be left out of any lesson or unit because of time limitations. These topics are well suited to student special interest projects.

Fig. 14–5. Illustrated are students engaged in special interest activities. (Photo by L. K. Olsen.)

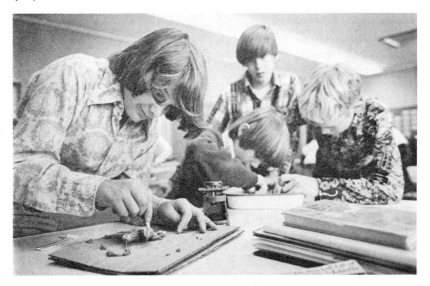

The teacher's role in this activity is to guide students through the process of defining and limiting the scope of the problem, developing outlines, gathering resources, and preparing their final reports.

When selecting a special interest topic, students tend to choose areas that are very broad in scope. It is important that they focus on a topic small enough to be dealt with in depth. Being an expert on a small topic is more rewarding than gaining a casual knowledge of several topics within a broad area of study. By urging students to focus on a specific topic area teachers can prevent the common student experience of turning an interesting activity into a laborious, frustrating experience that involves hours of copying down page after page of general information.

By narrowing the scope of a topic students can devote more time and energy to the development of useful writing skills. Since a focused topic does not require the hours needed to complete a several page report, students can be held responsible for the manner in which their report is constructed. For example, they can be asked to turn in outlines, keep a file of note cards, and even include a footnote system and bibliography in their final paper. Other means of reporting progress in a special interest topic should be encouraged. In lieu of or in addition to a written report, students can develop oral reports, psychodramas, skits, tape recordings, models, mobiles, posters, or other kinds of exhibits.

HEALTH SCIENCE FAIRS

A health science fair is a natural follow-up for special interest activities. The class can set aside a block of time and invite other classes and parents to take part in the fair. The fair would consist of booths and displays of the special interest projects. While the experience of getting up in front of a group to give a report can be good for the presenter, having to sit through consecutive reports by twenty to thirty classmates can be a disaster. The science fair allows students to get the satisfaction of showing their work to classmates and visitors, allows for a wider range of topics to be presented, and provides a unique break from the everyday routine.

MATERIALS CENTERS

Materials centers can be placed in individual classrooms or be designated areas in the school library. These centers are composed of library materials, displays, audiovisual aids, and audiovisual equipment. For example, a center can contain tape recorders, projectors, television receivers, slides, transparencies, books, pamphlets, and magazines.

The development of materials centers requires considerable effort on the part of the teacher. Collecting materials, record keeping, displaying items, and coordinating materials with the school library are time-consuming tasks. This type of activity can be facilitated with the assistance of teacher aids and the preparation time made available in a team-teaching situation. A well-equipped and carefully managed materials center can be the cornerstone of a successful health education program.

LEARNING STATIONS

Students of any grade level have a wide range of health skills, of knowledge and attitudes, of reading skills, and of learning abilities. Learning stations seem to be able to provide for these student differences.

In a learning station approach students move from station to station in groups or at their own pace. For a topic on nutrition, for example, the following stations can be set up: (1) nutrition and growth, (2) food selection, (3) obesity and health, (4) dietary essentials, (5) diagram of the digestive system, and (6) food fads and fallacies. At each station are the necessary books, pamphlets, and other materials. Students are taught to operate the overhead projectors, slide projectors, tape recorders, and other needed audiovisual equipment. For each station, students are given a series of study guide questions, programmed learning checklists, and other appropriate written and oral assignments.

This strategy does require extra preparation initially. The teacher has the organizational problems of collecting the necessary materials and equipment and developing the learning activities for each station. This self-paced activity combines individual attention from the teacher and the joy of pushing the buttons on the various pieces of audiovisual equipment. Students are given something to do with their hands, a chance to move around their room and to work with a group at their own pace. Depending upon the imagination of the teacher in terms of the types of activities at each station, health may well become the students' favorite subject.

STUDENT CONTRACTS

Contracts involve a cooperative effort between student and teacher in developing the student's goals. The teacher can determine the guidelines for the number, type, and quality of activities or have students determine their own pace, goals, assignments, and deadlines. The contract method fits easily into the pattern of classroom organization that includes materials centers, special interest activities, and learning stations.

Advantages The contract method can be said to possess the following advantages:

1. Students receive individual attention.
2. Students know where they stand in terms of grade and work to be completed.
3. Students gain experience in the acceptance and utilization of their limitations and strengths.
4. The program is noncompetitive.
5. Opportunity is available for the practice of self-direction and self-planning.

Disadvantages Disadvantages of the contract strategy include the following:

1. The work load of teachers increases in terms of counseling, grading papers, and planning.
2. Students tend to underestimate or overestimate their abilities and the time needed to complete a contract.
3. Many students will consistently work below their levels of ability.
4. Unless planned for, the students have a limited range of group interaction activities.
5. Paradise has been achieved for unmotivated students!

LANGUAGE ARTS

Many stories, plays, poems, and show-and-tell activities are pointed at health and safety topics. For example, a student showing and telling about a new cub scout knife, fishing pole, and the like, can provide a teachable moment concerning the safe use of such treasures. In addition, most of the stories read to students involve some human relations concepts and situation ethics that can be integrated into the areas of social and mental health.

The major advantage of having the regular classroom teacher guide students through health education is that an opportunity exists to integrate health topics into other subject areas. If school districts hire health experts who travel from school to school or from room to room, the opportunity to integrate and live health and safety is severely limited.

PROGRAMMED LEARNING

More and more schools are being equipped with computer terminals and with the now common programmed learning textbooks. The approach in either system is for the student to be exposed to some type of written statement and then be expected to answer questions about this statement. The text or computer informs the student if he is right or wrong, asks him to redo incorrect work, and offers more advanced activities if he is correct.

Programmed learning offers the advantages of student-paced learning and the chance to use a fascinating tool. The disadvantages are the cost and the yet unanswered questions concerning the total effectiveness of this approach. Programmed learning is designed to supplement the classroom teacher, not to serve as a replacement. Computer-based teaching in the cognitive domain will be expanded at a rapid rate in the near future. For example, computer programs are now available that pretest students, feed the results to the computer, and provide a readout offering unit objectives, teaching strategies, and resources for the topic to be taught.

DISPLAYS AND REALIA

National organizations such as the American Dental Association and the American Cancer Society have long been dedicated to a multimedia ap-

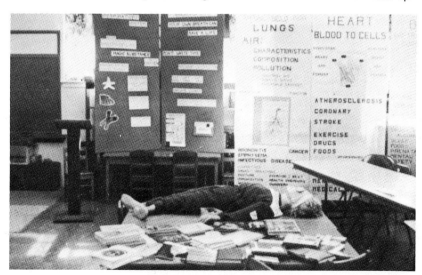

Fig. 14–6. Use of special displays and realia in the teaching of health education. (Photo by L. K. Olsen.)

proach in disseminating health information. The incredible number of posters, pamphlets, and realia these organizations have produced serve as a ready-made source of materials for bulletin boards and displays.

Bulletin board themes and displays are useful tools in a modern classroom. The key concepts presented offer a constant, colorful reinforcement for the objectives of the lessons being presented. In addition they serve as motivational devices, add color to a room, and provide an opportunity for student input. Students enjoy making these displays and gain insight into the subject matter presented. Students are often the best source for realia. Realia refers to actual pieces of equipment or material that are part of a health topic. For example, realia can be a stethoscope, a decayed or filled tooth, a petri dish, and the like. In general, a display should center around a single idea, be appealing, be easily read, be colorful, and be of good design.

VALUING STRATEGIES IN HEALTH EDUCATION

A value approach to teaching controversial issues is not new to health educators. Valuing and decision making have long been integral parts of "functional health teaching."[2] As indicated in chapter 12 functional health involves the development of health programs based on student needs, interests, and teacher-student planning, with emphasis on personalized student-centered activities.

Positive change in health attitudes is a major consideration within value activities. As suggested by Hochbaum and Rosenstock, a health decision or value judgment may involve the following factors:[3]

1. Students must perceive the issue as important.
2. Students must believe themselves susceptible to the problem.
3. Students must believe the problem is a serious one.
4. The intensity of the threat and resultant anxiety must not be so great as to paralyze one's ability to act.
5. There must be an action to take that the individual believes effective.

A value may be reconsidered when actions yield negative results and when the value is inconsistent with the values of society or respected associates. A value is reinforced when positive outcomes occur and when the value is found to be consistent with those of society and respected associates.[4] Horn and Waingrow suggest a valuing and decision-making model that requires motivation for change, perception of the threat, development and use of alternative psychological mechanisms, and factors facilitating or inhibiting continuing reinforcement.[5] In the attitude and value change models it is implied that the teacher may need to take an active role in convincing the students that a threat exists.

2. Howard S. Hoyman, *Functional Health Teaching* (Goshen, Ind.: McConnell School Map Co., 1949), 33–44.
3. G. M. Hochbaum, I. M. Rosenstock, and S. S. Kegeles, *Determinants of Health Behavior* (Washington, D.C.: White House Conference on Children and Youth, 1960).
4. Gus T. Dalis, and Ben B. Strasser, "The Starting Point in Values Education," *School Health Review* 5 (1974): 2–5.
5. D. Horn, and S. Waingrow, "Some Dimensions of a Model for Smoking Behavior Change." Paper presented at Forty-Third Annual Meeting of American Public Health Association, 20 October 1965, Chicago, Ill.

The strategies for value activities can be developed in two parts: (1) activities that are useful for generating value judgments and (2) various activities organized in a logical process for decision making. The following strategies or methods may be useful in formulating value judgments: rank order, voting, values continuum, and values whip activities; interviews; open-ended statements; devil's advocate role playing;[6, 7] Likert scale surveys;[8] role playing,[9] autobiography appreciation, and communication activities.[10, 11]

RANK ORDER
Students practice choosing among alternatives.

Example: Which of the following events do you feel would contribute most to mental health problems? Rank your choices.

Behind in school work	No friends
Mom and Dad fighting	Too much school work
Poor grades	Do not get along with brothers or sisters

VOTING
Depending upon the topic, students are asked to vote by a show of hands or secret ballot.

Example: Should anyone smoke?
Example: Should young people have to work for an allowance?
Example: Should good friends tell you when you are wrong?

VALUES CONTINUUM
This activity opens up a range of alternatives that surround a given issue.

Example: Is the role of the modern woman really changing?
Example: Can world famine be avoided?

VALUES WHIP
Individuals make a value judgment, but must also express how they arrived at their decision.

Example: What constitutes an other-person centered relationship?
Example: What is your strongest characteristic?
Example: What are the characteristics of a good friend?

INTERVIEWS
In this activity students actively seek the opinions of persons outside the classroom.

6. Sidney B. Simon, Leland Howe, and Howard Kirschenbaum, *Values-Clarification: A Handbook of Practical Strategies for Teachers and Students* (New York: Hart Publishing Co., 1972).
7. Louis E. Raths, Merrill Harmin, and Sidney B. Simon, *Values and Teaching* (Columbus, Ohio: Charles E. Merrill Publishing Co., 1966).
8. Renis Likert, "A Technique for Measuring Attitudes," *Archives of Psychology*, no. 140, 1932.
9. F. Shaftel, and G. Shaftel, *Role Playing for Social Values: Decision Making in Social Studies* (Englewood Cliffs, N.J.: Prentice-Hall, 1967).
10. Schmuck and Schmuck, *Group Process*, pp. 84–102.
11. Peter D. Cimini, "Humanizing as a Teaching Strategy," *School Health Review* 5 (1974): 15–21.

Example: What is your opinion about women's rights?
Example: What is wrong with today's children?
Example: Is there a real energy crisis?

OPEN-ENDED STATEMENTS

Students are to complete statements in this activity.

Example: The ideal sister or brother would . . .
Example: If my son or daughter took drugs . . .
Example: Friends are . . .

DEVIL'S ADVOCATE ROLE PLAY

A teacher or student role plays, taking a view in opposition to that of the class and argues with the class.

Example: The government should decide who is suitable to bear children.
Example: Disease can be eliminated.
Example: Our drug laws should be liberalized.

LIKERT SCALES

Students are forced to give an opinion in this type of survey. By weighting the choices 1, 2, 3, or 4 or vice versa, it is possible to generate a score which can be used in measures of central tendency. Therefore the scales can be used to measure attitudes and attitude changes between and among groups.

Example: Eight-to-twelve-year-old children are too immature to make "big decisions."
Strongly agree _____   Agree _____
Disagree _____   Strongly disagree _____

ROLE PLAYING

The teacher or class sets the scene, and selected students present the dramatization extemporaneously.

Example: You have borrowed a friend's bike and broken it.
Example: You are asking for a part-time job (the wrong way).
Example: You are arguing with your mother about cleaning your room.

AUTOBIOGRAPHY ACTIVITIES

Students are asked to write essays about themselves.

Example: Who am I and where am I going?
Example: My strengths are? My weaknesses are?
Example: These are my goals for today; for this week; for this term . . .

APPRECIATION ACTIVITIES

Emphasis is placed on students developing positive views of themselves and their surroundings. Students of this age have an intense interest in the human body. A number of appreciation activities can be utilized.

Example: Develop a Believe it or Not Book or Book of Records by listing some of the incredible details about the various systems of the body.

Example: Use classroom games and physical skills that involve short-term memory games, tongue twisters, balance, hand-eye coordination, and other body senses.

Example: Generate appreciation activities with discussions or position papers on such topics as: What good things happened today? How will I celebrate? Life's greatest pleasures are . . .

COMMUNICATION ACTIVITIES

Being able to give and receive information requires skill. Fortunately, students can be given the opportunity to practice communication skills.

Example: Role play and discuss nonverbal communication to suggest disgust, anger, hate, pleasure, and depression.

Example: Role play and discuss verbal communication for asking for something, making an apology, expressing anger, or expressing sympathy.

Example: Have two students come forward and stand with their backs toward one another. Hand one student a jacket and ask the other student to give explicit directions for putting the jacket on. The student putting the jacket on must follow the directions to the letter. Follow with a discussion on one-way versus two-way communication.

In addition to the nine activities described, the more traditional classroom activities are also effective. Activities such as student reports, special interest groups, demonstrations, guest speakers, panel discussions, discussions, debates, and buzz groups serve as useful tools for developing value judgments.

STRUCTURING VALUE ACTIVITIES

Most of the value activities involve discussion techniques. Since students have a difficult time trying to follow verbalizations, it is unreasonable to expect students to reach rational decisions from poorly comprehended information. Some system of structuring value judgments is needed. Simon, et. al. for example, suggest a values grid approach in which a student checks: (1) whether he has chosen his position freely without being forced; (2) whether he has made the choice from among alternatives; (3) whether he has made the choice after thoughtful consideration of the consequences of each alternative; (4) whether his choice was prized or cherished; (5) whether his choice was publicly affirmed; (6) whether his choice was acted on, and (7) whether his choice was repeated and became a pattern in life.[12]

As a follow-up to within-class value activities, it is useful to have students develop folders or notebooks that include the pros-and-cons of decisions they have reached and their final decision concerning each value judgment. Evidence or fact assembly sheets can be developed by the teacher as handouts for each student.[13] The handouts simply represent a form in which

12. Simon et al., *Values-Clarification*.
13. Lawrence Metcalf, ed., *Values Education*, Forty-First Yearbook (Washington, D.C.: National Council for the Social Studies, 1971), pp. 29–119.

the students indicate an area of concern, list the pros-and-cons for both sides of an issue in a factual manner, and indicate their final judgment. This type of checkoff form will greatly aid students with poor communication skills.

SUMMARY Teaching strategies in health education are similar to those utilized in other subject matter areas. A health lesson has the following requirements: (1) carefully planned introduction, (2) motivational devices, (3) student involvement, (4) lesson summation, and (5) careful choice of teaching strategy. One major difference between health lessons and lessons in other curricular areas lies in the relevance of most health topics for meeting the immediate needs of students. This relevance requires health teachers to emphasize student involvement and decision making in the learning process. Through the use of such strategies as role plays, discussions, experiments, problem solving, and student projects students can apply accurate health information to meet their own needs and problems.

Discussion Questions

1. Define the term *teaching strategy*.
2. Describe the commonalities of a good lesson.
3. What are some practical suggestions for improving classroom motivation in health education?
4. What is the role of student involvement in health education?
5. Why should one summarize a lesson?
6. Why should one teach a few things well?
7. Develop criteria for choosing a health education strategy.
8. List your strengths and weaknesses as a discussion leader. What are the characteristics of a good discussion leader?
9. Why are discussions emphasized in health education?
10. Rank the top ten strategies most suitable for decision making. Defend your ranking.
11. What is your favorite classroom strategy? Discuss why it is your favorite.
12. What have your experiences been with each of the strategies described in this chapter?
13. Do lectures have to be dull? Defend your response.
14. How can you incorporate student reports into your lessons without boring or confusing the rest of the class?
15. Why is problem solving an important strategy in health education?
16. Who is the most effective individual to demonstrate in the classroom?
17. Describe all the details needed to ensure a safe and useful field trip.
18. Why should special care be taken in organizing a health classroom?
19. What are the pros-and-cons of individual instruction, programmed learning, student contracts, and health science fairs?
20. Why should there be value activities in health education?
21. Develop a handout for students structuring a value-decision activity.

References

Cimini, Peter D. "Humanizing as a Teaching Strategy." *School Health Review* 5 (1974): 15–21.

Dalis, Gus T., and Strasser, Ben B. "The Starting Point in Values Education." *School Health Review* 5 (1974): 2–5.

Hochbaum, G. M., Rosenstock, I. M., and Kegeles, S. S. *Determinants of Health Behavior*. Washington, D.C.: White House Conference on Children and Youth, 1960.

Horn, D., and Waingrow, S. "Some Dimensions of a Model for Smoking Behavior Change." Paper presented at Forty-Third Annual Meeting of American Public Health Association, 20 October 1965, Chicago, Ill.

Hoyman, Howard S. *Functional Health Teaching*. Goshen, Ind.: McConnell School Map Co., 1949.

Likert, Renis. "A Technique for Measuring Attitudes." *Archives* of Psychology, no. 140, 1932.

Metcalf, Lawrence E., ed. *Values Education*. Forty-First Yearbook. Washington, D.C.: National Council for Social Studies, 1971.

Raths, Louis E., Harmin, Merrill, and Simon, Sidney B. *Values and Teaching*. Columbus, Ohio: Charles E. Merrill Publishing Co., 1966.

Schmuck, Richard A., and Schmuck, Patricia A. *Group Process in the Classroom*. Dubuque, Iowa: Wm. C. Brown Co. Publishers, 1973.

Shaftel, F., and Shaftel, G. *Role Playing for Social Values: Decision Making in Social Studies*. Englewood Cliffs, N.J.: Prentice-Hall, 1967.

Simon, Sidney, B., Howe, Leland, and Kirschenbaum, Howard. *Values-Clarification: A Handbook of Practical Strategies for Teachers and Students*. New York: Hart Publishing Co., 1972.

Chapter 15
STRATEGIES IN TEACHING MENTAL HEALTH, DRUG EDUCATION, AND FAMILY LIVING

Why are mental health, drug education, and family living considered controversial health education areas?

What are the most important topics in mental health, drug education, and family living?

Why should there be an emphasis on student decision making and valuing rather than on teacher opinion giving in these areas?

What philosophical issues are inherent in these areas of instruction?

How should students, parents and community members be involved in planning for instruction in these areas?

The discussions of mental health, drug education, and family living strategies are placed in a separate chapter because collectively they present similar problems in curriculum planning and philosophy. In addition, students, parents, and community members have an unusual interest in how these areas are taught. With the exception of mental health, which provides a basis for dealing with all health problems, these areas should *not* be considered more important than other major health education areas. Curriculum development committees should not dwell on these areas at the expense of other important health topics such as disease, safety, dental health, personal health and fitness, nutrition, consumer health, ecological concepts, and environmental quality

The choice of materials, content, and teaching strategies can be an emotionally charged issue, particularly in the area of family living. Persons who have attended an open meeting where concerned parents and community members discussed the sex education program can attest to the extremely strong opinions expressed and how emotionally involved some individuals can become in the ensuing deliberations. Issues such as teacher qualification, learning readiness, strategies, materials, content, and negative and positive effects of the program on children may be hotly debated.

Generally, such discussions occur when the program has not been developed according to certain established procedures. Community acceptance is perhaps the most crucial aspect in the development of a successful program. The public needs to be properly informed as to the aims, objectives, and aspirations of the sex education program. Careful planning at the local community level involving parents, teachers, clergy of various faiths, medical society, community leaders, and other groups is an essential prerequisite to program development.

The area of sex education as well as other controversial areas can present many challenges for present-day teachers, administrators, and boards of education. However, schools should not lag behind in their educational efforts because of fear of community reaction. To do so would be an injustice to the children, to the teaching profession, and to society in general.

The discussion of each of the following major health topics includes a brief description of the needs of students in these areas and a philosophical overview for presenting these particular health areas to students. Outlines and key questions are included for each major health education topic. In addition, examples of learning activities for each area are presented and grade placement is suggested.

It is not the intention to provide readers with a ready-made curriculum guide. Effective teaching and curriculum construction should not include the lifting of a published curriculum guide for Albany, New York, and inserting it in the guide for Los Alamos, New Mexico. To meet the specific health needs of a given class or community, planning must be individualized. Therefore, goals, objectives, time factors, specific units, and lesson plans have not been included. The purpose of this chapter is to provide teachers with a clear idea of the scope of each major topic area and the tools with which to generate individualized curriculum guides, units, and lesson plans.

MENTAL HEALTH

The need for mental health education in the elementary school can be pointed out in the following statistical analysis of the mental health problems of school children:[1]

1. An estimated 10 percent of our nation's fifty million school age children have moderate to severe emotional problems.
2. One out of three of the fifteen million children reared in poverty have serious mental and emotional problems.
3. An estimated one million school age children have personality problems.
4. In excess of 700,000 young people annually appear in court on criminal or antisocial acts.
5. While the adult mental disease hospitalization rate of one in fifteen has stabilized during the past decade, the number of children and adolescents in mental hospitals is increasing.
6. An estimated twelve million school age children come from broken homes.

A statistical analysis provides only a partial picture of the need for mental health education. The school may well be the only institution outside of the home capable of coming in contact with and dealing with the problems of almost all children. Careful observations of children by teachers and staff

1. Lealon E. Martin, *Mental Health/Mental Illness: Revolution in Progress* (New York: McGraw-Hill Book Co., 1970), pp. 67–76.

can often identify a large percentage of students with behavioral, emotional, or learning problems by the time these children have completed the second grade.[2, 3] Along these same lines, Abrams has pointed out the special problems of inner city children by suggesting that 48 percent of the white children and 76 percent of the black children compared to only 10 percent of the white middle-class children are educationally handicapped.[4] These figures compare unfavorably with a national average of 31 percent. There is no doubt that children tend to bring their mental and emotional problems with them to school. However, the school milieu does contribute to the problems of students through failure, boredom, peer pressure, rules, deadlines, and the like. Schools have a moral, if not a legal, obligation to detect and prevent the mental and emotional problems of students.[5]

In terms of a philosophy of teaching mental health, the key lies in generating a positive approach to meet the everyday social and emotional needs of students. In order to accomplish this, students and teachers must live mental health in the classroom in addition to taking part in sequentially planned mental health lessons.[6]

A review of textbooks and curriculum guides on mental health reveals a heavy emphasis on the negative aspects of classifying psychological disorders and detailing what can go wrong with the emotional and mental aspects of the human organism. Teachers should carefully avoid such a negative approach. Emphasis should be placed on activities that will aid students in achieving success in dealing with everyday personal, emotional, and social problems. As might be expected, the recommended teaching strategies in mental health center on discussions, problem solving, decision making, psychodramas, and valuing activities.

SCOPE AND KEY QUESTIONS OF MENTAL HEALTH

FRIENDSHIP

What is a good friend?

Why do we need friends?

How should people make friends?

What does other-person centered mean?

How do friends argue or disagree?

What if your friend or friends want to do something you do not want to do?

What things do popular people do? What things do unpopular people do?

Do friends force their friends to do something that might be risky?

Why do boys and girls seem to have difficulty being friends with one another?

Why do some people seem to have more friends than others?

What role does courtesy play in friendship?

2. Archie A. Silver, and Rosa A. Hagin, "Profile of a First Grade: A Basis for Preventive Psychiatry," *Journal of American Academy of Child Psychiatry* 11 (1972): 645-674.

3. John P. Glavin, "Persistence of Behavior Disorders in Children," *Exceptional Children* 38 (1972): 367–375.

4. R. S. Abrams, M. Vanecko, and I. Abrams, "A Suggested School Mental Health Program," *Journal of School Health* 42 (1972): 137–141.

5. W. C. Rhodes, "The Disturbing Child: A Problem of Ecological Management," *Exceptional Children* 33 (1967): 449–455.

6. Genelle K. Mantz, "Can Mental Health Be Taught?" *Journal of School Health* 42 (1972): 398–399.

What is it like to be a new student in school?
What things can be done to make a new student welcome?
Are brothers and sisters friends?
What is loyalty?
Should you have a few special friends or a lot of friends?
Do friends really tell everything to one another? Why? Why not?
How do you tell a friend something that might disappoint him?
How do friends decide what to do when they both have something different
      in mind?
What kinds of things do friends do that hurt your feelings?
How can friends be a good influence or bad influence on one another?
What role should your parents play in the choice of your friends?
What should you do if your parents do not appreciate your choice of friends?
What are the best and the worst things a friend can do to you?
Do friends give things and share things with one another?
What does it mean to try to buy friendship?

COMMUNICATION
What are some examples of good or bad communication?
How should one go about accomplishing the following acts?
      Criticizing someone
      Apologizing for something
      Thanking someone
      Telling people you are angry with them
      Asking for a favor
      Telling someone you do not want to do as suggested
How can one do a better job of following verbal directions?
Without talking how can you show you are happy, sad, jealous, angry,
      friendly?
How should you act when someone is angry with you?
Is there a generation gap? If so, who caused it?
How does one go about giving effective directions, writing a memo, writing
      a thank you note, writing a sympathy note?
How does one express sympathy?
How do you talk to someone who is very sad? who is dying? who is very ill
      or has recently lost a loved one?
How are we supposed to talk with someone who is very old?
When should we tell anyone our most secret thoughts?

PEER PRESSURE
What is meant by peer pressure?
How do your friends influence you?
What influence do you have on your friends?
How important is it for you to feel part of the group?
What should you do or not do to be accepted by a group?
How does the opinion of friends affect your decision making?
What is a clique?
What are the good and bad things about cliques?
Why do fads occur?
In what kinds of situations should people make their own decisions?
When should you go along with the group?

When should you not go along with the group?

What role do your parents play in your selection of a group of friends?

THE EMOTIONS

What are emotions?

How should we show our emotions?

How should we express our emotions positively?

When is showing our emotions good or bad for us?

Is there supposed to be a difference in how men and women react to emotional situations? What are these differences? Do you agree with these differences?

What physiological responses occur in regard to our emotions?

Can we put our emotions to good use?

What can we do if we feel our emotions are getting the best of us?

Should men cry? Why? Why not?

SELF-CONCEPT

Who am I?

What are my strengths and weaknesses?

How can one overcome feelings of distrust, guilt, fear, inferiority, and the like?

What are the characteristics of a mentally healthy person?

How does a mentally healthy person feel about himself, others, his past, his future?

How does a mentally healthy person plan ahead, adjust, and compensate?

How do you feel about growing old?

How do you accept failure?

When should someone give up and try something else?

What is your goal in life?

What is your philosophy of life?

What are your thoughts about death and dying?

What is meant by spiritual strength of character?

What are your greatest fears?

What are life's greatest rewards for you?

How do you seem to manage under pressure or crises?

LIFE'S ROLES

How would you describe the woman's role in modern society?

How would you describe the man's role in modern society?

How do the male/female roles seem to be changing?

What male/female role changes do you agree or disagree with?

How should you act when a person in authority such as a teacher, mother, father, or policeman is being angry with you for something you have done wrong? How would you react if this person is angry with you for something you did not do wrong?

How many different roles do we assume in a single day? What are some of these roles?

How do we talk to: a new student at school? someone we don't know? someone who is very ill or dying? an old person? someone who is confused? someone who is depressed or in a panic?

What is the role of a good leader? of a good follower?

How do we show that we like or love someone?
How do we show that we dislike someone?

PERSONALITY DEVELOPMENT
What is the meaning of the word *personality*?
What are the characteristics of a good personality? a bad personality?
What characteristics do you admire the most in others? the least?
What do you want to be remembered for?
How can persons change their personality or how others view them?
What influence do you have on the personality development of persons close to you?
How do persons close to you influence your personality?
Is everyone unique? Why?
How important are first impressions?
How do the following situations affect your personality and how you deal with others? stress, anger, fatigue, loss of face, problems at home, problems with someone close to you, success in school or sports, no success in school or sports?
Why does how we view ourselves seem to influence how we deal with others?
What are the emotional and physical needs of people?
How can we meet the emotional needs of people?
What are your most important emotional needs?

LIFE'S ALTERNATIVES
What is the role of relaxation in mental health?
How and when should people celebrate?
When do you really feel good?
What turns you on or off?
What is the best way to let off steam?
Which forms of entertainment are acceptable for people of your age group?
What is the role of the recreational use of drugs in mental health?
How do you view growing old? dying? being handicapped?
How does one determine what profession to pursue?
Why is attacking our problems considered good mental health practice?
What big decisions will you have to make today? this week? in your life?
How dependent or independent should we be?
What is meant by risk taking?
What kinds of things do you consider bad risks?
What is meant by a natural high?

MENTAL ILLNESS
What is mental illness?
How do you act toward someone you know has had or is having emotional problems?
What are some of the diseases of the nervous system?
What are some of the mental health problems of children?
What are some community mental health services?
How is mental illness treated?
What causes mental illness?
What is the role of drug usage in mental health?

STRATEGIES IN TEACHING MENTAL HEALTH,
DRUG EDUCATION, AND FAMILY LIVING

UNDERSTANDING THE NERVOUS SYSTEM

Why is it important to understand the nervous system?

Why is the nervous system considered the most important system in the body?

In relation to the other systems of the body, what is the role of the nervous system?

What is the special relationship between the nervous system and the endocrine system?

What are the functions of the nervous system?

What are the roles of food, drugs, exercise, rest, sleep, and tension in relation to the nervous system?

What are some diseases and disorders of the nervous system and how can they be prevented?

What kinds of things make one appreciate the nervous system?

ECOLOGY AND MENTAL HEALTH

What is the relationship between home and mental health?

How do children react to human relations problems in their home?

What does the pace of modern living contribute to mental health?

What are the ecological factors that influence mental health or illness?

What role does the school play in your mental health?

What influences do your friends have on your mental health?

Are human beings designed to be social animals? Why?

What is meant by inner or spiritual strength? How do people obtain or lose this strength?

Table 15–1. Suggested Grade Placement for Mental Health Topics

Topic	Grade Placement							
	K	1	2	3	4	5	6	7–8
Friendship	***	***	***	***	***	**	*	***
Communication	**	**	**	**	*	*	***	***
Peer pressure	*	*	*	*	*	**	**	***
The emotions	*	*	*	*	*	*	*	***
Self-Concept	*	*	*	*	**	***	**	***
Life's roles	***	***	**	*	*	*	**	***
Personality development	*	**	**	*	*	**	***	**
Life's alternatives	*	*	*	*	**	**	**	***
Mental illness					*	*	**	**
Understanding the nervous system					*	**	***	*
Ecology and mental health						*	**	***

Key: *** = major emphasis; ** = emphasis; * = touched upon or reviewed.

TEACHING STRATEGIES IN MENTAL HEALTH

Appropriate grade levels are suggested for each teaching strategy and appear in a key in the column at the right of each strategy. Use the key as follows:

P, most suited for the primary levels (kindergarten through grade three);

I, most suited for the intermediate levels (grade four through grade six);

U, most suited for the upper levels (grade seven and grade eight).

FRIENDSHIP

Choose a theme of friendship for each week. For example: sharing, asking, listening, and the like. Center the language arts activities around the friendship theme.   P

Select a historical example of a great friendship and analyze the characteristics of this relationship.   I U

Develop a make-a-new-friend campaign.   I U

Develop dramatizations, particularly role plays or puppet shows, that illustrate stress factors in a friendship such as not sharing, forcing a friend to take a risk, criticizing, and introducing yourself to someone new.   P I U

Develop bulletin board displays around a friendship theme.   P I U

Assign students to serve as special guides for new students. Have the class develop guidelines for serving in this capacity.   P I U

On a regular basis hold an appreciation ceremony in which students can openly express thank you to one of their classmates for a friendly gesture or special favor. This should be done on a voluntary basis   P I U

Have students complete and discuss open-ended statements such as the following:
> Friends usually . . .
> Friends should never . . .
> How do you feel when a good friend . . . .   P I U

Through buzz groups or class discussion have students develop their own ideas about the role of friends, making friends, sharing, reacting to hurt feelings, and the like.   P I U

Collect songs, essays, and poems dealing with friendship.   P I

Utilize valuing activities in which students rank the top characteristics of a good friend and defend their choices.   I U

Develop problem-solving activities around such topics as the following: What do you do if your friend wants to do something you do not feel you should do?
What should you do if you are a new student and would like to make friends?
Do friends argue? How? How do they work things out?
How do you tell people you are unhappy with them?   P I U

COMMUNICATION

Role play and discuss the following scenes:

Asking for something	Being criticized
Criticizing someone	Asking for a date
Refusing something	Giving directions
Apologizing	Introducing someone P I U

Utilize dramatizations showing how people physically show anger, doubt, concern and sadness.   P I U

Demonstration: The following humorous activities can serve to illustrate the advantages of two-way communication over one-way communication.
> Two students come forward and stand back-to-back so that they cannot see one another.
> Student A is given some article of clothing.

Student B must give the directions for putting this article of clothing on.

Student A must follow B's directions explicitly. More humorous results occur when A receives the article of clothing upside down or inside out.

Once the task has been completed, have the same two students or two others try the activity again, but allow student A the opportunity to ask questions and give clarifying responses.

Follow this interesting activity with a discussion of the whys and hows of two-way versus one-way conversation.   P   I   U

Language arts: Have students practice giving directions and following directions. Also, have them practice giving appropriate responses to the following situations:

Expressing sympathy
Asking for a favor
Thanking someone
Congratulating someone   P   I   U

Develop posters or bulletin board displays illustrating communication scenes such as body language, facial expressions, and types of conversation.   P   I   U

Problem solving: In groups, as a class, or individually have students analyze a classroom or school communication problem area. Develop a plan of action to improve this communication problem and put the plan in action.   I   U

PEER PRESSURE

Have students complete a personal survey in which they list those persons close to them who seem to influence them the most and those who try to influence them the most. Have students tell how much they wish to comply with these people.   I   U

Develop a display of fads that have occurred over the years. Discuss reasons why fads occur.   I   U

Have a fad day in which students rummage through closets at home and bring or wear a bit of nostalgia to school.   P   I   U

Hold class discussions on the following topics:

How do our friends influence us?
Why do fads occur?
Why do people do things in groups they would not do alone?
Do good friends try to change you?
What are the characteristics of (1) a leader, (2) a follower, and (3) a loner?

Hold a panel discussion on the good and bad points of belonging to a close group of friends   I   U

Peer pressure game: Without telling why, have students stand beside their desks, facing forward. Tell them they cannot talk or look at the other members of their "team" behind them. Have them stand with their arms straight out from their shoulders with their palms up. Begin timing them as if it were a contest. Remind them that if their arms drop or if they talk or turn around their row will be disqualified and they will have to sit down. Once a winning row has been determined, utilize the following key questions to lead into a discussion of peer pressure:

    1. How did those of you in the front feel about the activity?
    2. Did you feel a responsibility for the other members of your group? Why?
    3. Were any of you angry at losing? Why?
    4. Why did you people participate in this activity?
    5. Why did some of you quit while others did their best?
    6. How many of you felt foolish but kept going anyway?
    7. How does peer pressure influence us in other ways?   I U

Problem solving: Have individuals or groups develop solutions for the following everyday peer pressure problems:

    While walking home your friends dare you to throw a rock through the window of an unoccupied house.

    You are with your close group of friends on a summer outing in a nearby forest preserve. They offer you some marijuana.   I U

    Your best friend is having an argument with someone. The argument becomes very heated, and your friend asks you to side with him. Unfortunately you think the other person is in the right.

    Your friends want you to skip school.   I U

Comic situations: Have students relate embarrassing things that have happened to them. If someone has just come in late to class, ask him how he feels or what he is thinking about.   P I U

Language arts: Select stories that reflect peer pressure situations, qualities of leadership, loyalty, and being a good follower.   P I U

Have students make a personal list of the positive ways and negative ways their friends influence them. Have them rank these ways.   I U

Have students relate situations in which they made their own decision rather than follow the group and reflect on the consequences of their personal decision.   P I U

THE EMOTIONS

Develop dramatizations which include plays, role plays, or puppet shows illustrating how individuals display emotion. Follow each with a discussion on the appropriateness of the expression of the emotion and how people should respond to outbursts of emotion from others.   P I U

Set scenes with the use of photographs, slides, movies, or filmstrips that depict emotional responses. Have the students judge what emotion is being expressed, whether or not the response is appropriate, and the alternatives to the illustrated responses.   P   I   U

Generate class discussion concerning the role of emotions and when it is appropriate to express them. Also discuss society's view of appropriate emotional responses for men and for women.   P   I   U

Illustrate through a diagram or slide the actions of the sympathetic and parasympathetic nervous systems in an emotional situation. Discuss why and how the reactions occur.   I   U

Emotion grab bag: In a paper bag have students place anonymous slips of paper on which are written descriptions of real-life situations in which they had expressed strong emotion. Place additional slips in the bag, on which are written such questions as Do boys cry? Should emotions be pent up? and the like. At appropriate times draw a slip from the bag and discuss the situation described on the slip.   P   I   U

Have students complete the following open-ended statements:
When I feel sad . . .
When people are jealous of me . . .
. . . makes me sad/happy/jealous/angry . . .   P   I   U

SELF-CONCEPT

By lot, a student is chosen to wear a badge marked Our Great and Noble Leader. During the school day other students are to treat this individual as their leader by asking advice, permission, and directions. At the end of the school day Our Great and Noble Leader must explain his feelings and how he thought others viewed him. The class enters into a follow-up discussion on self-image.   P   I   U

As an autobiographical activity, ask students to list in order their strengths, weaknesses, goals, and problems.   I   U

Have students select an item they are least pleased with about their self-image. Ask them to develop a plan for improving this item. Also, these items could be listed on slips of paper and placed in a box anonymously and used for surveying self-image problems, problem solving, and class discussion.   I   U

Have the class develop a self-test on self-image.

	Never	Rarely	At Times	Often	Always	
I feel secure	___	___	___	___	___	
People make fun of me	___	___	___	___	___	
I have confidence	___	___	___	___	___	I U

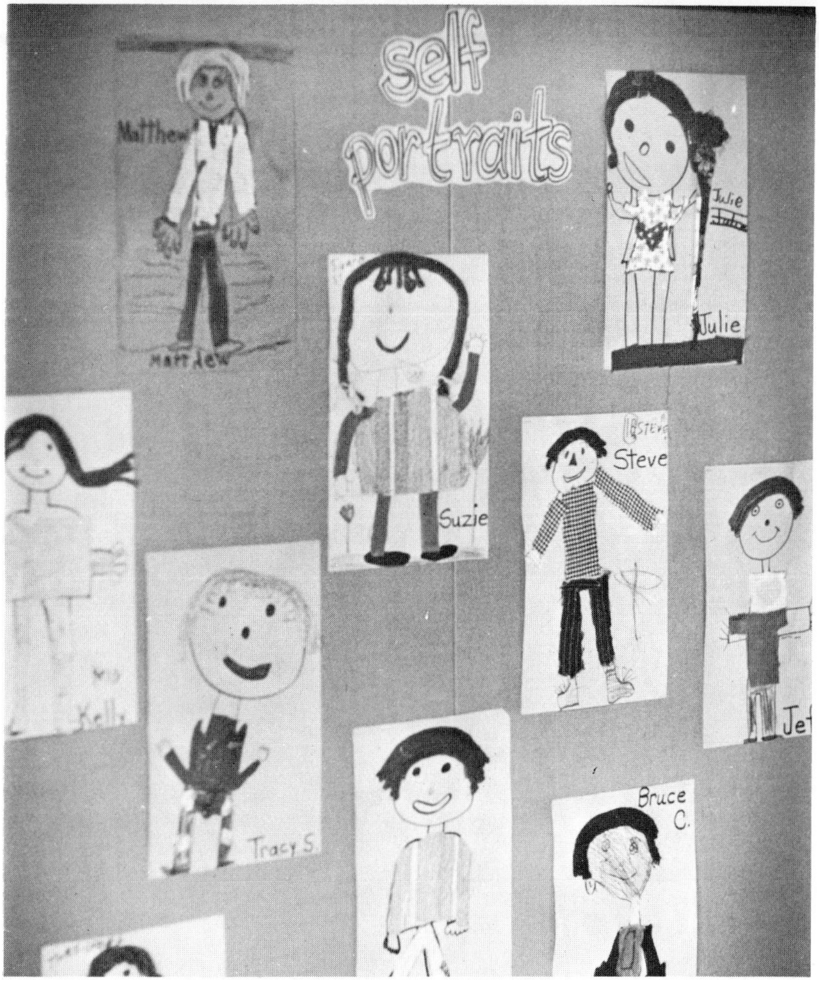

Fig. 15–1. Student display illustrating the health topic of self-concern.

Have students complete open-ended statements such as:
    If I could be . . . .
    If I could do something over, it would be . . . .
    My strengths are . . . .   P   I   U

Guide students to stories or plays that involve the following situations:
        Overcoming feelings of inferiority
        Thinking positively
        Trying or doing one's best
        Making mistakes, accepting them, and profiting from
            the experience   P   I   U

Have class discussions on the following topics:
    When can making mistakes help one progress?
    How does one overcome feelings of failure, insecurity, fear
        of not having people like one, and the like?

What is the role of success in self-image?

When should someone quit and try something else?

Why do some people have more self-confidence than other people?   P I U

In buzz groups or individually have students try to find solutions for the following problems:

     Overcoming failure

     Shyness in meeting new people

     Fearing failure

     Gaining confidence

     Telling people how you feel

     Overcoming other types of fears

     Accepting ourselves   I U

LIFE'S ROLES

Have a debate or panel discussion on male/female roles in society, home, school, sports, business, and politics.   U

Have a class discussion or buzz group on a student's role in such special situations as:

     Speaking to an ill friend or a friend who is dying

     Accepting the death of a family member or friend

     Dealing with people who have such severe problems that they are not themselves

     Talking to someone who has just had a personal tragedy   I U

Have students develop displays depicting life's special roles such as being old, women in sports, parents, and the like.   P I U

Conduct a survey on such topics as:

     What is a good parent?

     What is a good friend?

     How do you feel about aging?

     What is your view of death and dying?

     When someone confides in you, how should you respond?   I U

Have students make value judgments by ranking and defending their choices on such factors as:

Long life, pleasure, health	Money, health, pleasure
Love, money, pleasure	Brains, beauty, money
Career, good children, health	Adventure, peace, love

     P I U

Have students determine their personel expectations in terms of being a parent, husband, wife, friend, and counselor and being very ill or handicapped.   I U

PERSONALITY DEVELOPMENT

Provide stories, plays, or films that depict different types of personalities and people who have changed their self-image.   P I U

Through class discussion define personality, role of personality, what the characteristics of good and bad personalities are, and whether or not personality is how we view ourselves.   I U

Have students list in order their three greatest personality strengths and weaknesses. Without having the students reveal their names, collect these statements, tabulate them, and use them for class discussion. I U

Develop panel discussions or buzz group discussions around what constitutes a personality that is pleasant, real, phony, or unpleasant. I U

Have students complete open-ended statements such as:
I feel that others view me as . . .
If I could change one part of my personality, it would be . . .
I am happy as I am because . . . I U

Utilize role plays to depict how not to go about selling yourself to someone you have just met; about being a gracious winner or loser; about accepting congratulations; and about having a job interview or selling something. P I U

Develop and administer a survey on what constitutes a good or poor personality. Utilize the results for class discussion. P I U

Have students develop stories or displays depicting the different types of personality characteristics people have. Generate themes around such topics as Gloomy Gus, Silly Sal, and Mean Manfred. P I U

LIFE'S ALTERNATIVES

Utilize everyday situations for individual or group problem solving such as the following:
At the end of a successful day, how will you celebrate?
John S. feels he has been picked on by Sam S. all day.
What are John's alternatives and consequences. I U

Have students develop statements on the following topics:
What turns me on?
What things I get the most or least enjoyment from.
If I had my choice I would . . .
What is meant by life's simple pleasures? P I U

Survey parents and friends on such topics as the following:
What turns you on?
What is great about our school? our friends? our town? our country?
What is your favorite recreation?
What are some of life's most beautiful moments?
What is the best way to relax? I U

Hold class discussions on such subjects as the following:
What do you do when you are worried? tense? happy?
What is great about life?
What are life's simple pleasures?
How can we best relax?
What is the role of drug use as a means to any end? I U

Have students complete autobiographical items detailing what they enjoy most in life; what they can do when they are sad, mad, or happy; what they regret the most; and the like.   P I U

Have a panel discussion or debate on entertainment, life's pleasures, or the recreational use of drugs.   I U

Have a theme for each day of the week depicting one of life's simple pleasures.   P I U

After a survey asking other members of the school or class about what turns them on, have the class make a bulletin board or other display illustrating the kinds of things their classmates really enjoy doing.   P I U

Have students give reports on their favorite sport, recreation, or hobby.   P I U

MENTAL ILLNESS

Have group or individual reports on the various community agencies dealing with mental health.   U

In a brainstorming or buzz group session have students develop ideas concerning how to treat or act toward someone who has had a mental illness.   I U

Bring in a guest speaker who is acquainted with the kinds of treatments given to individuals having mental health problems.   U

Have student reports or special interest activities concerning such topics as mental retardation, mental disorders, drug-caused mental disorders, and the legal aspects of mental illness.   U

Describe and demonstrate first-aid techniques for someone who is extremely upset.   I U

UNDERSTANDING THE NERVOUS SYSTEM

Use any or all of the following appreciation activities:

Memorization game: Have teams come forward and try to memorize a wide variety of items placed on a tray. Set a time limit for reviewing and returning to their places and recording the miscellaneous items.   P I U

Hold a food-tasting party.

Play games that disrupt the senses such as pin the tail on the donkey, balance on one leg with eyes open and then with eyes closed.

Have students stand on their head and drink water.

Collect and display optical illusions.

Have students identify their optical blind spot.

Have students determine their dominant eye to prove that the brain has hemispheres.

Have lipreading contests.

Have reading contests in which the upper half or lower half of each word is covered.

Illustrate genetic traits by seeing who in class can role the tongue over.

Try patting the head and rubbing the stomach at the same
time.   P I U

On a series of cards write down each of the parts of the nervous
system. Hand out the cards so that each student has a part.
On an outline of the human body have students come up
and place the parts where they should go.   I U

Develop a series of three-to-six learning stations. At each station
have materials such as filmstrips, tapes, books, and pamphlets
describing certain parts of the nervous system. Also at each
station have study guide questions. Have the students rotate
through each learning station.   I U

Have a Believe It or Not or Book of Records display of all the
strange and interesting facts about the nervous system.   I U

Have students generate reports or special interest activities about
specific parts of the nervous and endocrine systems.   I U

Develop a carefully prepared presentation on drug interactions
with the nervous system.   I U

Generate class discussions on such topics as:
What are some individual differences?
How important is the nervous system?
What does the nervous system do for one?
How have you used your nervous system in the last half
hour? (brainstorming)
How do sleep, rest, and nutrition influence the nervous sys-
tem?   I U

ECOLOGY AND MENTAL HEALTH

Have students develop displays around such topics as The rat
race and mental health; The modern life style and ecological
factors that influence mental health such as space, weather,
and economic conditions.   I U

Have buzz groups discuss the roles of the following ecological
factors and mental health: school, weather, culture, politics,
population, and nutrition.   U

Have students develop a philosophical statement concerning the
role of inner or spiritual strength and mental health.   U

What is the role of drugs in mental health? This can be a teacher-
led discussion about people who are allergic to specific substances, followed by a discussion of individual differences
and individual tolerances. This should be followed by a discussion of the safe use of medication. Eventually the discussion leader should investigate the short- and long-range uses
of drugs on a recreational basis.   I U

The drug problem in the United States clearly includes the use of all drugs
rather than the current focus on the use of illicit street drugs by some young
people. Because such a high percentage of the population is involved in

DRUG EDUCATION

the recreational use of drugs, drug educators are making a serious blunder by placing so much emphasis on the use by adolescents and young adults of street drugs such as marijuana, barbiturates amphetamines, LSD, and heroin. In terms of a health problem, a much larger proportion of our population is heavily involved with the use of psychotherapeutic medications and in the recreational use of drugs such as alcohol and tobacco. For example, in 1970 Americans spent $15.7 billion for alcoholic beverages, $9 billion for tobacco, and $3.2 billion for caffeine beverages, accounting for an astounding total of $27 billion.[7] The rate of prescriptions filled in the United States is slightly more than five prescriptions per person per year. Of these prescriptions, 17 percent are for psychotherapeutic drugs.[8]

Sex, as well as age, is a factor in drug abuse. While men seem to have at least six times the alcoholism rate of women, women, especially those between the ages of thirty and sixty years, have a much higher use of prescription drugs. Women account for 63 percent of the barbiturates used, 68 percent of the tranquilizers, and 80 percent of the amphetamines.[9]

Another factor indicating that the drug problem is not limited to the streets or to young people can be found in Fort's observations that the average "straight" American consumes three to five mind-altering drugs a day.[10] Included in this list of mind-altering drugs are alcohol, caffeine, and nicotine. The most serious drug problem is the abuse of alcohol. Of the 94,000,000 users of alcohol in the United States, an estimated 9,000,000 are classified alcoholics. The misuse of alcohol costs an estimated $25 billion annually.[11]

The information in regard to drug use by elementary children is limited. However, a large number of surveys have focused on the drug-taking patterns of junior and senior high students. A summary of these surveys indicates that between 39 and 68 percent of secondary school students use or have used marijuana, and there is a similar but lower-range usage of amphetamines, barbiturates, and LSD. If these surveys were to include alcohol, the percentage of drug usage might be as high as 70 to 80 percent. One incomprehensible figure is that an estimated 432,000 teenagers were arrested for drug offenses during the period of 1969–1971. Figures for drug-related deaths and overdoses are not available on a national scale, but a trip to any major hospital center will provide a startling picture of drug-related emergencies and emotional trauma.[12]

Drug usage on the level that is now concerning most Americans is not new. In fact, Brecher points out that in the nineteenth century the percentage

7. Summary of 1970 Consumer Expenditures," *Supermarketing* 26 (1972): 39.

8. American Medical Association, *Health Education Services for Schools and Colleges* 12 (1972): 1.

9. Task Force on Prescription Drugs, *The Drug Users* (Washington, D.C.: Government Printing Office, 1969), p. 33.

10. Joel Fort, *The Pleasure Seekers: The Drug Crisis, Youth and Society* (Indianapolis, Ind.: Bobbs-Merrill Co., 1969).

11. National Clearinghouse for Alcohol Information of the National Institute on Alcohol Abuse and Alcoholism, "Second Special Report Updates Alcohol Knowledge," NIAAA Information and Feature Service, 20 October 1974.

12. Select Committee on Crime, *Drugs in Our Schools* (Washington, D.C.: Government Printing Office, 1973).

of drug abuse was probably higher than our current estimates because of the availability of opiates.[13] There is some evidence to indicate that mass media, by sensationalizing the use of marijuana, LSD, and glue sniffing, brought about the more rapid increase in drug use. In any case, the billions of dollars poured into drug advertising serve to reinforce the thousands of years of our mystical faith in herbs and nostrums and our current acceptance of the belief that we can now take a pill for most everything. Commercials claiming veritable blood transfusions or suggesting that we all deserve an aspirin break have helped create beliefs and behavioral intentions that are difficult for any drug education program to overcome. Blum suggests that school drug education programs are in a weak position to overcome drug-taking behavior because it is the family that shapes attitudes toward drug usage in the home through use of medications and recreational use of drugs.[14] Blum further states that the quality of home life in such areas as life goals, values, humor, respect, and communication is an indicator of who will be most likely to abuse drugs.[15]

Drug education is not without its detractors. In a recent study of 1,300 students and 168 teachers, 68 percent of the teachers and 75 percent of the students stated that they did not feel drug education prevented drug use. This study also found, however, that most drug education teaching strategies utilized traditional scare tactics and did not teach drug education within a health context.[16] In addition to the negative reaction of teachers and students is the concern experts have expressed over the quality of drug education materials and curriculum plans. A review of curriculum plans in drug education gives the distinct impression that curriculum committees simply copy from one another. In addition, many of the plans are replicas of drug education unit plans developed more than twenty years ago. DeLone suggests that errors can be found in 80 percent of the current published drug education materials and that existing drug education curricula have not been tested for effectiveness.[17] Along these same lines the National Commission on Marihuana and Drug Abuse has recommended a moratorium on the production and dissemination of new drug information materials to enable the government to develop standards for accuracy and concept.[18]

Drug education is not a panacea and should not be expected to stop the use of all drugs. Recreational, religious, and medical uses of drugs have been part of man's culture for thousands of years, and if the results of a recent survey indicating that 73 percent of the teenagers using drugs do so only for fun are accurate, a similar pattern of drug use will continue.[19] Along

13. Edward M. Brecher, *Licit and Illicit Drugs* (Boston: Little Brown & Co., 1972), pp. 3–46.
14. Richard Blum, "Schools Are Not Effective in Drug Education," *Drugs and Drug Abuse Newsletter* 3 (1972): 1.
15. Ibid.
16. Macro Systems, Inc., *Evaluation of Drug Education Programs: Main Report,* (Silver Spring, Md.: Macro Systems, Inc., June 1972).
17. Richard H. DeLone, "The Ups and Downs of Drug Abuse Education," *Saturday Review* 11 November 1972, pp. 27–32.
18. Second Report of National Commission on Marihuana and Drug Abuse, *Drug Use in America: Problem in Perspective* (Washington, D.C.: Government Printing Office, 1973), p. 355.
19. Macro Systems, *Evaluation.*

these same lines, teenagers not using drugs for recreational purposes were found to base their decision on erroneous beliefs.[20] Rather than try to stop the use of recreational drugs, drug education should emphasize the rational use of drugs through an approach based on decision-making and valuing activities.

Elementary teachers should avoid a drug education approach based only on the presentation of facts concerning the legal, historical, and pharmacological aspects of drugs. The emphasis in drug education should be on learning activities designed to build drug value concepts within health topics such as nutrition, growth and development, safety, prevention and treatment of disease, mental health, and human relations.

As expressed in Table 15–2, drug education programs appear to be based on either a hard-sell or soft-sell approach.

Table 15–2. Hard Sell Versus Soft Sell Approach to Drug Education

Hard Sell: Emphasis on	*Soft Sell: Emphasis on*
Information gathering	Value activities, knowledge and clarifying responses, decision making
Nomenclature and drug "menus"	Concern for student needs and readiness
Legal, historical, and pharmacological drug facts	Role of drugs in health and disease
Categorizing drugs: nondrugs, drugs, hard, soft, over-the-counter, street drugs, etc.	All drugs have side effects
Negative aspects of drugs	Life's natural highs
Special drug education teachers	Prepared secondary school health education teachers and regular classroom elementary teachers
Teacher moralizing	Teacher remains unbiased
Crash programs with all disciplines teaching drug units	Planned K-12 drug educaiton units within a K-12 districtwide health education program
Large assemblies with special guest speakers	Drug concepts taught within health education classes with an emphasis on small group activities
Special drug units taking place of other health topics	Drug topics integrated with health concepts in nutrition, human growth, disease, and mental health

Source: James D. Brown, "Illinois Trends in Elementary School Drug Education: The Soft Sell," *Journal of Drug Education*, vol. 3, no. 2 (1973). Copyright © Baywood Publishing Company, Inc. 1973. Used by permission of Baywood Publishing Company, Inc.

Drug units with primary emphasis on categorizing and describing the legal, historical, and pharmacological aspects of drugs seem to be patterned after many teacher preparation courses in drug education. This type of organization presents an enormous amount of factual information in a logical sequence and facilitates the memorization of the information. However, while teachers may take comfort in students' committing an impressive

20. Edward A. Wolfson, Marvin A. Lavenhar, Richard Blum, Mark A. Quinones, Stanley Einstein, and Donald B. Louria, "Survey of Drug Abuse in Six New Jersey High Schools: Methodology and General Findings," in *Student Drug Surveys*, ed., Stanley Einstein (Farmingdale, N.Y.: Baywood Publishing Co., 1972), pp. 9–32.

amount of drug information to memory, the gathering of facts does not necessarily lead to student decision making.[21] The assumption that people make decisions based on facts alone ignores the enormous influence social pressure has on decision making. It also appears that knowledge does not significantly influence attitudes and behavior in the use of drugs.[22] Educators also need to be concerned with the attitudes, fears, and knowledge children already have about drugs.

One pattern of drug education that should be discouraged is the development of exceptionally long lists of generic names and street-slang terms for the available drugs. These endless lists of mild, dangerous, exotic, and even legendary drugs may be fascinating and impressive, but some serious doubts exist concerning their effectiveness in developing rational drug-taking behavior.

Halleck suggests that vast knowledge of the physical and psychological effects of a seemingly endless list of medical and street drugs is unlikely to help people make a moral decision on whether or not to inhale, ingest, or inject a substance into their body.[23] It seems possible that the ubiquitous "drug menu" may be of use only to that certain percentage of students already heavily into drugs who are looking for new experiences and the means for dealing with or avoiding undesirable drug reactions.

Yolles and Levy point out the importance of value activities, teachers with unbiased views, and student involvement in the decision-making areas of drug education.[24, 25] The all too common pattern of employing special drug education teachers, mass assemblies, and crash programs that do not build drug education into a health concept ignores the suggestions of drug education leaders.

The following scope of drug education differs from that for other health topics presented previously. In developing the critical pattern of building drug education into a health concept, what follows is a set of guidelines for placing most of the major drug education topics into lessons dealing with other health topic areas. For example, a logical place to discuss the safe use of medications and the fact that all drugs have side effects is within a unit on disease and the treatment of disease. Similarly, consideration of recreational use of beverage alcohol might better be handled in a lesson on the mental health aspects of releasing tensions, on escapism, or on determining appropriate responses to life's alternatives. Although most of the drug education topics can be covered in other health areas, there remains a need for a decision-making type of drug unit that can tie the related drug topics together.

21. Educational Policies Commission, *The Central Purposes of Education* (Washington, D.C.: National Education Association, 1961).
22. Godfrey M. Hochbaum, "How Can We Teach Adolescents About Smoking, Drinking and Drug Abuse?" *Journal of Health, Physical Education and Recreation* 3 (1972): 2.
23. Seymour Halleck, "The Great Drug Education Hoax," *The Progressive* (Madison, Wis.: 1970), p. 2 (reprint).
24. Stanley Yolles, "Managing Mood Changes," *Journal of Drug Education* 1 (1971): 104–105.
25. Marvin R. Levy, "Background Consideration for Drug Programs," in *Resource Book for Drug Abuse Education*, PHS publication no. 1964 (Washington, D.C.: National Clearinghouse for Mental Health Information), p. 3.

SCOPE AND KEY QUESTIONS OF INTEGRATED DRUG EDUCATION

Note that most of the major drug education topics are integrated into other health education areas.

TOPICS IN MENTAL HEALTH

What is the role of peer pressure in drug decision making?
How does the nervous system react to drugs?
What are the psychological effects of medications and street drugs?
What are some of life's natural highs?
Are drugs used to combat a problem or for fun?
Is drug abuse an emotional disease?
Can drugs cause personality and psychological problems?
How can stress be handled without the use of drugs?
What will the role of drugs be in your life?
When are drugs a psychological or social crutch?
Why do friends turn on their friends to drugs?
What is meant by the concept that all drugs have side effects?
When can drugs cause neural and psychological damage?
Under what conditions can psychotherapeutic drugs serve a useful purpose?
Why is there emphasis on individual differences in terms of drug tolerance?

TOPICS IN SAFETY EDUCATION

How can household chemicals be used safely?
What kinds of household fumes are dangerous?
Why is the medicine chest considered dangerous?
What are the first-aid procedures for poisoning?
How can children be protected from harmful encounter with household chemicals and medications?
What are the first-aid procedures for drug overdose?

TOPICS IN CHRONIC AND COMMUNICABLE DISEASE

What are the dangers of self-medication?
Why do the miracle drugs seem to cure some people but bring about fatal allergic reaction in other people?
Why should medications be used only when needed?
How important is the concept that all drugs have side effects?
What is the role of tobacco, alcohol, and street drugs in body defenses, disease, disease recovery, and life expectancy?
Is drug abuse a disease?
How does stress affect the body's resistance?
What drugs lower the body's defense against infections?

TOPICS IN NUTRITION

How are drugs absorbed into the system?
How are drugs metabolized in the body?
What is the role of food additives in health?
Can drugs be effectively used in weight control? How?
Is alcohol a food or a nonfood?
What digestive disorders are related to drug use?
What nutritional disorders occur with extended drug use?

TOPICS IN CONSUMER HEALTH

What is the role of advertising in our current attitude toward drugs?
What are the hazards of self-medication?
What are some guidelines for the safe use of over-the-counter drugs?
Are physicians sometimes guilty of overprescribing drugs? When?
What are the legal aspects of using prescription drugs?
What are the laws concerning possession and sale of legal and street drugs?
How is the quality of prescription and over-the-counter drugs controlled?
Is there any quality control for street drugs?
What are some highlights of the history of medications?
What drugs are the most dangerous?
What effects do drugs have on learning ability, weight control, and skill in sports?

TOPICS IN FAMILY LIVING

Under what circumstances does drug taking such as smoking, drinking, and using street drugs become a personal decision?
How do parents influence your drug-taking behavior?
Does how your parents use drugs such as sleeping pills, tobacco, and alcohol influence your use of drugs?
How would you react if you had a son or daughter who acted as follows:
  Used drugs
  Had drugs in the house
  Was a pusher
  Had a serious drug problem
  Was arrested on a drug charge
  Was straight
How can you have an influence on the drug-taking behavior of your brothers or sisters?
Drug problems occur in what kinds of families?
How is family life changed when a parent has a drug problem such as alcoholism?
What agencies can offer assistance to families with drug problems?
What influences can drug taking have in a dating relationship?
What dictates a couples' drug-taking behavior?
What is social drinking?
Why should a person booze at parties?
Should people urge others to smoke, drink, or use street drugs? Why? Why not?

It is suggested that a carefully developed drug education unit be taught during the sixth grade and again during the seventh or eighth grade. The emphasis in these units should be on bringing together the key concepts and personal decisions from the drug topics already covered in other areas of health and safety education. The key goals for these units can be as follows:

SEPARATE DRUG EDUCATION UNITS

1. To realize that all drugs have side effects.
2. To reduce the damage done by drugs.
3. To emphasize responsible medical and recreational use of drugs.

4. To develop an awareness of alternatives to chemicals as a means of recreational endeavor and in handling stress situations.
5. To create an accurate perception of causes and consequences of drug abuse: psychological, physiological, social, and legal.

SCOPE AND KEY QUESTIONS OF A SEPARATE DRUG UNIT

DRUGS IN THE HOME

What role has the family played in the current overuse of over-the-counter drugs?

What are the characteristics of an intelligent consumer of over-the-counter medications?

How do advertisements influence home consumption of drugs?

Why do authorities state that they can predict who might be a potential drug abuser by the drug patterns of parents and the quality of home life?

How do the attitudes of your friends differ in terms of smoking and drinking if their parents do not smoke or drink?

How should parents react if they found drugs in their child's room?

How are parents affected by the drug-taking behavior of their children?

If your son or daughter was arrested for a drug offense, how would you react?

What is the effect of heavy alcohol use on home life?

How do you influence the drug-taking behavior of your brother or sister?

What are some safety suggestions for the storage and use of potentially dangerous medications?

What kinds of common medications are considered dangerous?

Why should one person not take another individual's prescriptions?

Why should there be smaller dosage levels of medication for younger people?

THE BIG TWO—TOBACCO AND ALCOHOL

Why do people smoke?

What are the physiological and psychological effects of smoking?

What are the rights of smokers and of nonsmokers?

How do people get started smoking?

What are the health and monetary costs of smoking?

How do nonsmokers and older students view smoking by very young students?

In light of the overwhelming information against smoking, why do people start or continue to smoke?

What is emphysema? What is lung cancer?

What is alcohol and how has it been used for thousands of years?

What are the psychological, physiological, social, and legal factors associated with alcohol?

How can appropriate drinking behavior be taught?

What is a social drinker?

What is abuse of alcohol?

Who uses alcohol and why?

Why is age a factor in the drinking of alcoholic beverages?

How does alcohol abuse influence family relationships?

What is alcoholism? What are the treatments for alcoholism?

What role should alcohol play in your life?

SOCIETY'S VIEW OF DRUG TAKING

Why have alcohol, tobacco, and medications been considered nondrugs, while pot, heroin, barbiturates, amphetamines, and LSD been considered drugs?

Do we have a drug epidemic? Why?

What are your school's policies and procedures on use of drugs?

If we made our drug laws stronger, would drug abuse stop? How?

What should young people know about the legal aspects of drug possession, use, and sale?

What sociocultural factors seem to be involved in drug use and abuse?

How do you view the use of the different drugs?

What kinds of drug use does society reject?

What kind of drug-taking behavior does society seem to accept?

THE STREET DRUGS

Why are marijuana, amphetamines, heroin, hallucinogens, and barbiturates called street drugs?

Why do we have street drugs?

What are the characteristics of the local drug scene?

Why is age a factor in drug usage?

What are the psychological, social, physiological, and legal aspects of these drugs?

What are your beliefs about the use of pot, speed, heroin, alcohol, LSD, and barbiturates?

What are arguments for and against legalization of marijuana?

What are the legal risks involved in the use of drugs?

What are the benefits of using recreational drugs?

What is the quality of street drugs?

What is your personal decision concerning the use of pot, heroin, and other street drugs?

What is the role of drugs in learning ability, relaxation, creativity, physical skill, motivation, and achievement?

What are the characteristics of persons who use drugs?

THE COMMUNITY AND DRUGS

How is your community organized to assist persons with drug problems?

What are the emergency care procedures for a drug overdose victim, and how is your community organized to assist in these emergencies?

What agencies in your community are dealing with alcohol and drug problems?

How would a community be organized to combat or prevent drug abuse?

How is alcoholism treated?

How are the school and community cooperating to prevent drug abuse?

How do crisis centers function?

How are your local law enforcement officials reacting to drug problems?

RECREATIONAL AND OTHER APPLICATION OF DRUGS

Since social drinking is accepted by at least 60,000,000 Americans, what kinds of drinking behavior are appropriate?

How can a host who serves alcoholic beverages protect the safety of his guests?

What kinds of guidelines should people follow for the drinking of beverage alcohol?

When is an individual mature enough to use drugs such as alcohol?

What kinds of behavior by persons under the influence of a drug do most people feel are offensive?

What are the signs and symptoms of an individual with a drug problem?

What turns you on?

What are the alternatives to the use of drugs for recreation or as a means of escape?

Why does peer pressure play a large role in our decisions concerning drug use and our patterns of drug use?

What are the psychological, physiological, social, and legal factors involved in use of drugs for these reasons or purposes?

> To relieve pain
> To diet
> To relieve emotional tension
> To enhance learning ability and study efforts
> To ease fatigue
> To increase physical skill
> To increase athletic ability

Why do tolerance and individual differences play such an important role in drug usage?

Who should avoid the use of drugs?

What are the basic functions of the nervous and endocrine systems and how do drugs affect the neural mechanism?

Table 15–3. Suggested Grade Placement for Drug Education Topics

Topic	Grade Placement							
	K	1	2	3	4	5	6	7–8
Drugs in home	***	***	***	***	***	**	**	***
Tobacco and alcohol		*	*	*	*	**	**	***
Society's view of drug taking					*	*	*	***
Street drugs					*	*	**	***
Community and drugs						*	*	***
Recreational and other application of drugs					*	**	**	***

Key: *** = major emphasis; ** = emphasis; * = touched upon or reviewed.

TEACHING STRATEGIES IN DRUG EDUCATION

The key for suggested grade level use of the following teaching strategies is explained on page 288.

DRUGS IN THE HOME

Group activity: Divide the class into groups. Have each group responsible for bringing in advertisements for health foods, over-the-counter drugs, vitamins, alcohol, and tobacco. Have students evaluate the ads after developing criteria for the evaluation of health advertising. Determine what the ads are implying about drug use.

I   U

Language arts: Have students develop advertisements for fake health aids. Have them include imaginary testimonials and several false claims for their imaginary product. Rather than draw the advertising posters, students could write and perform television commercials for their classmates. Follow with a discussion of the types of advertising seen on television. I U

Develop a display illustrating guidelines for the safe use and storage of medications in the home. Include empty prescription bottles and mock medicine cabinets showing the right and wrong ways to store drugs. I U

Problem solving: Have students find solutions to some of the following problems:

> Your younger brother or sister has begun to use drugs.
> How could you get Mom or Dad to stop smoking?
> Friends offer you marijuana.
> You find someone who appears to have taken a drug overdose.
> You are a parent who finds drugs in your child's room. I U

Panel discussions: Organize the class into groups and assign the following topics for panel discussion:

> Why should we have drugs in our society?
> What is meant by the modern pill culture?
> How can drug usage affect the home? I U

Classroom discussions: Provide the following topics for general class discussion:

> Your home and your friends.
> What is your influence on the drug habits of your brothers, sisters, and parents?
> Will your parents' drug-taking habits influence your drug usage?
> As a parent, how would you react to your child's use of drugs?
> How does advertising influence the use of drugs in the home? U

Debate: Have students debate the following issue:

> Parents who expect their children not to use drugs should not drink alcoholic beverages or smoke. I U

Have students make a list of all the drugs that can be found in their home. Discuss the dangers of having these drugs around and the hazards of self-medication. I U

Buzz groups: Divide the class into small groups and have the groups discuss the following topics:

> What would you tell your son or daughter about drugs?
> What would you tell your parents about drugs?
> What is a generation gap?
> What kinds of things can children do to upset their parents?
> What kinds of things can parents do to upset their children?
> What are the good things about home? I U

THE BIG TWO—TOBACCO AND ALCOHOL

Student projects and reports: Assign projects or reports on the following topics:

What are the hazards of secondhand smoke?

Emphysema

Health hazards associated with smoking

Diseases related to the abuse of alcohol   I U

Surveys: Have the class conduct surveys asking such questions as:

Why do people smoke?

When did you start smoking and why?

Have you tried to stop?

Why do you not smoke?

Is it impolite to smoke in front of persons who are non-smokers?

(Similar questions could be asked concerning the use of alcohol)   P I U

Debates: Plan debates on the following topics:

Smoking should not be allowed in public places.

Legal drinking ages should be lowered.   U

Discussions: Have students develop discussions on the following topics:

Why do people smoke?

Why do people not stop smoking if they feel it is hazardous to their health?

What constitutes rational drinking behavior?

Who should or should not drink?

What is abuse?

How do you refuse a drink or a cigarette?

How do you feel about smokers who cannot seem to quit even though they want to?

At a party, how do people really view a drunk?

Should people be taught how to drink?

What are some suggestions for persons who plan to drink?   I U

Guest speakers: A number of highly qualified guest speakers are available who can speak on alcoholism, on family problems associated with alcoholism, and on all aspects of smoking and disease. Consult a telephone directory for the names of organizations involved in these areas.   I U

Teaching-learning stations: Have students complete study guide questions and other activities while rotating through such stations as understanding the respiratory system, physiological effects of smoking, emphysema, lung cancer and smoking and health. Learning stations for alcohol could include alcohol and the nervous system, alcohol absorption, physiological effects of alcohol, diseases and alcohol, what is alcohol?   I U

Display: Collect advertisements on alcohol and tobacco and post them with student-made advertisements. Note: A number of

humorous posters and antismoking posters are available from
the American Cancer Society.   P   I   U

Hot box: Have student volunteers who are smokers or nonsmokers
face a barrage of difficult questions from the rest of the
class.   U

Role play: Assign role-playing activities on such topics as the following:
> Ask someone to stop smoking on a bus or in a small
> room.
> Refuse a drink or offer of a cigarette.
> Try to sell someone on how great it is to smoke or drink
> and have that individual try to counter your argu-
> ments.   I   U

Demonstrations: A number of demonstrations are available for
smoking. These include: smoking machines that can collect
tars; volunteers who can inhale cigarette smoke and then ex-
hale into a clean tissue; a swab from the windshield of a
smoker's car (simply wipe the inside of the windshield with
a clean white handkerchief); and a before-and-after blood
pressure reading from a volunteer smoker.   U

SOCIETY'S VIEW OF DRUG TAKING

Role plays: The following topics make fine role-playing scenes:
> The offer and refusal of an unknown substance
> Archie Bunker describing today's drug takers
> Two members of the drug-taking culture discussing the state
> of the world
> Two "straights" discussing the drug scene at school
> A role play panel discussion in which selected students as-
> sume the roles of a panic-stricken housewife, a police-
> man who is waging a one-man war against the drug
> scene, a with-it teacher, an archconservative parent, a
> concerned parent, and a former drug user now working
> in a drug crisis center   U

Debates: Plan debates around the following topics:
> Should the laws against the use of marijuana be liberalized?
> Is there a real drug abuse epidemic?
> Can drug abuse be controlled through the use of strict drug
> laws?   U

Panel discussions: Hold panel discussions on such topics as the
following (try generating more enthusiasm by having students
role play being policeman, parents, and the like):
> Why is there an increase in drug usage?
> Why is our culture called a "pill culture"?
> Define drug abuse, drug use, and drug use in moderation.
> Who is most likely to have a problem with the use of
> drugs?
> How can drug usage be reduced?
> What role should age play in drug usage?   I   U

Buzz groups: Have small groups discuss the following topics:

Describe the scope of the local drug scene.

Define abuse and moderation in drug taking.

Rank order the following drugs in terms of their potential for abuse and danger: heroin, pot, LSD, barbiturates, alcohol, and amphetamines. Make this ranking in light of your opinions, and list the drugs again in the order you feel your parents would make.

What are the characteristics of the drug abuser; of the drug user; and of the drug nonuser?   U

Collect, post, and discuss newspaper and magazine stories on drugs.   I   U

Have students generate stories about drug-taking situations. Leave the endings of these stories blank so that the rest of the class can provide appropriate endings through class discussion.   I   U

Open-ended statements: Provide these statements for students to complete:

I feel that society views drug taking as . . .

Our drug laws should be . . .

My parents would view my use of drugs as . . .   I   U

Study projects and reports: Have students develop projects and reports on the following topics:

Legal aspects of drug taking

A review of some of the surveys made on the scope of drug use

The school's policies and procedures concerning drug use   I   U

Guest speakers: Have as guest speakers: experts who can present society's concern with and the legal aspects of the drug scene such as persons who work in drug rehabilitation programs, juvenile authorities, policemen, and knowledgeable attorneys.   I   U

Problem solving: Present the following situations for students' consideration:

What do you do if you are at someone's house and the police make a drug raid?

What do you do if someone begins using drugs in your home and you do not want him to?   U

THE STREET DRUGS

Discussion: Have students discuss such topics as the following:

What are the street drugs?

Who uses street drugs?

What is the quality of street drugs and how does one know what he is purchasing or being given?

Where do the drugs come from?

What are the legal implications of possession and sale of illicit drugs?

How prevalent is the local use of street drugs? of school use
of these drugs?
What are the effects and hazards of these drugs?
Why do people use these drugs?
Which drugs seem to be the most dangerous? Why?   I   U

Debate: Have students debate the issue of marijuana versus alcohol.   U

• *Teaching-learning stations:* Have a station with appropriate study
guide question-and-learning activities for each of the major
street drug classifications: hallucinogens, uppers, downers,
heroin, and marijuana.   I   U

Displays: Using artwork, pamphlets, and student-prepared posters, organize a display around a street drug theme that the
students select.   I   U

Position statements: Have students develop opinions on the fol-
lowing topics:
Dope pushing—a crime without a victim?
Which drugs would you use? not use?
You accidentally discover drugs in your thirteen-year-
old's room. What will you do? Defend your actions?
Rank the available drugs in the order you perceive them
to be in terms of hazardousness.   I   U

THE COMMUNITY AND DRUGS

Guest speakers: Many communities have highly developed drug
rehabilitation and prevention programs. Guest speakers are
available from such sources as Alcoholics Anonymous, half-
way houses, youth groups, crisis houses, juvenile authorities,
and church-related groups. The theme of their talks should
relate to community drug intervention, prevention, and
rehabilitation services.   I   U

Student reports can be generated by having students visit the various agencies in the community that deal with drugs and report to the class the organization and services of these
agencies.   I   U

Demonstrations should be given on the emergency care procedures for accidental poisoning and drug overdose. Particular care should be taken to explain that seeking medical attention for a drug overdose does not make one open for
criminal prosecution.   I   U

RECREATIONAL AND OTHER APPLICATION OF DRUGS

Student reports can be developed on the following topics:
Drugs for pain
Drugs for diet
Drugs for mental problems
Drugs for learning
Drugs for skill
Drugs for fatigue
Drugs for athletics   I   U

Have students complete open-ended statements such as these:

>To reward myself I . . .
>I feel guilty when . . .
>I feel terrific when . . .
>Drunks are . . .
>Taking drugs is . . .
>People take drugs because . . .   I   U

Autobiographies can be used for developing such ideas as the following:

>My favorite pleasures are . . .
>How do my friends influence me?
>The following are the things that turn me on to life . . .   I   U

Have students develop surveys to find out what turns people on to life and to compile a list of life's natural highs.   P   I   U

Buzz group topics can include the following:

>Guidelines for the recreational use of alcohol, tobacco, and other drugs.
>Who is mature enough for the recreational use of drugs?
>How should one celebrate?
>What is the role of peer pressure in the recreational use of drugs?
>What are some good ways to reduce tension and to get away from life's pressures for awhile?   P   I   U

The following topics can be utilized for classroom discussions and panel discussions:

>Should drugs be used for recreational purposes?
>Should you offer a friend a drug? Why? Why not?
>What kinds of drug-taking behavior do you find offensive?
>Why is individual tolerance an important factor in drug usage?
>What is the quality of street drugs?
>Who is ready for drugs?
>What are the reasons for the use of drugs? for the non-use of drugs?
>What is your personal decision concerning the use of medications, tobacco, and alcohol?   I   U

FAMILY LIFE EDUCATION

The major emphasis in family life education is on the issues of human relationships within the family unit, heterosexual interpersonal relationships, views of male and female roles, and guidelines for establishing and maintaining pair-bond relationships. The focus is on rational expectations within a framework of other-person-centered human relationships. In light of the major topics just mentioned, human reproduction, human growth, and the role of sex in our society account for only a small portion of family life education.

If one takes into consideration the fact that in some communities almost 30 percent of the adult population oppose the teaching of sex education in the schools,[26] it becomes evident that our young people are confronted with an enormous array of confusing and conflicting information upon which they must make very important decisions.

The following list presents reasons why family life education should be developed in the public schools.

1. The news and entertainment media have gone to great lengths to ignore the joys of the everyday human relation aspects and more usual characteristics of human sexuality. For monetary reasons, newspapers, magazines, television, and films inundate us with accounts of unusual and often bizarre behavior. While innovative nude photography, emphasis on the sexual act, and countless essays and articles devoted to fringe sexual and sex role groups are matters of individual taste, this kind of mass inoculation does have its side effects. Our young people now have a much wider and more confusing array of information upon which to base very important and rational decisions concerning family living, sex roles, and human sexuality.

2. The following statistical information builds a strong case for family life education:

   a. Slightly over 50 percent of a sample of young men and 65 percent of young women studied received sex information exclusively from friends, not from parents.[27]

   b. One-third of all marriages in the United States end in divorce. Well over half of all teenage marriages will end in divorce.[28]

   c. In his summary of statistics on venereal disease, Bender indicated that in the United States over 2,000 teenagers contract a venereal disease each day and that over 90,000 cases of syphilis and 1.4 million cases of gonorrhea are treated each year.[29]

   d. Even though birth control measures can be over 90 percent effective, more than 300,000 illegitimate births occur each year,[30] and 7,000 to 10,000 of the pregnant girls are between the ages of ten to fourteen years.[31]

THE FAMILY UNIT

What can children contribute to the home?
What is meant by other-person centered home living?
What kinds of stresses does modern society put on a family unit?
What is a definition of a good home?
Is the concept of family living becoming obsolete? Why? Why not?

SCOPE AND KEY QUESTIONS OF FAMILY LIFE EDUCATION

26. James L. McCary, *Human Sexuality* (New York: D. Van Nostrand Co., 1973), p. 17.
27. J. H. Gagnon, "Sexuality and Sexual Learning in the Child," *Psychiatry* 28 (1965): 212–228.
28. Arlene Skolnick, and Jerome Skolnick, *Intimacy, Family, and Society* (Boston: Little, Brown & Co., 1974), p. 4.
29. Stephen J. Bender, *Venereal Disease* (Dubuque, Iowa: Wm. C. Brown Co., Publishers 1971), pp. 1–4.
30. A. F. Guttmacher, "How Can We Best Combat Illigitimacy," *Medical Aspects of Human Sexuality* 3 (1969): 48–61.
31. Benjamin A. Kogan, *Human Sexual Expression* (New York: Harcourt Brace Jovanovich, 1973), p. 172.

How can relationships between brothers and sisters be improved?
How are family patterns changing?
What is the purpose of a home?
Who runs the home?

HUMAN GROWTH AND DEVELOPMENT

Why do people grow physically at different rates?
What causes growth and physical change?
Are there any emotional changes that are part of puberty?
What kinds of physical characteristics are genetic?
Which glands and hormones are involved in human growth and development?
What are the structures and functions of the male and female reproductive systems?
How important are the physical characteristics of the reproductive organs to an indivdiual's self-image?
How does conception take place?
How are sperm cells produced? What are nocturnal emissions?
What are the characteristics of the menstrual cycle?
What is sexual tension?
What are the major systems of the body?
What are the purposes of, location of, main organs of, importance of, and health problems of each of the major systems of the body? (Note: The major body systems are digestive, skeletal, muscular, circulatory, endocrine, respiratory, excretory, reproductive, and nervous systems.)

SOME CONSIDERATIONS CONCERNING BOY-GIRL RELATIONSHIPS

How do boys differ from girls in their views concerning the following factors:
Appearance
Play
Sports
Male/female roles
School
The boys . . . the girls in our class . . .
Friends
Things they like to do?
Which is the weaker sex?
How are the roles of men and women in our society changing?
How and when can a boy or girl have a friend of the opposite sex without there being a romantic attachment?
What is right or wrong with the boys/girls in our class?
Why do girls mature more quickly?
What are the advantages and disadvantages of being a boy? of being a girl?
How do boys and girls differ in their views of aging?
How can one be a good conversationalist with a person of the opposite sex?
Is it important to have friends of the opposite sex? Why?
How does home life for a boy differ from that for a girl?
What kinds of things do boys and girls think about the most?
How are emotional needs for boys different from those for girls?

DATING

Why should one date?

Who should date?

When should dating begin?

What is expected on a date?

How does one go about asking for, accepting, or refusing a date?

Should Mom or Dad be around when you have a group of people to your house?

Does or should your family influence whom you date? Explain.

How do you let someone know that you like him?

What should you do if someone expresses a romantic interest in you but you are not interested in that person?

What different types of dating patterns are there and how do you feel about them?

What role does money play in dating?

Why do older boys usually date younger girls?

What is wrong or right with the dating practices in our school?

What attracts people to one another?

What constitutes a good dating partner?

HUMAN SEXUALITY

Is there a sexual revolution? Defend your response.

What are the sexual standards of your age group?

How have values and standards concerning sexual behavior changed?

Who is responsible for the level of sexual activity in a relationship?

What is a meaningful versus an exploitive activity for the boy? for the girl?

How is promiscuity viewed in today's society?

What is the role of sex in casual dating, going steadily, long-term love relationships, marriage?

How does one know whether or not a relationship is based on sexual attraction or on other factors?

What factors are the most important to base a relationship on?

How do parents view the sexual behavior of their children?

What is your view about pornography?

What is your view concerning free love and the more unusual sexual patterns reported in the news media?

What factors are involved in sexual response?

How does the male view the role of sex? How does the female view the role of sex?

Why is there pressure on the male to "prove himself"?

What is homosexuality? How does society view it?

What factors should a couple consider before progressing to higher levels of sexual activity?

What are the specific methods of birth control?

How can venereal disease be prevented?

FAMILY LIVING

What kinds of adjustments do all members of a family have to make?

How can the roles of the modern wife and husband be described?

How important is religion in the home?

Do opposites attract? Do marriages between opposites end in divorce courts? Explain.

What are your expectations for marital decision making concerning the raising of children, finances, housing, professional responsibilities, social obligations, and housekeeping duties?

What are the characteristics of a good husband and father?

What are the characteristics of a good wife and mother?

When is a person ready for marriage?

Why is there a high divorce rate among people who marry before they are twenty-one?

How do in-laws and other relatives influence a marriage?

What influence do poor health, financial difficulty, and parent-child difficulty have on the home?

What special problems are there when there is only one parent in the home?

What adjustments must be made when both parents are working?

How should people communicate with one another in the home?

What kinds of problems do most people have with their parents?

What kinds of problems do most parents have with their children?

What kinds of responsibilities should children have in the home?

Table 15–4. Suggested Grade Placement for Family Life Education Topics

Topic	Grade Placement							
	K	1	2	3	4	5	6	7–8
Family unit	*	*	*	*	*	*	*	***
Family living	*	*	*	*	**	**	**	***
Some considerations concerning boy–girl relationships	*	*	*	*	**	**	**	**
Human growth and development	*	*	*	*	*	*	**	***
Dating								***
Human sexuality								***

Key: *** = major emphasis; ** = emphasis; * = touched upon or reviewed.

TEACHING STRATEGIES IN FAMILY LIFE EDUCATION

The key for suggested grade level use of the following teaching strategies is explained on page 288.

THE FAMILY UNIT

Surveys: Have peers make a list of the good things they contribute to their homes. Ask parents and grandparents to compare whether or not it is now more difficult to maintain a stable home and give the reasons for their answers.　I　U

Position papers: Students develop a brief essay using their own opinions on such topics as these:
The purpose of a family is . . .
Being other-person centered at home is . . .
Is the family unit becoming obsolete?　I　U

Display: Collect pictures and stories depicting things that families do together and problems a modern family might have.　P　I　U

Picture/Discussion: Collect a series of large pictures or drawings depicting family scenes. Ask students to discuss what is occur-

ring and what the members of the family in the pictures are
thinking.   P I

Role play: Have students depict a scene in which Dad comes home
and tells the family they must move out of state because of
a terrific new job opportunity. Another scene can be a family discussion about adjustments that will have to be made
because Mom has taken a nine-to-five job.   P I U

Problem solving: In groups have students develop a list of suggestions (1) for making new friends after a move, (2) for helping
at home if one parent is missing, and (3) for making special
adjustments if mother is working.   P I U

Discussion topics: Provide the following topics for class discussion:
> What does other-person centered mean?
> Compare the home life of previous generations as
>   depicted on television programs with the home
>   life of today.
> What kinds of problems can a family have?
> What are the good things about a home?   I U

HUMAN GROWTH AND DEVELOPMENT

Teacher-learning stations: Have students rotate in groups and
perform specific assignments for the following stations:
> Station 1. Diagrams of the male reproductive system
> Station 2. Diagrams of the female reproductive system
> Station 3. The endocrine system
> Station 4. Growth patterns
> Note: Each station should have appropriate filmstrips,
>   transparencies, study guides, and the like.   I U

Teaching-learning stations can also be used for studying the major systems of the body: digestive, skeletal, muscular, circulatory, endocrine, respiratory, excretory, reproductive, and
nervous systems. Study one system at a time by setting up
stations for studying the purpose of the system, the structure of the system, the importance of the system, and the
disorders of the system.   I U

Through classroom discussions, investigate the importance of
each of the major body systems. Have students rank the systems in order of importance (in their opinion). Also stress
the interrelatedness of the body systems and how the mal-
function of one system can disrupt function of the other
body systems.   I U

Using large pieces of brown wrapping paper, have groups of students draw in an outline of the human torso by tracing the
outline of one of their members. Without giving instruction
on the body structures, have the groups try to draw in and
label all the parts of the body. After there has been instruction on the body systems, have the groups repeat this exercise.   I U

As students study a body system have them develop crossword puzzles, anagrams, acrostics, synonyms, and antonyms for the various body structures and functions.   I U

Demonstrations can be utilized in family life education. For example, a concept of the population growth curve can be illustrated by having the teacher or students inoculate a petri dish and leave the dish (covered) in the sunlight for several days. Students will observe that the population of organisms increases dramatically and then dwindles and almost disappears when the food source is used up because of overpopulation. Another effective demonstration for developing a concept of reproduction is to raise live breeding fish or some type of rodent in the classroom.   P I U

Films and filmstrips: A number of excellently prepared audiovisual aids are available that describe the reproductive systems, birth process, and human growth. School boards and curriculum committees often wish to preview this type of visual aid; therefore, it is often advisable to check to determine which films and filmstrips have been judged acceptable. Also, preview these films before showing them. Films are available that range from the traditional diagrams and charts to very frank illustrations using live models.   I U

Displays: Develop a family photograph album using photographs of class members as toddlers, first graders, and the like. Develop a chart showing typical growth patterns. Another idea for a display is to focus on inherited characteristics.   P I U

Guest speakers: Guest experts are available to discuss human reproduction, birth control, and venereal disease. Teachers must be careful, however, not to rely on these guests for all of the instruction in these areas. Prepare the students well in advance with lessons in these areas and follow through on reviewing the material covered by the guest speakers.   I U

Question box: Students are often reluctant to ask questions regarding sexuality and the reproductive system. If students turn in specific questions (of any nature) anonymously, a wider range of information can be developed. Teachers using this technique will be amazed at the kinds of misconceptions students have as well as the kinds of things that worry them about human sexuality.   I U

SOME CONSIDERATIONS CONCERNING BOY-GIRL RELATIONSHIPS

Debate: Using the guidelines of an interscholastic debate, have students debate the following motion: Resolved: Men are the weaker sex.   I U

Position papers: In their own words have students develop both sides of and present their views on the following issues:

What is the best and the worst about being a boy? about being a girl?

The best things about boys/girls are . . .
The worst things about boys/girls are . . .
What is your view of masculinity?
What is your view of femininity?   I   U

Discussion questions that can be utilized for panel discussion,
large groups, or buzz groups include the following:
Who is the weaker sex?
What are the characteristics of a good friend of the op-
posite sex?
What are the different interests of boys and of girls?
What kinds of advantages are there in being a boy? in be-
ing a girl?   P   I   U

Displays: Have groups of students determine the role of men and
women in society. Have them illustrate their views by using
drawings, posters, photographs, and stories.   P   I   U

DATING

Drama: Have students write and present scenes depicting dating
problems, parents and dating, asking for a date, dating courtesy, and other dating situations.   U

Advice to the Lovelorn: Have students write to a class panel of
experts regarding dating problems and practices. The teacher
will need a sense of humor and should be prepared for anything with this strategy.   U

Role playing scenes are probably the most effective means of
illustrating some of the communication and human relations aspects of dating. Have students role play how to ask
for, accept, or refuse a date; how to introduce your date to
your parents; getting home later than your parents wanted
you to after a date; trying to discourage someone whom you
are not interested in.   U

Panel discussions: Separate the class into several small groups and
have them discuss the following topics:
How do we know that we are ready for dating?
The role of parents in dating
What to do on a date
The male versus the female view of dating practices   U

Discussion topics that are appropriate for large or small group dis-
cussions include:
How do you feel about the different types of dating
patterns?
Who should make the decisions in a dating relationship?
What are the characteristics of a good date?
What are some suggestions for dating courtesy?   U

Surveys can provide a basis for several interesting discussions. Sur-
vey questions can include the following:
The three things I like to do most on a date
The three things I like to do least on a date
How much to spend on a date

The female view of the characteristics of a good date
The male view of the characteristics of a good date
Things that most attract boys to girls
Things that most attract girls to boys U

Autobiography topics can include topics such as:
I date because . . .
I like to be with someone who . . .
My parents view of dating is . . .
As a dating partner my strengths are . . . and my weaknesses
are . . . U

Problem-solving buzz groups can attempt to develop guidelines
for how to host a party, how to talk to a parent about dating
problems, how to get asked for a date, what to do on a blind
date, and other specific dating problems. U

HUMAN SEXUALITY

Have a guest panel of community experts or have students assume
the role of experts on the role of sex in dating, serious dating,
and marriage. U

Question box: Students often have questions that are too personal
or that they feel would be too embarrassing to ask in front of
their peers. Simply have students write down their questions
and put them unsigned in a designated question box. The
teacher may then discuss the questions at the end of each lesson. I U

For a problem-solving activity have students develop a series of
real-life situations that demand decision making in regard
to ethics, other-person-centered solutions, and sexual behavior. U

Role play a scene in which parents are in the process of telling
their son or daughter what is expected of them in terms of
sexual/moral behavior. U

Utilizing both small and large group discussions, have students
express opinions concerning such topics as the role of sex,
how to define an exploitive relationship, the male view versus the female view of sexual behavior, who is responsible for
the level of sexual behavior in a relationship, society's view
of homosexuality, pornography laws, parental view of the sexual behavior of their children, promiscuity, and the modern
view of sexual behavior. U

Guest speakers can be very effective in discussing family planning,
agencies that assist unwed mothers, problems of being an
unwed mother, venereal disease control and prevention, and
problems of teenage marriage. U

FAMILY LIVING

Survey: Have students collect opinions on the power structure of
a marriage such as who should make the decisions concern-

ing financial matters, housing, furniture, raising children, employment, circle of friends, and housekeeping duties.   U

Panel discussions: Panel discussions can be particularly effective when such issues as the following are under consideration:

      Parent-child relationships

      Modern roles of husbands and wives

      Family planning

      Characteristics of a good marriage

      Adjustments children have to make in single-parent homes

      Working mothers and the responsibilities children should have in the home

Note: Be sure to involve all class members in the discussions.   I   U

Problem solving: These activities can include topics such as these:

      You feel your parents are not giving you enough trust or freedom. What can you do?

      Your son or daughter has been found to have drugs in his or her room. What would you do?

      Your brother or sister is in with the wrong crowd.

      You are in a family in which divorce proceedings are in progress.

      Your parents do not like your circle of friends.

      No one listens to you at home.

      Your mother and father both work until 6:00 P.M. everyday.

      You do not get along with your brothers and sisters.   P   I   U

Valuing activities: Ask students to evaluate these situations:

      What are the ten best things about home? the ten worst things?

      What are your expectations of your parents?

      How do you perceive how a dad, mom, brother, or sister should be?

      How can you contribute to your family?   P   I   U

Role plays and dramas: Have groups of students portray real-life family scenes. Follow each dramatization with a class discussion concerning the human relationships illustrated and the implications of each alternative manner for handling the various problems.   P   I   U

Lively classroom discussions can revolve around such topics as the following:

      What bugs children about home?

      How do children bug parents?

      How are you treated differently from your brothers or sisters?

      What are some of the worse things that children can do at home? How would you react to these things if you were a parent?

      What can you do if one of your parents is sick or injured?

      Should children just receive an allowance? or earn it?

      What does being a good son or daughter mean?

How can children get their parents to listen?

How should your friends act when they are in your home?

How much privacy should people have in their own home?   P I U

References

Abrams, R S., Vanecko, M., and Abrams, I. "A Suggested School Mental Health Program." *Journal of School Health* 42 (1972): 137–141.

American Medical Association. *Health Education Services for Schools and Colleges* 12 (1972): 1.

Bender, Stephen J. *Venereal Disease.* Dubuque, Iowa: Wm. C. Brown Co., 1971.

Blum, Richard. "Schools Are Not Effective in Drug Education." *Drugs and Drug Abuse Newsletter* 3 (1972): 1.

Brecher, Edward M. *Licit and Illicit Drugs.* Boston: Little, Brown & Co., 1972.

Brown, James D. "Illinois Trends in Elementary School Drug Education: The Soft Sell." *Journal of Drug Education* 3 (1973): 157–163.

DeLone, Richard H. "The Ups and Downs of Drug Abuse Education." *Saturday Review,* 11 November 1972, pp. 27–32.

Educational Policies Commission. *The Central Purposes of Education.* Washington, D.C.: National Education Association, 1961.

Fort, Joel. *The Pleasure Seekers: The Drug Crisis, Youth and Society.* Indianapolis, Ind.: Bobbs-Merrill Co., 1969.

Gagnon, J. H. "Sexuality and Sexual Learning in the Child." *Psychiatry* 28 (1965): 212–228.

Glavin, John P. "Persistence of Behavior Disorders in Children." *Exceptional Children* 38 (1972): 367–375.

Guttmacher, A. F. "How Can We Best Combat Illegitimacy." *Medical Aspects of Human Sexuality* 3 (1969): 48–61.

Halleck, Seymour. "The Great Drug Education Hoax." *The Progressive.* Madison, Wis., 1970.

Hochbaum, Godfrey M. "How Can We Teach Adolescents About Smoking, Drinking, and Drug Abuse?" *Journal of Health, Physical Education and Recreation* 3 (1972): 2.

Kogan, Benjamin A. *Human Sexual Expression.* New York: Harcourt Brace Jovanovich, Inc., 1973.

Levy, Marvin R. "Background Consideration for Drug Programs." In *Resource Book for Drug Abuse Education.* PHS Publication no. 1964. Washington, D.C.: National Clearinghouse for Mental Health Information.

McCary, James L. *Human Sexuality.* New York: D. Van Nostrand Co., 1973.

Macro Systems, Inc. *Evaluation of Drug Education Programs: Main Report.* Silver Spring, Md.: Macro Systems, Inc., June 1972.

Mantz, Genelle K. "Can Mental Health Be Taught?" *Journal of School Health* 42 (1972): 398–399.

Martin, Lealon E. *Mental Health/Mental Illness: Revolution in Progress.* New York: McGraw-Hill Book Co., 1970.

Rhodes, W. C. "The Disturbing Child: A Problem of Ecological Management." *Exceptional Children* 33 (1967): 449–454.

Second Report of National Commission on Marihuana and Drug Abuse. *Drug Use in America: Problem in Perspective.* Washington, D.C.: Government Printing Office, 1973.

Select Committee on Crime. *Drugs in Our Schools.* Washington, D.C.: Government Printing Office, 1973.

Silver, Archie A., and Hagin, Rosa A. "Profile of a First Grade: A Basis for Preventive Psychiatry." *Journal of American Academy of Child Psychiatry* 11 (1972): 645–674.

Skolnick, Arlene, and Skolnick, Jerome. *Intimacy, Family, and Society.* Boston: Little, Brown & Co., 1974.

"Summary of the 1970 Consumer Expenditures." *Supermarketing* 26 (1971): 39.

Task Force on Prescription Drugs. *The Drug Users.* Washington, D.C.: Government Printing Office, 1969.

Wolfson, Edward A., Lavenhar, Marvin A., Blum, Richard, Quinones, Mark A., Einstein, Stanley, and Louria, Donald B. "Survey of Drug Abuse in Six New Jersey High Schools: Methodology and General Findings." In *Student Drug Surveys,* ed. Stanley Einstein. Farmingdale, N.Y.: Baywood Publishing Co., 1972.

Yolles, Stanley. "Managing Mood Changes." *Journal of Drug Education* 1 (1971): 104–105.

Chapter 16
SELECTED
AREAS
OF
HEALTH
INSTRUCTION

By grade level, what are the needs of students in the major areas of health education?

What are some philosophical considerations for selecting teaching approaches in certain health education areas?

What is a suggested scope for each major topic area in health education?

What key questions are available for each topic area?

What specific teaching activities are available for each topic within the major health education areas?

The offerings in this chapter are designed to generate ideas and to form a philosophical base for teaching the following major health education areas: dental health, nutrition, safety, personal health and fitness, consumer health, ecological concepts and environmental quality, and communicable and chronic disease. As in chapter 15, the purpose of this chapter is to provide teachers with a clear idea of the scope of each major topic area and the tools with which to generate individualized curriculum guides, units, and lesson plans.

DENTAL HEALTH

Dental caries, periodontal disease, and loss of teeth are major health problems for all age groups. Even a conservative estimate finds that 90 percent of the population of the United States have some type of dental disease.[1] Approximately 25 million people are without natural teeth.[2] Some important statistics in regard to school age children include:[3]

1. Upon entering school the average child has three decayed teeth.
2. Children usually have eleven decayed teeth by age fifteen years.
3. About one in four children loose teeth because of caries.

1. American Dental Association, *Survey of Needs for Dental Care* (Chicago: American Dental Association, 1965), p. 38.
2. J. C. Green, "Dental Health Needs of the Nation," *Journal of American Dental Association* 84 (1972): 1073–1075.
3. Ibid.

4. Fifty percent of our population suffer from malocclusion, and 25 percent of those suffering from malocclusion have serious problems.

Dental health is a complex science involving genetics, nutrition, economics, prenatal care, professional service, and home care. Heredity, for example, plays a role in that a few individuals are free of caries in spite of poor oral hygiene practices. Dietary deficiencies, poor food selection, and sugar intake have proved to be major factors in dental disease.[4] Also, lack of calcium in the diet of the mother can seriously influence the prenatal dental development of the fetus.[5] It has also been found that improved economic conditions influence positively the number of people seeking professional dental care. However, the fact remains that 42.6 percent of the nation's preschool children never visit a dentist.[6] Home care and diet appear to be the most significant factors in dental health.

Considering what is known about the causes and prevention of dental disease, one of the more obvious preventative measures lies in expanding dental health education. Elementary and preschool dental health education may provide one of the most effective approaches to reducing dental disease.[7] Research supports the effectiveness of elementary school dental health education. For example, Friedman found that schools can effectively reduce caries and improve dental health practices, while Stolpe et al. discovered that a passive dental health program did not yield positive results.[8, 9]

Dental health is one of the health topics that needs to be emphasized several times throughout a kindergarten through grade twelve curriculum.

Table 16–1.   Suggested Grade Placement for Dental Topics

Topic	K	1	2	3	4	5	6	7–8
Structure and function of oral structures and teeth	*	*	*	*	***	**	**	***
Dental caries and periodontal disease	*	*	*	*	***	**	**	***
Prevention	**	**	***	**	***	***	***	***
Malocclusion and other disorders					*	**	**	***
Dental health services and selection of dental aids		*	*	*	*	*	*	**
Attitudes toward dental health	**	**	**	**	**	**	**	**

Key: *** = major emphasis; ** = emphasis; * = touched upon or reviewed.

4. Henry W. Scherp, "Dental Caries: Prospects for Prevention," *Science* 173 (1971): 1199–1205.
5. Ibid.
6. U.S., Department of Health, Education, and Welfare, *The Health of Children* (Washington, D.C.: Government Printing Office, 1970).
7. Donald H. Masters, "The Classroom Teacher . . . Effective Dental Health Education," *Journal of School Health* 42 (1972): 257–261.
8. Lawrence A. Friedman, "Impact of Teacher-Student Dental Health Education," *Journal of School Health* 44 (1974): 140–143.
9. J. R. Stolpe, R. E. Mechlenberg, and R. L. Lathrop, "The Effectiveness of an Educational Program on Oral Health in Schools for Improving the Application of Knowledge," *Journal of Public Health Dentistry* 31 (1971): 30.

Fortunately the topic includes laboratory-type activities that students enjoy, and the key points needed to understand structure, function, causes and prevention of dental disease are not difficult to grasp. In general, the methodology of dental health education should emphasize the development and performance of oral hygiene skills and the existing oral examination techniques.

SCOPE AND KEY QUESTIONS OF DENTAL HEALTH

STRUCTURE AND FUNCTION OF ORAL STRUCTURES AND TEETH

Why are the teeth considered part of the digestive system?
What is the role of the salivary glands?
What is mastication? How does mastication work?
What kinds of teeth are in the mouth? What are their functions?
How is a tooth constructed?
What causes people to lose their teeth?
What kinds of bacteria are in the mouth?
How can teeth be replaced?
What is the role of heredity in the formation of teeth?
What are the taste buds? Where are they?
What are the functions of the tongue?

DENTAL CARIES AND PERIODONTAL DISEASE

What is the role of diet in dental disease?
How do bacteria cause dental disease?
What is the role of sugar in dental caries?
What is dental plaque?
What role does saliva play in tooth decay?
What causes gingivitis?
What occurs if periodontal infections are left untreated?
What are the treatments for dental caries and periodontal diseases?

PREVENTION

How can plaque be controlled?
How often should individuals visit a dentist for a checkup and professional cleaning?
What are the directions for flossing and brushing the teeth?
What foods are the best to eat? the worst?
What is the role of fluorides in dental health?

MALOCCLUSION AND OTHER DISORDERS

What causes malocclusion?
How can proper care of primary teeth prevent malocclusion?
What kinds of habits cause malocclusion?
What are the long-range effects of not correcting malocclusion?
How does an orthodontist correct malocclusion?
What is trench mouth and how can it be prevented or treated?
What are the symptoms of oral cancer?

DENTAL HEALTH SERVICES AND SELECTION OF DENTAL AIDS

What are the educational qualifications of a dentist?
How often should one visit a dentist?
What does a dentist have to do to repair one's teeth?

What kinds of toothpastes are best? worst?
How does one select a toothbrush properly?
What kinds of medications work best on sores in the mouth?
What do you do if you have a toothache? Should one seek professional attention for each toothache?
How do you prevent bad breath?
What causes bad breath?
Do mouthwashes help reduce the bacteria in the mouth?
What kinds of things irritate the mouth and gums?

ATTITUDES TOWARD DENTAL HEALTH
Why do not people take better care of their teeth?
Why is it important to study dental health?
What is your opinion of people who have bad teeth?
How do you view persons with braces on their teeth?
How do you feel about going to the dentist?
Who influences you the most to take care of your teeth?
Why do not people brush their teeth after every meal?
How do you feel about your teeth?
Why do not people floss their teeth regularly?
Why do not people control their intake of candy and sweets when they know it causes tooth decay?

Appropriate grade levels are suggested for each teaching strategy and appear in a key in the column at the right of each strategy. Use the key as follows: P, most suited for the primary levels (kindergarten through grade three); I, most suited for the intermediate levels (grade four through grade six); U, most suited for the upper levels (grade seven and grade eight).

TEACHING STRATEGIES IN DENTAL HEALTH

STRUCTURE AND FUNCTION OF ORAL STRUCTURES AND TEETH

Organize teaching-learning stations where students can study the function and structure of the teeth and the digestive system. At each station have appropriate models, filmstrips, checklists, and other visual aids.   I   U

Develop a bulletin board or other display illustrating the structures of the mouth.   P   I   U

Form a realia center in which actual teeth, orthodontia models, dental aids, and dentistry equipment are displayed.   P   I   U

Organize a food-tasting party after showing where the taste buds are located in the tongue.   P   I   U

Demonstrate the action of saliva by having students chew a piece of bread until it becomes sweet.   P   I   U

Discuss the functions of different types of teeth and ask the students to develop a list of problems caused by poor oral hygiene.   P   I   U

DENTAL CARIES AND PERIODONTAL DISEASE
Realia: Have displays of the following items:
    Dentist tools
    Decayed teeth

Xrays
Orthodontia models
Athletic mouth protectors
Dental floss
Toothbrush   P I U

Demonstrate how bacteria grow in the mouth by inoculating a
    sterilized petri dish with a sample from the mouth of a stu-
    dent. Have another petri dish serve as a control. Any small,
    covered plastic or glass container can be used in place of a
    commercially prepared petri dish. The media for culturing
    the bacteria can be made from gelatin slightly sweetened
    with sugar. Sterilize the dishes with the media in them by
    placing them in an oven at 120 degrees for one hour. After
    inoculation, place them upside down in a warm place.   P I U

Illustrate the importance of tooth enamel by puncturing the skin
    of an apple to show how rapidly the flesh decays after the
    skin has been punctured.   P I U

Obtain a guest speaker such as a dentist or hygienist. These peo-
    ple often have specially prepared presentations for school
    groups.   P I U

Allow students to develop individual studies or student reports
    on the different aspects of dental caries and periodontal
    disease.   I U

Place a donated primary tooth in a glass of soda pop to illustrate
    how acid destroys enamel. A similar but more rapid disin-
    tegration occurs when an egg is placed in a bowl of vinegar.   P I U

Develop a series of cartoons around a character such as Phidius
    Plaque to illustrate how plaque is formed and prevented and
    the role of plaque in gingivitis.   P I U

PREVENTION

Have the students design and give a survey asking students and
    adults to honestly report how they care for their teeth. In
    addition ask the subjects to identify the number of teeth they
    have had filled or have lost due to caries. Follow with a class
    discussion of the results of the survey.   I U

Interview students and adults about their brushing and flossing
    habits.   I U

Bring in enough toothbrushes for all class members and have
    demonstrations and practice sessions on the proper way to
    brush teeth. Also teach how to floss in this manner. Using
    disclosing tablets and mirrors, have the students check to
    see how well they brush and floss. Note: Disclosing tablets
    can be purchased at many pharmacies.   P I U

Have students make their own tooth powder from baking soda,
    salt, and peppermint flavoring. Follow with a discussion
    on the role of toothpaste in preventing dental caries.   P I U

Develop bulletin board displays and charts illustrating how to brush and floss. Also display the proper tools for caring for teeth.   P I U

Plan a field trip to a dentist's office and if possible arrange for all the students to have a dental inspection.   P I

Dramatizations: Role play scenes such as going to the dentist's office, interviewing someone who doesn't brush his teeth, and reacting to bad breath commercials.   I U

Post a daily checklist for students to record the brushing and flossing of their teeth.   P

Demonstrate the effectiveness of the proper choice of foods by using the following activity: Select four subjects. Have each student chew a disclosing tablet. Then have one subject eat a cracker; one, a carrot; one, an apple; and the fourth, some soft candy. Compare the results. Have all students eat a cracker and later a piece of celery or carrot to compare how clean their teeth feel.   P I U

For a period of time have all students brush their teeth after lunch or midmorning snack. Check for proper brushing technique.   P I

MALOCCLUSION AND OTHER DISORDERS
Through a lecture/discussion carefully explain other disorders such as oral cancer, broken teeth, and infections.   I U

Illustrate through drawings or by demonstration the kinds of habits that can contribute to malocclusion.   P I U

DENTAL HEALTH SERVICES AND SELECTION OF DENTAL AIDS
Through class discussion, develop criteria for the selection of dental services.   U

Have students bring in advertisements for dental aids. Analyze these ads and have students develop criteria for evaluating health advertising.   I U

Have students do individual reports on the training of dentists and dental hygienists.   I U

ATTITUDES TOWARD DENTAL HEALTH
Hold class discussions on the following topics:
How do you feel your teeth influence your appearance?
Who influences you to care for your teeth?
How do you feel about going to the dentist?
Why do not people care for their teeth?
How important is a good smile?   P I U

Have students complete such open-ended statements as the following:
I brush my teeth only . . .
The dentist . . .

My teeth are important to be because . . .
I don't brush my teeth when . . .   I   U

What do you do when the following situations occur?
    You cannot brush your teeth.
    You have a toothache.
    You have run out of toothpaste.
    You have broken or chipped a tooth.   P   I   U

NUTRITION

Although a large portion of the world is starving, at least 10 percent of the children and 25 percent of the adults in the United States are overweight. In addition, Americans spend an estimated half billion dollars a year on food supplements, weight control nostrums, and food fads.[10] Furthermore, approximately 9 percent of the population with income over $10,000 maintain poor diets.[11] The need for nutrition education is evident in the tragedy of the obese child, in the increased threat of heart disease, in medical problems due to poor nutrition, in the prevalence of food fads, in the practice of quackery, and in the rapidly rising food costs. [12,13]

The emphasis in nutrition education should be on decision-making activities pointed at meeting the basic nutritional needs of the students. Being a good consumer, role of diet in health, weight control, and world food production are the kinds of topics that students enjoy. Students are also interested in food fads and fallacies. Conservation of our human and natural resources should be an underlying theme. It is important that teachers not continue to have students memorize the traditional nutritional information concerning dietary essentials, recommended dietary allowances, unusual nutritional deficiencies, and the basic four food groups. Emphasis should be placed on understanding and decision making.

Table 16–2.   Suggested Grade Placement for Nutrition Topics

	Grade Placement							
Topics	K	1	2	3	4	5	6	7–8
Understanding digestive system	*	*	*	*	**	**	***	**
Dietary essentials	*	*	**	**	**	**	**	***
Overweight, obesity, and weight control					*	**	**	***
Diet and disease	*	*	*	*	*	**	*	***
Food fads and fallacies				*	**	**	**	***
Food selection	**	**	**	**	**	**	**	**

Key: *** = major emphasis;   ** = emphasis;   * = touched upon or reviewed.

10. Jean Mayer, *Health* (New York: D. Van Nostrand Co., 1974), pp. 115–152.
11. U.S., Department of Agriculture, *Dietary Levels in the United States, Spring, 1965* (Washington, D.C.: Government Printing Office, 1968).
12. Myron Winick, "Childhood Obesity," *Nutrition Today* 9 (1974): 6–12.
13. Alex Comfort, "Eat Less, Live Longer," *New Scientist* 53 (1972): 689.

UNDERSTANDING THE DIGESTIVE SYSTEM

What is metabolism and what are the energy requirements of the body?

What are the roles of carbohydrates, fats, proteins, and water in the metabolic process?

What are the major parts of the digestive system and their function?

What are the major digestive juices and enzymes?

How is food absorbed into the bloodstream?

How is food moved through the digestive system?

How is food eliminated from the system?

What kinds of factors upset the digestive system?

How are drugs absorbed and eliminated from the body?

DIETARY ESSENTIALS

What are the functions of the following six dietary essentials?

Fats

Carbohydrates

Proteins

Water

Vitamins

Minerals

Should people take vitamin supplements? when? what kinds?

What is the vitamin C controversy about? What is your stand on this issue?

OVERWEIGHT, OBESITY, AND WEIGHT CONTROL

What are the causes of obesity?

What is obesity? overweight?

Why are medical authorities concerned about overweight children?

Does heredity play a role in obesity?

What are the health consequences of being obese? of being overweight?

What are the social consequences of being obese? of being overweight?

Are overweight people carefree?

What is the role of activity in obesity?

Why is food selection so important in weight control?

What are some of the fad diets? Why do medical authorities dislike these diets?

How does one go about gaining or losing weight in a healthful manner?

Why is it that two people can eat the same foods and one gains weight and the other does not?

Why should we count calories?

What kinds of foods should people trying to lose weight not eat?

How effective are diet aids?

DIET AND DISEASE

How does the digestive system react to stress?

What kinds of diseases are caused by improper diet?

What is the relationship between diet and heart disease?

What is an ulcer?

What are the symptoms of a digestive disorder?

What is meant by food poisoning? by food infection?

What is botulism?

How can one tell if food is spoiled?

What are the rules for the storage of food?

What kinds of health problems can occur from improper food handling?

Should people use over-the-counter remedies for digestive disorders?

What are the long-range effects of improper diet?

Who needs special diets?

What is constipation and how can it be avoided?

FOOD FADS AND FALLACIES

Does anyone need vitamin and mineral supplements?

What are some of the old wives' tales about food? Which ones are true?

What is the truth about organic foods?

What is a macrobiotic diet?

What is the truth about vegetarianism?

Do athletes need dietary supplements?

What kinds of quackery occur in nutrition?

Are modern foods overprocessed?

In regard to food production and processing, what are the consumer-protection agencies?

FOOD SELECTION

What are your eating patterns, caloric intake, and intake of vitamins and minerals?

Do your patterns of eating change on weekends?

What are the Basic Four Food Groups?

How does exercise influence the kinds of food one should eat?

What are some guidelines for the purchase of food?

What kinds of foods should be selected for snacks?

Why should we eat a good breakfast?

What constitutes a good breakfast?

How can you determine what is a good buy in a grocery store?

What are empty calories?

What are the special dietary needs of growing children?

What is the function of each of the Basic Four Food Groups?

What are the causes of the current increase in food costs?

Should students drink caffeinated beverages?

What are some simple rules for reducing food waste?

TEACHING STRATEGIES IN NUTRITION

The key for suggested grade level use of the following teaching strategies is explained on page 327.

UNDERSTANDING THE DIGESTIVE SYSTEM

Drawing: In groups have students try to draw in the digestive organs on an outline form prior to studying the digestive system. Have a list of the organs on the board.   I   U

Puzzle: Have an outline of the digestive system on a large chart. Give each student a label for one of the organs of the digestive system. One at a time, ask them to come up and place the label in its proper place. The class could be divided into teams, and this activity could be scored as a game.   I   U

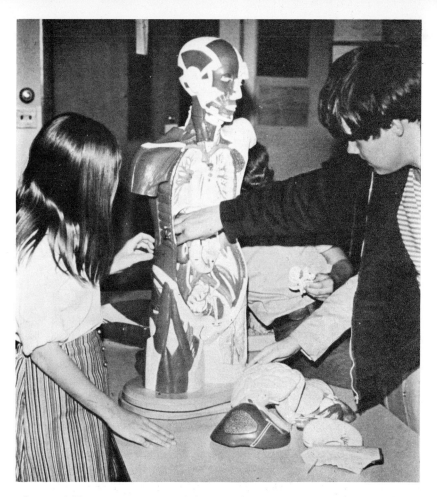

Fig. 16–1. Students at a learning station organized around the health topic understanding the digestive system. (Photo by L. K. Olsen.)

Films and filmstrips: Because of the complex nature of trying to illustrate how food gets from the stomach to the cells and how waste is eliminated, teachers should try to procure films that can provide a visual picture of these complex digestive activities.   P I U

Fish game: Place paper-clipped tags with the names of the organs in a large basket. Provide the students with a fishing pole with a small magnet attached. Divide the students into teams and keep score as they draw a name and try to identify the function of the organ named.   I U

Experiments: Arrange for the following experiments:

  1. Swallowing: Illustrate peristaltic action by having a head-stand expert swallow water while standing on his head. P I U

  2. Mastication: In separate glasses of water place a ground-up cube of sugar and a whole lump of sugar. Note how much of the ground-up cube of sugar dissolves. Follow with a discussion on the importance of ample chewing of food.   P I U

3. Food to the cells: Illustrate that certain foods can pass through cell walls more easily than others by performing this experiment: Fold a four-by-four-inch piece of paper towel to act as a filter cone; place the cone in a glass of water; put equal parts of salt and cocoa in the filter. Note by tasting that the water is salty but does not have the taste of cocoa. Follow with a discussion of how chemicals pass through the stomach and cell walls. I U

4. Food energy waste: Burn a sugar cube, noting that heat is given off and waste is accumulated. Follow with a discussion of heat and energy and how the body has to eliminate the waste products. P I U

5. Have students chew a piece of bread until it becomes sweet. This illustrates the effect of the enzymes in saliva. Follow with a discussion of the digestive juices and enzymes. I U

Have student reports and individual projects on the parts of the digestive system. I U

DIETARY ESSENTIALS

Develop riddles so that students can identify the purpose and function of the dietary essentials. I U

Have students develop scrapbooks or displays in which they can have pictures of sources of the dietary essentials. P I U

Have students give individual reports on the different dietary essentials. I U

Survey the class for their favorite food within the four basic food groups. Have them analyze this food in terms of calorie, protein, fat, carbohydrate, vitamin, and mineral content. I U

OVERWEIGHT, OBESITY, AND WEIGHT CONTROL

Have students prepare confidential statements concerning their view of overweight people, the problems of being overweight, physical self-image, and how people should look. I U

Select some of the current fad diets and analyze them for vitamin and mineral content, and the like. I U

Discuss best ways to lose or gain weight, role of activity in weight control, views of an obese person, selecting the right kind of snacks, who should or should not diet, and why balanced meals are important for growing bodies. I U

Have a survey of the class to list their favorite snack foods. Check these foods for caloric content on a large chart. I U

Interview adults of different ages to find out how they keep their weight down and why. I U

At random, select six different students for a detailed diet study. In the study include all food eaten for three days, and analyze the food intake for the dietary essentials and recommended daily intake. Discuss the differences. Make a special effort to protect the obese child from embarrassment. I U

Develop a poster campaign against empty calories. I U

Obtain a guest speaker from a Weight Watchers or Tops Club. Note that the emphasis is on balanced meals and counting calories, not on starvation or diet aids. I U

Collect advertisements for diet aids. Discuss cost, fine print, truth in the advertising, and effectiveness of the aids. Make special note of the mechanical devices and their hazards. I U

DIET AND DISEASE

Have students read stories about food-related epidemics. Also have them bring in newspaper stories about contaminated water supplies as a result of natural disasters. U

Discuss the effects of food poisoning after asking if anyone has had an attack or heard of the circumstances in which an attack occurred. Follow with a discussion of proper food handling. I U

Discuss how the digestive system responds to stress. Explore the implications of the responses. P I U

Set up student-learning stations or assign student reports on the parts of the digestive system and related disorders. At each station should be appropriate study guide sheets, filmstrips, books, models, and pamphlets. I U

Schedule a trip to a facility that specializes in food preparation. P I U

Have students prepare checklists to take home in regard to food handling and storage. Include how to prevent spoilage in home-canning operations I U

FOOD FADS AND FALLACIES

Have the class prepare a list of food myths and fallacies. Have them quiz adults and other students. Discuss the findings. I U

Have a panel discussion or a debate on the current emphasis on organic foods. U

Role play a high-pressure quack food or fake elixir pusher. Discuss why people fall for such terms as *subclinical deficiency*. I U

Do an analysis of one of the more dangerous fad diets. U

On separate days, bring in a guest speaker from a local organic food store and a speaker from an agency such as the National Dairy Council. U

FOOD SELECTION

National food patterns: Have students discuss or describe their favorite foods and an unusual dish their family enjoys.

Christmas is an excellent chance to have students bring samples of different pastries for tasting. P I U

Have secret observers make a check of the kinds and amounts of food uneaten during lunch hour. Decide how to solve this problem of waste. Perhaps a checklist or poster campaign might be the answer. P I U

Develop a poster or display of the Basic Four Food Groups. Use photographs of actual food. Ideally, this can be combined with a tasting party. P I U

Divide the class into seven groups and have each group plan menus for a week. Include breakfast, lunch, supper, and snacks. I U

Visit a grocery store and have students with shopping lists in hand bargain shop for the best possible values. They simply record the price of what they would buy, with no actual purchases being made. Upon returning to class compare how each group did. I U

Have an animal nutrition study in which one animal in a group of the same species is fed an inferior diet for a short period of time. Record the weights of the animals and keep a careful list of all food eaten. P I U

Have students do a detailed self-diet study. Each study should include caloric, protein, and vitamin intake, and analyses and conclusions should be made. I U

Have students write for materials and pamphlets from agencies dealing with food production, handling, and promotion. I U

Have a food of the week. Include a description of the nutritive value of the food and have a tasting party. P I

Have the students plan and prepare a well-balanced lunch for visiting parents. P I

Have students choose a nutrition problem. Help them define the problem, narrow the topic, and proceed toward a solution of the problem. I U

On a prepared checklist have students record the foods their family wastes in a single day. Follow this with a discussion of world food production and famine. P I U

Plan field trips to dairies, food-processing plants, and well-organized farms and retail agencies. Interview each about food processing and ask for opinions about rising food costs. Compare responses upon return to class. P I U

Hold a class discussion on whether people need vitamin pills. Include a discussion on the organic foods and vitamin C controversies. U

Have students indicate their favorite snack foods. Follow with an analysis of cost and nutritive value of the snacks. Offer alternatives if necessary. P I U

Chapter 16

Discuss the dietary needs of special groups such as athletes, dia-
betics, babies, and others who require special diets.   P   I   U

Accidents are the most important health problem of elementary school
children. Accidents account for more deaths of school age children than all
other causes combined.[14] The grim statistics include an annual loss of
approximately 8,400 children. Included within this figure are 2,000 pedestrians, 500 pedacyclists, and 1,700 motor vehicle fatalities; 1,400 drowning
and 650 fire victims; 600 firearm accidents; and 200 suffocation and 200 fall
victims. Although accurate statistics are not available, the number of injuries each year is enormous. For example, toys alone have been estimated to
cause 700,000 injuries per year,[15] and school injuries have been estimated
at 800,000 each year. The statistical evidence clearly indicates that safety
should be the number-one health concern in the elementary school. Schools
have a moral, as well as a legal, obligation to protect and teach children in
a safe environment.

The philosophy of safety education is to have students live safety, not
to just make students aware that safety rules exist. Living safety represents
day-to-day emphasis on performing all activities in a safe manner, protecting others, and appreciating that safety skills enhance the enjoyment of
life. Table 16–3 illustrates some of the do's and don'ts of safety education.

SAFETY

Table 16–3.   Do's and Don'ts of Safety Education

Do's	Don'ts
Have students develop safety rules.	Simply post or relate the rules.
Say Do this and you will be less likely to hurt yourself or others.	Say Don't.
Safety is a group activity.	Safety is only for oneself.
Tell the why of the rule.	Just give the rule without explanation.
Teach through doing.	Just show or verbalize the rule.
Emphasize living safely each day.	Have periodic safety lessons.
Develop the concept that safety skills lead to more adventure.	Make safety just another set of rules.
Explain that safety is for the protection of others.	Risk taking is a personal thing.
Safety is for greater enjoyment.	Safety is freedom from injury.

Table 16–4.   Suggested Grade Placement for Safety Topics

Topic	*** Grade Placement K	1	2	3	4	5	6	7–8
School safety	***	***	***	***	***	**	**	**
Safety at home	*	**	*	**	*	**	**	**
Psychology of accidents				*	*	*	**	***
Traffic safety	***	***	***	***	**	**	**	***
Fire safety	**	**	**	**	**	**	**	**
Farm safety (if appropriate)	**	**	**	**	***	***	**	***
Work safety	**	**	**	**	**	**	***	***
Outdoor safety	**	**	**	**	***	***	***	***
First aid	*	*	*	*	*	**	***	***

Key: *** = major emphasis; ** = emphasis; * = touched upon or reviewed.

14. *Accident Facts* (Chicago: National Safety Council, 1974). Unless
otherwise noted, all safety statistics cited are drawn from this source.
15. *School Safety* 5 (1969): 26.

SCOPE AND KEY QUESTIONS OF SAFETY EDUCATION

SCHOOL SAFETY

Why should there be school safety rules?

Who is responsible for safety in the school?

What kinds of hazards exist in the school and its surroundings?

Is safety other-person centered?

What is your safest route to school?

Why should primary students have a separate playground?

How have you or your classmates been injured at school?

What do you do if someone is injured at school?

Why is clutter considered a safety hazard?

What are some safety rules for going to and from school?

What are the fire drill regulations for your school?

SAFETY IN THE HOME

How many hazards are there in your home?

Why is the home considered the most unsafe place to be?

What do you know about safe use of electricity?

Why are tools dangerous? Which ones are the most dangerous?

Which room in the house is the most dangerous?

Do you know the emergency telephone number for the police department? for the fire department?

How does one "baby proof" a house?

Are there special rules for safety with animals?

What are the rules for cooking safely?

Can a home be made safe from falls?

How should medications, poisons, and household chemicals be stored?

Does your family have a safety plan in case of a fire or tornado?

How have you been injured in the home? How could this accident have been prevented?

How are electrical, chemical, and other fires extinguished?

Where do you live? What is your telephone number? Where can your parents be reached if they are not at home?

What are some safety rules for baby-sitting?

Should you have friends in the house when your parents are not home?

PSYCHOLOGY OF ACCIDENTS

Why is judgment an important factor in accidents?

What does it mean to be accident-prone?

Do emotions play a role in causing accidents and injury?

Who seems to have the most accidents?

Do people get hurt just to get attention?

What is the multiple-causation theory of accidents?

Under what types of conditions are accidents most likely to occur?

What is the role of peer pressure in causing accidents?

TRAFFIC SAFETY

What are the rules of the road for pedacycles?

How does one cross a street which has a traffic light? which does not have a traffic light? which has a crossing guard?

What are the safety rules for being a passenger in a bus, car, train, airplane, boat, motorcycle, and other vehicles?

Are there any special rules for being a pedestrian on a street or road without sidewalks?

What kinds of things can one do to become a visual pedestrian?

How do traffic accidents occur?

What are the rules for school bus safety?

If an accident occurs, what should you do?

Should pedacyclists be given traffic violation tickets?

What is your safest route to and from school?

How is a safety check done for pedacycles?

FIRE SAFETY

Does your family have a fire escape plan? What should it be?

What are the causes of fires?

How does one extinguish chemical, electrical, oil, and wood fires?

Why are smoke, fumes, and superheated air the greatest hazards in a fire?

How can one avoid the smoke, fumes, and hot air of a fire?

What are the safety rules for storing paints, chemicals, and rags?

What is spontaneous combustion?

What are the fire safety rules for camping?

What special fire precautions must be taken during the winter and at Christmastime?

Which is more dangerous, a full can of gasoline or an almost empty can? Why?

How dangerous are aerosol cans?

What are the rules for burning trash and leaves?

Are your clothes flame retardant?

What are the most dangerous kinds of clothing to wear around fires?

How do electrical fires start? How can they be avoided?

What are your school's fire safety rules?

How should matches be stored and used?

Have you ever been burned? How did it happen?

FARM SAFETY

What special precautions must be taken when farm machinery is operated?

When are farmers most likely to be injured?

Which piece of farm machinery is the most dangerous?

What are the safety rules for operating tractors, combines, corn pickers, corn choppers, and other pieces of farm equipment that might be dangerous?

What are the special dangers to children on the farm?

What farm animals are dangerous and how should they be handled?

What special fire precautions must farmers take?

Why is noise a hazard on the farm?

Do farmers need to take any special precautions from the sun?

In spite of the safety hazards, why is farming considered a healthy and fulfilling life?

What kinds of farm accidents have you had?

Why is it important to put tools away after they have been used?

WORK SAFETY

Why has industry worked very hard to reduce the occurrence of accidents?

What are the factory safety rules regarding these situations?

Handling tools
Moving and lifting heavy objects
Keeping work areas clean
Wearing protective equipment
Protecting other workers

Why is noise a safety hazard and how can you protect yourself from noise?
Why are fumes and dust safety hazards? How can they be avoided?
Have you ever been hurt while working with tools? How did the accident happen?
Who is responsible for the safety of persons at work?
What types of work are the most dangerous?
What is the safety color code?
What kinds of safety rules do offices, hospitals, and other businesses have?

OUTDOOR SAFETY

What are the safety rules for both outdoor and indoor sports?
What are the special safety precautions for outdoor winter sports such as sledding, skiing, snowmobiling, and skating?
Why are there so many drownings?
What are the water safety rules for swimming, diving, rescuing, and boating?
How can a campsite be made safe from forest fires, insects, poisonous plants, and storms?
How can one avoid injury while handling knives and axes?
What special precautions must hikers and climbers take?
How can firearm and hunting accidents be avoided?
How are fishermen usually injured?
Family outings and picnics can result in injury. How can the number of such injuries be reduced?
What is the difference between heat exhaustion and heatstroke?
How can heat exhaustion and heatstroke be avoided?
Why is conditioning important in avoiding injury?
Which sports are the most dangerous? Why? How can the number of injuries in these activities be reduced?

FIRST AID

What are the "hurry up" cases?
What should you do when you arrive at the scene of an accident?
What is a definition of first aid?
What are the emergency care procedures for the following events?
Bleeding
Shock
Choking
Victim not breathing
Burns
Victim unconscious
Broken bones

Who is capable of giving first aid?
What are the first-aid procedures for poisoning?
How does one approach someone who is emotionally upset?
What are the first-aid procedures for someone who has taken an overdose of medication, alcohol, or other drug?

What kinds of first-aid equipment should one have in his home, car, outdoor sports gear, and place of business?

What kinds of first-aid mistakes do people commonly make?

When should an accident victim not be moved? How can victims be transported safely?

If someone is seriously injured, how does one get help?

What are the first-aid procedures for minor cuts and abrasions?

The key for suggested grade level use of the following teaching strategies is explained on page 327.

TEACHING STRATEGIES IN SAFETY EDUCATION

SCHOOL SAFETY

Walk for school safety: Have students tour the building and playgrounds removing hazardous articles and noting the types of equipment and activities that are potentially dangerous   P I

Develop a school safety theme for the week: These themes can involve posting safety rules, cartoons, and actual pictures of the hazards and include a discussion of each problem. The themes could be playground, halls, pedacycle, and classroom hazards; people to contact in case of an accident; safe use of tools; why is safety for others; role of storage and clutter in safety; and safety to and from school.   P I U

Safety detective groups: Divide the class into detective groups so that they can study unsafe practices throughout the school. For example, one group might study unsafe practices on the playground; another, safety at crosswalks, etc. Each group keeps a record of the unsafe practices and reports them to the rest of the class. A problem-solving approach concerning how to eliminate the unsafe practices would be a logical follow-up activity.   I U

Have students make storage boxes for the tools in the classroom. Discuss the importance of carefully returning tools to their place.   P I

Have safety demonstrations on the following: safe use of tools; pedacycles at school; crossing the street; playing on the playground equipment; safety in recess and classroom games; storage; lifting heavy objects; and falls. Be sure that students observe how safe habits are formed and then have a chance to try the safety skills.   P I

Develop poems and limericks about school safety practices.   P I U

Using a problem-solving approach have students generate safety campaigns and suggestions for the various aspects of school safety.   I U

Promote a school or classroom Junior Safety Council. The activities of the council can be to organize safety patrols, to have a safety theme for the month, to assist in the development of safety rules, and to organize safety campaigns.   I U

Safety show and tell: Have students relate the kinds of accidents or near misses they have had and why these accidents occurred.　　P　I

During activities appoint a safety director as part of the class leadership program.　　P　I

If possible give a group of students access to the school's accident reports. Allow them to develop and report a statistical picture of where, when, and how accidents occur in their school.　　I　U

Hold a cartoon, slogan, or poster contest with safety themes.　　I　U

Generate a series of stories about the safety misadventures of a fictitious character such as Charlie B. Hurt .　　P　I　U

Have a dramatization or role play on themes such as the following: safety judgment; daring someone to take a risk; what to do at the scene of a school accident; and how to ask someone to stop a potentially dangerous activity.　　P　I　U

SAFETY AT HOME

Survey: Have students do a home survey of all the unsafe or potentially dangerous situations in their home. In the survey have them include hazards in their yard and street as well.　　P　I　U

Discussions: Have students discuss the following topics:
Why is the home considered the most unsafe place to be?
What area of the home is the most dangerous?
Why do people take unnecessary chances in the home?
What is the role of clutter in causing accidents?　　P　I　U

Demonstrations: Demonstrations can be used to show the following safety practices:
　　Safe use of tools, electrical equipment, and cooking equipment
　　Safety in mowing the lawn
　　Safe use of knives and other sharp instruments
　　Safe storage practices
　　Safe use of ladders
　　Safe participation in yard games　　P　I　U

Practice lifting heavy objects by using empty cardboard boxes.　　P　I　U

Have a safety poster contest.　　P　I　U

Bulletin boards and artwork: Develop bulletin board themes and art displays around such topics as these:
　　Safety cartoons using the characters Mr. and Mrs. Calamity
　　Photographs of existing hazardous conditions
　　Newspaper stories of home accidents　　P　I　U

Have show and tell sessions on personal experiences with home accidents.　　P　I

Play charades in which students try to portray or guess unsafe acts in the home.　　P　I　U

Design a *Safety Christmas Tree* with suggestions and slogans for a safe holiday season.   P I U

Have students design and distribute home safety checklists.   I U

Have students develop dramatizations about safety in the home.   P I U

Problem solving: Set up hypothetical unsafe conditions in the home; include pictures if possible. Ask students to identify the unsafe conditions and ask them how the conditions can be corrected. Also include situations in which emergencies have occurred and ask students to react to these emergencies.   P I U

Through special interest projects or teaching-learning stations have students develop checklists for preventing falls, poisonings, electrical burns or shock, other burns, and the like.   P I U

PSYCHOLOGY OF ACCIDENTS

Problem solving: Design situations in which students are forced to make judgments. Include first-aid situations, emergency situations, peer pressure risk situations, and reaction in order to avoid an accident.   I U

Using descriptions of real accidents have the students analyze each accident from a psychological point of view and in light of multiple causes.   I U

Investigate accidents in light of the good or bad judgments made and search for all the causes of the accidents.   I U

Hold class discussions on some of the following topics:
Accident-proneness.
The role of emotions in accidents.
Who seems to have the most accidents? Why?
What is the multiple-causation theory of accidents?
Do some people get hurt to get attention?
What is the role of peer pressure in accidents?
Discuss stories of persons who have taken calculated risks after careful preparation, for example, stunt drivers.   P I U

Open-ended statements: Have students complete the following statements:
When I have been hurt I . . .
When people give me sympathy . . .
When someone I know has been injured . . .
If I have hurt someone . . .   I U

Have students develop cartoons or stories about Mr. and Mrs. Calamity illustrating the multiple-causation theory of accidents.   I U

Have students develop position statements about the concept of safety for greater adventures.   I U

TRAFFIC SAFETY

Relate stories about calculated risk takers such as race car drivers and stunt men and how long and carefully they prepare themselves and their equipment to eliminate risks. P I U

Safety Town: Using cardboard boxes for houses and tape or chalk to outline the streets, sidewalks, and crosswalks, have the students learn how to be pedestrians. Also have a traffic light and crossing guards. P I

Have students plan and memorize their safest route to school. P

Organize a pedacycle safety campaign to include posters, school regulations, rules of the road, safety inspections, and safe-driving contests or exercises on the playground. P I

Many states have manuals on pedacycle rules of the road written for the elementary level. Have students study the manual and take written and on-the-road driving tests. Older students could take turns being examiners. P I U

Have students construct traffic signs. Generate self-tests on these signs and then hold the class responsible for being 100 percent accurate in recognizing each sign. I U

Discussion: Develop class or buzz group discussion around the following topics:
> What is a good passenger?
> Why should automobiles have seat belts?
> How can bus rides be made safer?
> Should one accept things from strangers?
> What are the pedestrian and pedacycle rules of the road? P I U

Problem solving: Using signs, drawings, pictures, and scenes have students depict a hazardous setting and suggest how it may be made safer. P I U

Have students develop an alphabet of safety slogans. For example: *A* is for *alert; B* for *beware;* and so forth. P I U

Have students try to put the finishing touches on unfinished limericks. For example:
> A man from Mars
> > Would walk in front of cars
> Of course he didn't know
>
> _____ I U

Have students show and tell about accidents and near misses as pedestrians and as bike riders. Relate what happened and how the situation could have been avoided. P I

Have a group of students stand on the busiest street corner nearest the school and count the number of motor vehicle and vehicle and pedestrian violations. I U

Invite the local police department to provide a traffic safety guest speaker. P I

Organize a display or bulletin board display on different traffic
safety themes. This makes an excellent group project. Have
one group try to display graphically accident statistics.   I   U

FIRE SAFETY

Demonstrations: Have students give demonstrations of the following safety practices:

        The three types of fires and how to extinguish them

        The three needs of fires: heat, fuel, and oxygen (A glass
jar placed over a candle will illustrate the need for
oxygen.)

        Safe use of matches

        Starting charcoal fires, camp fires, camp stove fires, and
putting the fires out.   P   I   U

Design special holiday themes on fire safety. For example, burning leaves and fire problems at Christmas. This could include
checklists incorporated into greeting cards that are taken
home, a bulletin board display, and a schoolwide campaign.   P   I

Guest speakers: Local fire departments often have prepackaged
programs for elementary schools. Usually included are the
types of fires and how to extinguish them, electrical safety,
escape routes in a home fire, and other fire prevention tips.
Normally they also have some clever demonstrations to present. Insurance companies also often provide similar
services.   P   I   U

Fire drills: Have the fire escape routes posted and carefully explained. Try to have a few fire drills in which obstructions are
placed in the hall and a sign warning of thick smoke and high
heat. This will allow students to react to a more realistic fire
situation. Follow each fire drill with a discussion and review
of key points.   P   I   U

Organize a home fire safety week. Have students prepare and take
checklists home, perform a home fire inspection, draw up the
floor plan of their home, and develop a home fire escape plan.   P   I   U

Problem solving: Have students form judgments on the following
issues:

        How to react to certain types of fires

        What to do if you do not have a fire extinguisher

        Imaginary fire situations such as blocked halls, fire on the
upper floor of a hotel or motel, car fire, forest fire,
tent fire, and clothing fire

        How to treat burns

        Fire in a neighbor's house   P   I   U

Take a field trip to the fire department or through the school to
determine all the fire precautions taken. Follow with a discussion of the why and how of public building fire protection.   P   I

Realia: Collect and display fire fighting equipment, frayed exten-
sion cords, blown fuses, items that have accidentally caught

on fire, empty gasoline cans, aerosol cans, and other fire
hazards.　　　　　　　　　　　　　　　　　　　　　　　　P　I　U

Discussions: Have students discuss the following topics:
    Close calls or actual accidental fire experiences
    How to prevent home, school, work, outdoor, and farm fires
    When fires are most likely to occur
    Daily fire dangers　　　　　　　　　　　　　　　　P　I　U

Make a fire extinguisher:
    Students can make a carbon dioxide fire extinguisher by using
        these procedures:
                3 tablespoons of vinegar
                1 teaspoon of baking soda
                1 cork
                1 drinking straw
                1 heavy-duty bottle
                1 piece of thread
                1 piece of thin cloth
    Pour the vinegar into the bottle; wrap the soda in the piece
        of cloth; tie up the bundle of soda and suspend the bun-
        dle from the cork inside the bottle. Insert a straw through
        the hole in the cork so that the straw rests one-fourth
        inch from the bottom of the bottle. When the bottle is
        inverted, the vinegar reacts with the baking soda, and
        carbon dioxide pours through the straw. Do not shake
        the bottle. To extinguish a flame simply point the straw
        at the fire.　　　　　　　　　　　　　　　　　　　I　U

Have students develop stories or dramatizations regarding care-
    less fire safety behavior　　　　　　　　　　　　　P　I　U

FARM SAFETY

Using a brainstorming session have students list on the blackboard
    all the danger spots on a farm.　　　　　　　　　　P　I　U

Consult the National Safety Council for farm injury statistics and
    discuss the frequency of injuries, where they occur, and when
    they are most likely to occur.　　　　　　　　　　　　I　U

Discussions: The following topics can be handled in buzz groups
    or as class discussion:
        Weather hazards on a farm
        Livestock safety
        Proper use of farm machinery
        Safe use of chemicals
        Spontaneous combustion
        Special problem of child safety on a farm　　　　I　U

In groups, have students develop safety checklists for all the ma-
    jor safety areas on the farm.　　　　　　　　　　　　I　U

Develop displays and stories around the major farm safety areas.　P　I　U

WORK SAFETY

Organize a field trip to a nearby industrial plant. Provide checklists of things to look for and questions to ask of the safety supervisor. Follow with a class discussion.   I U

Guest speakers: As part of a safety unit or a unit on choosing a profession, invite professionals to explain their work, training, and safety precautions. Particularly effective are such guest speakers as a professional stunt man and persons in high-risk professions such as a high-rise construction engineer or utility lineman.   P I U

Discussion: Have students discuss the following topics:
Why children should stay away from construction sites.
What are the safety rules for your parent's occupation?
When and how were you injured while working?
Why do industrial plants insist on safe work habits and conditions?
Why is safety considered other-person centered?
Why is noise a hazard?
Why are dust and clutter dangerous?   P I U

Demonstration: Have students become expert in the safe use of common tools. Have them demonstrate to the class safe handling of these tools.   P I U

Collect some of the safety slogans and posters from local industries and post them around the classroom.   P I U

Have students correctly identify the safety color codes of industry and hospitals and use these colors for making pictures of industrial safety.   I U

OUTDOOR SAFETY

Discussions: Students can discuss the following topics on outdoor safety:
Why are family outings sometimes dangerous?
What kinds of close calls have you had in outdoor recreation?
Which outdoor sports are the most dangerous? Why?
What are the safety precautions for winter sports?
What are safe swimming and boating practices? dangerous practices?
What are the roles of physical fitness and knowledge of the sport in preventing sporting injuries?   P I U

Organize a display around a sport theme. Include posters, cartoons, slogans, and realia concerning a given sport. This makes a particularly good group project and can be coordinated with the physical education program.   I U

Through the Junior Safety Council organize schoolwide campaigns concerning outdoor recreation safety.   P I U

If possible visit a swimming pool and have the students participate in water safety instruction. P I U

Have the boy scouts in the school organize and present a program on camping safety. I U

Develop problem-solving situations around outdoor sports. Students are expected to solve the problem and include alternative solutions. I U

Seek guest speakers who have special interests in gun and hunting safety, water safety, and camping safety. I U

Search through magazines that feature sport adventure stories and have students relate the safety problems that arose, how they could have been avoided, and the precautions the experts take. Follow with a discussion of the meaning of safety for greater adventure. I U

FIRST AID

Develop an art display of drawings or posters from the local American Red Cross showing different first-aid techniques. Organize the display around a first-aid technique for the week. P I U

Guest experts are particularly helpful in this area. Most communities have trained first-aiders. I U

Have demonstrations and practice sessions on "hurry up" cases such as unconsciousness, severe bleeding, stoppage of breathing or heartbeat, shock, and poisoning. P I U

Discuss the more simple first-aid techniques of handling minor wounds. P I U

Have show and tell activities on real stories of first-aid situations. P I U

Problem solving: Problem-solving activities are ideal to develop first-aid training. Ask students to solve such situations as the following:

First aid for an unconscious victim with an empty bottle of sleeping pills
First aid for a victim of a fall who complains of severe neck pain
First aid for a seizure victim. I U

With the aid of specially trained student experts, teaching-learning stations could be set up for each of the major first-aid problems. I U

Make sure that all students know what to do if they come on the scene of an injured victim in terms of seeking help. Role play the theme calling for help on the phone. Make sure students know whom to call and how to give the correct information. P I U

Personal health and fitness education involves the study and care of the body senses, the care of the skin, hair, and nails, and the role of posture, exercise, and rest in health. The health problems in these areas concern debilitating conditions, rather than lethal conditions. However, vision, hearing, skin, and sleep disorders have an influence on a person's life-style, potential, and self-image. Most individuals are affected by one or more of these health problems. Fortunately, knowledge and simple health practices can often prevent the possibility of lifelong disability.

The following statistics illustrate the scope of personal health problems:

1. Nearly one-tenth of children ages six to eleven years have been found to have visual abnormalities or disease in one or both eyes. In addition, an estimated 100,000,000 children and adults need eye glasses in the United States.[16]
2. It has been estimated that 12,000,000 people in the United States have suffered a hearing loss. Approximately 70 percent of these hearing losses could be prevented.[17]
3. Almost all adolescents have skin disorders. While a few may never even develop a pimple, others suffer through skin conditions that can be physically and emotionally damaging.[18]

Table 16–5. Suggested Grade Placement for Personal Health and Fitness Topics

Topic	Grade Placement							
	K	1	2	3	4	5	6	7–8
Care of senses	*	*	**	**	**	**	**	**
Role of sleep and relaxation in health	**	**	**	**	*	*	*	**
Care of skin, hair, and nails	**	**	**	*	*	**	*	***
Exercise, posture, and health	*	*	*	*	*	*	*	**

Key: *** = major emphasis; ** = emphasis; * = touched upon or reviewed.

CARE OF THE SENSES

How important are the eyes?

How is the eye constructed and how does it function?

What are some of the common eye disorders and how can they be prevented?

What are some rules concerning protection of the eyes?

Why do some people refuse to wear glasses?

What are the emergency care procedures for eye injuries?

Many blind people lead full and productive lives. How do they manage this?

What makes a good listener?

16. U.S., Department of Health, Education, and Welfare, *Eye Examination Findings Among Children in the United States,* DHEW Publication no. 721057 (Washington, D.C.: Government Printing Office, 1972).

17. C. L. Anderson, *Health Principles and Practice,* 5th ed. (St. Louis: C. V. Mosby Co., 1972), pp. 253–254.

18. Marjorie Bauer, "Skin Diseases and the Adolescent," *Journal of School Health* 5 (1970): 236–238.

What is the structure and function of the auditory system?
How does loud noise damage hearing?
How can loss of hearing be prevented?
Have you had auditory and vision examinations?
What are the recommended steps for removing wax from the ears?
In addition to hearing and vision, what are the other body senses and how
do they function?

ROLE OF SLEEP AND RELAXATION IN HEALTH

Why do we sleep?
What are some of the modern theories about why we sleep and dream?
How much sleep should people receive?
What kinds of things can people do to help in falling asleep?
What is tension and how is it caused?
What kinds of things influence how we sleep on a given night?
What happens when we do not get enough rest?
What are some tips for learning how to relax?
Why is relieving tension important to health?
How should people unwind after a difficult day or week?

CARE OF SKIN, HAIR, AND NAILS

What are the structure and function of the skin, hair, and nails?
What kinds of skin injuries occur? How should they be treated?
Can people avoid skin problems by diet alone? Why? Why not?
What are some tips for preventing skin disorders?
What are some suggestions for using cosmetics?
What kinds of diseases occur when poor cleanliness practices are followed?
How often and how should we go about washing the hair?
What are the proper techniques for caring for fingernails and toenails?
What kinds of skin, hair, and nail disorders are associated with athletics?
Which medical specialties deal with the treatment of skin, hair, and nail
disorders?

EXERCISE, POSTURE, AND HEALTH

Why should one exercise?
How does one develop strength, flexibility, agility, endurance, and physical
skill?
What is the difference between isotonic and isometric exercise?
Why do experts believe that the most beneficial exercises are those that pro-
mote cardiorespiratory endurance?
How much exercise do you need?
What will the role of physical activity be in your life?
What is the role of posture in health?
What are some of the postural disorders? How can they be avoided?
How can we avoid injuries while lifting heavy objects?
What are the proper techniques of walking, running, sitting, and lifting?
What causes foot problems? How can these problems be avoided?
Quackery in fitness aids is common. Do you agree or disagree with the
statement? Why?

The key for suggested grade level use of the following teaching strategies is explained on page 327.

CARE OF THE SENSES

Valuing activities: Have student volunteers try being blindfolded for part of the school day or pretend to be unable to hear, touch, smell, or talk. Ask them to relate their experiences to the class. Ask students to decide which of the body senses they would least like to lose and have them defend their choice.   P I U

Student or group reports: Have students investigate and report to class on the necessary precautions to take in avoiding injury to the various body senses. Other reports could be on the means of detecting deficiencies in the senses, available medical personnel, and available treatment.   I U

Have students develop displays on each of the body senses, illustrating safety precautions, detection of deficiencies, treatment, and what these senses do for one.   P I U

Demonstrations: The following demonstrations can be used to illustrate the importance of the senses:
    Find the blind spot in the eye
    Determine the dominant eye
    How the pupil of the eye adjusts to light
    How a camera and its lens (or lenses) amplify and distort images
    How sound amplification and reception work   P I U

Appreciation activities could include having students sit as quietly as possible with their eyes closed and try to recognize all the various sounds they hear. This can be particularly enjoyable in an outdoor park setting. For appreciation of the eyes have students quickly scan a photograph, the room, or some other scene and then relate all they have observed. Games such as pin the tail on the donkey and tasting parties, children blindfolded and holding their noses, standing on one foot with the eyes closed, or performing simple tasks with the eyes closed also build appreciation of the body senses. P I U

Classroom discussions can involve such topics as appreciation of the body senses; what the body senses are; what it would be like without some of these senses; and how to protect the body senses. Also include discussion of acceptance of wearing glasses.   P I U

Have students participate in auditory and vision screening tests.   P I U

ROLE OF SLEEP AND RELAXATION IN HEALTH

Discussion questions could include such topics as:
    Why do we need to sleep?
    What happens to us if we do not get the right amount of rest?

How long should we sleep?

What are the physiological reactions during sleep?

Why and how do we dream? What do dreams mean? P I U

Class surveys can be useful for determining how long people sleep, special tricks for getting to sleep, and situations in which it is usually difficult to get to sleep. P I U

With the aid of a physical education teacher hold a demonstration and practice session on how to relax the various muscle groups of the body. Illustrate the best sleep positions for maximum relaxation and emphasize the role of concentration in relaxing the muscle groups, particularly those muscles that build tension around the head and neck. P I U

Have students develop an analysis of their sleep patterns by keeping track of the hours they have slept including naps. Have them reflect on how they felt socially, emotionally, and physically (1) after a good night's rest; (2) after experiencing an irregular sleep pattern over a period of days such as on a vacation trip, and (3) after very little sleep during a camping trip or a slumber party. P I U

Buzz group discussions followed by large group interaction can be utilized for consideration of the following situations:

The role of relaxation and sleep in mental health

At the end of a tough but rewarding day, how should one relax?

What will be your attitude toward the recreational use of drugs such as alcohol in your life?

What is the role of tension in health? How do we generate emotional tension?

When is stress healthy?

What is your favorite recreation?

What turns you on? I U

CARE OF SKIN, HAIR, AND NAILS

Organize teaching-learning stations so that six groups can rotate from station to station where charts, diagrams, slides, and study guide questions are located. Three stations can be utilized for the structure and function of the skin, hair, and nails and three stations for the care of the skin, hair, and nails. I U

Guest speakers can be very effective in this area. A list of guest speakers and their topics could include the school nurse on care of injuries and prevention of such skin infections as impetigo and ringworm; a dermatologist on the care of acne, rashes, and allergies; a beautician on the care of the hair and nails; and a public health worker on the dangers of venereal diseases. I U

Classroom demonstrations can be utilized for illustrating the proper care of skin, hair, and nails. In many cases several students should have the opportunity to perform the activities. P I U

Individual and group reports can include topics such as teenage skin problems and care, allergies, nail biting, baldness, choice of cosmetics and over-the-counter medications, special tips for suntanning, and medical specialties in these areas.   I   U

Utilizing groups, have students bring in advertisements concerning the care of skin, hair, and nails. Put these ads on display and discuss the factors involved in being a good consumer and how to avoid quackery in this area.   I   U

Hold class discussions on such topics as these:
How to care for the skin, hair, and nails
What about nail biting?
The role of cleanliness in the spread of disease
The role of good grooming in winning friends and influencing people
Improper personal care—a self-destructive process?   I   U

EXERCISE, POSTURE, AND HEALTH
Value activities should concentrate on the why of physical fitness and posture. For example, have students discuss their view of why one should be fit, the role of exercise in their health and personal appearance, and how they feel about physical exertion.   I   U

Discussion topics can include the following:
Why should one exercise?
Who is physically fit? Why are they physically fit?
What are the relationships between exercise, posture, and health?
Can fitness prevent disease? Defend your opinion.
What are some safety suggestions for exercising?
What is the relationship between exercise and weight control?
Why should strength, endurance, and flexibility be combined in exercise?
Why do people not get more exercise?   I   U

Have students collect stories and articles about famous people and their fitness attitudes and practices.   I   U

Have students indicate their favorite sport and then have a follow-up exercise on developing a training schedule for the sport that includes exercise, the skills to practice, and their goals for this activity. Have them report to the class.   I   U

In conjunction with studying the heart and respiratory system, have students learn to take their own heart and respiration rates. Illustrate the effects of exercise on the cardiorespiratory system by having students determine their resting heart and respiration rates and then have them run in place for one minute. Students then check their rates immediately after exercising and again after two and five minutes. Follow with a discussion of the training effect of endurance activities on the cardiorespiratory system and why the development of endurance is important for all age groups.   I   U

With the aid of a physical education teacher or a group of student experts have students explore the different types of exercises, their purpose, and how they should be performed. Note: do not make this a strenuous activity. Simply have students learn how to perform the exercises properly.   P I U

With the use of bulletin boards and group reports have students discuss the development of skills for and the safety aspects of their favorite physical activities.   I U

On a large sheet of paper have students draw the outline of their partner's posture. After illustrating the proper ways of walking and standing, have students analyze their posture.   P I U

CONSUMER HEALTH

Americans spend an incredible amount of money on health aids and services. An annual expenditure of over $1 billion on nonprescription drugs, $28 billion on recreational drugs (alcohol and tobacco), and an estimated $2 billion on fake health aids is a clear indication of the need for consumer health education.[19] Educators will have to continue to contend with the skills of advertising agencies. Advertising inundates us with inducements to buy miracle cosmetics, diet aids, cold remedies, antacids, and other health aids. For example, Kime reports that over $100 million are spent each year in advertising headache remedies alone.[20]

Self-diagnosis, fad diets, and use of remedies suggested by friends are common behaviors of teenagers as well as of adults. A quick perusal of media advertising reveals that a great amount of advertising is directed toward teenagers. While many sales appeals are designed for adults, adolescents do consume over-the-counter prescriptions, cosmetics, and diet aids. Dealing with their specific needs can help establish good lifelong consumer health practices.

In addition to being able to cope with their own consumer health problems, young people need to be aware of other dimensions of consumer health. Since medical costs in the United States rose from $25 billion in 1962 to $83 billion in 1972, students should be made aware of the major problems in our present health-care delivery systems.[21] In addition, an understanding of advertising practices, quackery and consumer protection should be developed.

Table 16–6.   Suggested Grade Placement for Consumer Health Topics

Topic	Grade Placement							
	K	1	2	3	4	5	6	7–8
Young people and consumer health					*	**	**	***
Nostrums, fads, and fallacies				*	*	*	**	***
Health advertising				*	*	**	**	**
Health quackery and consumer protection						*	**	***
Modern health care systems								**

Key: *** = major emphasis; ** = emphasis; * = touched upon or reviewed.

19. Summary of the 1970 Consumer Expenditures," *Supermarketing* 26 (1971): 39.
20. Robert E. Kime, *Health: A Consumer's Dilemma* (Belmont, Calif.: Wadsworth Publishing Co., 1970), pp. 2–3.
21. Gus Alevizos, Robert Walsh, and Phil Aherne, eds., *Socioeconomic Issues of Health* (Chicago: American Medical Association, 1973), p. 87.

YOUNG PEOPLE AND CONSUMER HEALTH

What kinds of health products and services do young people buy?

Why are young people considered a market for health products?

What kinds of health products and services do young people seek without the advice of parents?

What would you do if you had a health problem such as a venereal disease and you did not want your parents to find out about it?

What prompted you to buy certain health products?

How can you go about being a wise health consumer?

NOSTRUMS, FADS, AND FALLACIES

What are some of the old wives' tales? Are they reliable sources?

What are some of the food fads and how can they influence health?

Where can one get relief for the common cold?

Why do fads and fallacies exist?

Which well-known health products do you think are worthless?

Why do people continue to purchase ineffective health products?

HEALTH ADVERTISING

How can you effectively evaluate health advertising?

Why do manufacturers sometimes participate in misleading advertising?

What advertisements are pointed directly at young people?

What is the cost of advertising to you?

For health products and services, what are your most accurate sources of information?

HEALTH QUACKERY AND CONSUMER PROTECTION

What is quackery?

How are we protected from false claims and quackery?

Why does quackery continue?

Who is most susceptible to quackery?

What can you do if you suspect something is wrong with the medical services you are paying for?

What agencies protect the consumer?

Why do unreliable treatments sometimes seem to bring about miraculous cures?

MODERN HEALTH CARE SYSTEMS

What medical services should young people be aware of?

How does one go about selecting medical services?

Why are the costs of medical services rising?

What emergency services are there in your community?

Why is there an increasing congressional trend toward federal support of the cost of medical services?

When should people seek the services of a physician?

What are the dangers of self-diagnosis and treatment?

What are the pros-and-cons of a national health insurance plan?

How do medical services vary from community to community and from neighborhood to neighborhood?

Where and how can one receive low-cost medical service?

What kinds of careers are there in medical science?

What can you do if you cannot afford medical services?

TEACHING STRATEGIES IN CONSUMER HEALTH

The key for suggested grade level use of the following teaching strategies is explained on page 327.

YOUNG PEOPLE AND CONSUMER HEALTH

A number of surveys can be conducted. These surveys can be done by individuals or groups and can include the following topics:

> The number of students who have purchased their own health products
> The kinds of health products students purchase and use
> The cost of the health products
> The reasons for purchasing health products   I   U

Through a brainstorming technique list health problem areas on the board such as acne, colds, coughs, and the like and have the students identify all the remedies they know for each ailment. Discuss why there are so many over-the-counter remedies. Explore the effectiveness of some of these health aids.   I   U

Problem solving: Select a major student health problem. In groups have the students determine the following: (1) whether medical counsel should be sought, (2) whether the medical problem is hazardous, (3) whether over-the-counter remedies are available, (4) the cost of medical attention, and (5) where medical attention can be received. As the groups report their findings, the teacher must correct erroneous information and explore the implication of self-diagnosis and self-treatment.   I   U

Role playing or dramatization: Several topics on consumer health can make informative as well as humorous dramatizations. Some of the topics are visiting the doctor or dentist, things one should or should not say to someone who is ill, self-medication, spreading of fads and fallacies, and use of another person's medication.   I   U

Have students check their medicine chest at home for products that should be thrown away or replaced. Have the class follow through by making a list of over-the-counter health aids that should be in the average home.   I   U

Through a class discussion develop criteria for the purchase of health aids and services. Note that health aids for this age group include cosmetic aids and dental products as well as other medications.   I   U

NOSTRUMS, FADS, AND FALLACIES

Student reports can be given on many of the old wives' tales in health (e.g., feed a cold and starve a fever). Included in each report can be a survey concerning who believes these tales and a factual account of the scientific accuracy of the statements.   I   U

Have the class design and administer a test on nostrums, fads, and
   fallacies.   U

Topics suitable for role playing include the following:
   How not to cure the common cold
   A visit with Aunt Nostra and her fabulous cure-alls
   George the super vitamin pill salesman
   Selling your favorite fad   I U

After making a listing of the many fads and fallacies in the area
   of health, have students discuss the scientific accuracy of
   each fad and fallacy and determine why they continue to be
   believed by so many people.   I U

HEALTH ADVERTISING

Have students bring examples of health advertising to class. In
   groups have them develop criteria for judging advertising and
   apply these criteria to the health advertisements.   I U

Ask students to develop their own advertisements for imaginary
   health products and services. This can be done in groups and
   can involve a series of improvised commercials.   I U

Generate displays and bulletin board themes around false advertising, rules for evaluating advertising, imaginary false advertising, and listings of the types of ads written for this age
   group.   I U

Through class discussion investigate the following topics:
   Sources of accurate health information
   Why well-known products are sometimes misadvertised
   How advertising is paid for
   What kinds of products for young people are advertised
   Why advertising increases the profits of the product makers   U

Over a period of one week have students make a list of all the advertisements they see that are pointed at a health problem of
   their age group. Discuss the accuracy of these advertisements
   and the effectiveness of the products advertised.   I U

HEALTH QUACKERY AND CONSUMER PROTECTION

Develop class discussions around such topics as the following:
   What is quackery?
   Why does quackery continue to exist?
   Who is most susceptible to quackery?
   What is the cost of quackery to consumers?
   How can consumers be protected?
   What can you do if you feel a legitimate physician is in error?
   Why do people give testimonials for various commercial
   products?   I U

Invite guest speakers from the local medical society and Better
   Business Bureau to discuss ways of preventing medical fraud.   U

Through group reports have students study the types of frauds that have occurred in some of the major health problem areas.   I U

Have students construct fraudulent medical apparatus, develop advertisements for their products, and place them on display.   I U

Allow students to write and present a drama illustrating the scene of a con man and an unsuspecting victim.   I U

MODERN HEALTH CARE SYSTEMS

Ask students to survey parents and relatives concerning the costs of specific medical services. In addition, have them ask parents and relatives to explain (1) why medical costs are rising, (2) their view of the current universal health insurance plans before the United States Congress, and (3) their plan for reducing medical costs.   U

Invite guest speakers from local medical service and welfare agencies to explain the problems of medical costs and the procurement of low-cost medical services.   U

Through a problem-solving technique have students determine how to solve specific medical problems in terms of who to seek medical attention from, when to seek medical attention, and what to do if they cannot afford medical assistance.   U

Have individual reports concerning medical careers, medical specialties, medical insurance, and local medical agencies.   U

ECOLOGICAL CONCEPTS AND ENVIRONMENTAL QUALITY

Man is the most dangerous factor in the earth's environment. By making use of his intelligence and the tools of science man has been able to manipulate the environment with remarkable skill and in many instances with incredible ignorance. Motivated by a combination of self-improvement and greed, man has destroyed vast areas of land and sea and wasted a large portion of the natural resources.[22] Fortunately, in response to or in spite of the prophets of doom, industrialized nations have made successful efforts in environmental reclamation and conservation. Our future depends upon an all-out effort toward protecting the delicate balance of life on the planet earth.[23]

Table 16–7. Suggested Grade Placement for Ecological Concepts and Environmental Quality Topics

Topic	Grade Placement						
	1	2	3	4	5	6	7–8
Ecological cycles and systems	*	*	*	*	*	**	***
Some major ecological problems	*	*	*	*	*	**	**
Student's role in the environment	**	**	**	**	**	**	**
Some future considerations		*	*	*	**	**	***

Key: *** = major emphasis; ** = emphasis; * = touched upon or reviewed.

22. Barry Commoner, *Science and Survival* (New York: Ballantine Books, 1963), pp. 11–33.

23. René Dubos, *So Human An Animal* (New York: Charles Scribner's Sons, 1968), pp. 3–30.

While elementary and middle school students may have difficulty understanding the complexities of the ecosystem, they can make personal decisions about conservation, population control, use of natural resources, pollution, and moral obligations to future generations. By carefully developing ecological concepts and positive attitudes toward protecting the environment we can help prepare this generation for the complex and difficult decisions that must be made to avoid future ecological disasters.[24]

ECOLOGICAL CYCLES AND SYSTEMS

How can the terms *ecosystem, environment,* and *biosphere* be defined?
Of all the factors in the environment, which are the most important?
How would you describe the "spaceship Earth" concept?
Why are ecological problems worldwide in scope?
What is the difference between a microsystem and a macrosystem?
What are the principle characteristics of such ecological systems as (1) capture of energy, (2) population, and (3) hydrological cycles and genetic coding? What are some of the other systems?
Why is man considered the most dangerous factor in the ecosystem?
Why is it important to understand that the various ecological systems are interconnected?

SOME MAJOR ECOLOGICAL PROBLEMS

What are the major ecological problems?
How has man contributed to these ecological problems?
Why is life-style considered an ecological problem?
What are the characteristics of the following ecological problems: air pollution, water pollution, waste disposal, waste of energy, population growth, unwise use of living space, waste of natural resources, genetic control, and negative side effects of scientific advances?
How are some of these ecological problems being solved?
What are our chances of improving the environment rather than destroying it?
How is your community organized to protect your water supply, disposal of waste, and environmental quality?
How is your community health department organized?
What are the voluntary and public health organizations in your community and what are their functions?
What are the implications of ignoring environmental problems?

STUDENT'S ROLE IN THE ENVIRONMENT

How do young people contribute to ecological problems?
What are some day-to-day activities that all people can do to aid the environment?
What kinds of sacrifices will we have to begin to make to ensure a healthful environment for future generations?
What does a healthy environment mean to you?
What are your feelings about the predicted ecological disasters?
Can you think of ways we can avoid the predicted ecological disasters?

24. Alvin Toffler, *Future Shock* (New York: Random House, 1970; Bantam Books, 1971), pp. 371–487.

SCOPE AND KEY QUESTIONS OF ECOLOGICAL CONCEPTS AND ENVIRONMENTAL QUALITY

SOME FUTURE CONSIDERATIONS

Why is change in life-style considered a major factor in our survival?

How will present forms of consumption have to be altered to avoid further environmental problems?

What is meant by the "throwaway culture"?

How do you personally feel about the future?

What kinds of obligations do we have to future generations?

Who is responsible for the quality of the environment?

How have scientific advances created ecological problems?

How can science be used to improve and restore the environment?

How do the environment and stress influence mental health?

Which ecological problems should we concentrate on solving first?

How can we get people to protect the environment?

What is your stand on population control?

TEACHING STRATEGIES IN ECOLOGICAL CONCEPTS AND ENVIRONMENTAL QUALITY

The key for suggested grade level use of the following teaching strategies is explained on page 327.

ECOLOGICAL CYCLES AND SYSTEMS

Charts, diagrams, and displays can be developed by individual students or groups to illustrate ecological systems and such concepts as biosphere, hydrological cycles, nitrogen cycle, and others. Included within these displays should be descriptions of these cycles and how man can improve or destroy these ecological factors.   I   U

An experiment in this area can utilize two fish tanks and some inexpensive goldfish. In one fish tank follow all the necessary procedures for ensuring the proper temperature, plant life, cleanliness, oxygen content, salinity, and the like. In the other tank provide the opposite environment. Have students keep a daily log of observations and comments concerning the status of each tank and why differences occur. A similar experiment can be conducted using terrariums.   P   I   U

Discussions should concentrate on the importance of understanding that all the factors in the environment are interdependent. Discussions can include such topics as the following:

    All the environmental controls and systems needed in a spaceship

    The factors involved in the nitrogen cycle, hydrological systems, and other cycles and systems

    Why should we conserve energy?

    The implications of a population explosion

    How ecological problems interact

    The international problems of environmental protection   I   U

Open-end stories: Have students relate all the repercussions from such actions as a walk in the woods and a careless match, an industrial plant polluting a nearby stream, a farmer trying to increase his crop yield by the use of a potent pesticide, and the like.   I   U

Ecological factors can be investigated through field trips to a local water works, sewage treatment plant, and industrial plant that is making an effort to control pollution. Have students study all the factors involved in protecting other areas of the environment at each visitation   P I U

Have students write a position paper on the ecological cycle or system they think the most important.   I U

Language arts activities can include reading stories and essays on environmental issues. Science fiction can be included. Also, students can be asked to write their own stories or dramas concerning these problems.   I U

SOME MAJOR ECOLOGICAL PROBLEMS

Displays and models of the major ecological problems can be an excellent student activity. Perhaps a display and model for each major problem such as air pollution, water pollution, and noise pollution could be put up each week. In each display suggest solutions to the problem.   I U

Because of the enormous amount of material available, each major ecological problem can be assigned each student or student group. Within each project include a display, an oral report, and a suggested class activity. Within each report include the causes, consequences, and possible solutions to the problem.   I U

After investigating the efforts of the various community agencies toward improving environmental quality have the class write sample laws for protecting the environment.   U

Class debates or panel discussions can effectively cover such topics as these:

> Is there really an energy crisis?
> Who is responsible for the environment?
> Which of the environmental problems are the most serious?
> Should we support starving nations at our own expense?
> What is the price of not using pesticides? of using pesticides?
> Why is environmental protection a worldwide problem?
> Should we have more laws?   I U

Problem solving: As a class project have students define all the environmental problems within the school; suggest ways of controlling these problems; suggest rules and develop a schoolwide campaign to combat these problems.   I U

Teacher-learning stations can be utilized for each of the major ecological problems. At each learning station have the appropriate materials: visual aids and study guides for defining the problem, and for indicating the causes of the problem; short- and long-range effects of the problem; problem solutions; and students' role in the ecological problem.   I U

Have students generate information from surveys by asking adults and other students such questions as the following:

Is there an energy crisis?

Who caused the crisis?

What are some of the solutions to the problem?

What is the most important environmental problem?

Can the environment be saved?

Would you pay more taxes to save the environment?   I   U

Valuing activities in this area can include having students determine their role in the solution of ecological problems, their moral responsibility to future generations, and their stand on the controversial aspects of the environmental issues.   U

STUDENT'S ROLE IN THE ENVIRONMENT

Have students present dramas or role plays dealing with such issues as asking a neighbor, industrialist, or governmental agency to stop pollution.   I   U

Through a brainstorming technique have students generate the ways they contribute to environmental problems and the ways they can assist in protecting the environment.   I   U

Develop panel and class discussions on such topics as these:

Ways we contribute to environmental problems

What a healthful environment means to us

Our role in protecting future generations

The kinds of sacrifices we should make to protect the environment.   I   U

Have the class decide on a community service project related to protecting the environment and have them follow through on the activities.   P   I   U

Have the class develop and post rules that each student can follow to protect the environment.   P   I   U

Organize a schoolwide campaign against pollution, waste of energy, and conservation of national resources.   P   I   U

Invite guest speakers from agencies dealing with environmental issues.   P   I   U

SOME FUTURE CONSIDERATIONS

Through a brainstorming technique have students list the difficult decisions that will have to be made in order to ensure the survival of future generations. For example: population control, vast reduction in the use of natural resources by industrialized nations, and the like.   U

From the list of difficult personal decisions that will have to be made to protect the environment have the students develop a position on their personal decisions and the repercussions from their decisions.   U

Using buzz groups have students list the kinds of adjustments that should be made in life-style in order to protect the environment. | I U

In class discussions have students reach a decision concerning issues such as the concept of the current "throwaway culture," the enormous use of rapidly depleting natural resources, and our moral obligation to other nations and future generations. | I U

Have panels and debates on the most difficult decisions that will have to be made in order to protect the environment. | U

Have students contact community agencies involved in environmental protection and ask for their opinions on decisions for a future healthful environment and report on the kinds of activities each agency is involved in. | U

Develop stories and displays on what life will be like in twenty, forty, and sixty or more years hence. | I U

Communicable and chronic diseases are serious health hazards for elementary and middle school children. Since this age group is highly susceptible to skin disorders and respiratory infections, a basic understanding of prevention and care of these problems can be of immediate need. Students require more than just an understanding of communicable disease prevention. Lifestyle, heredity, environmental factors, and detection are important aspects of communicable and chronic disease prevention. The increasing incidence of cancer and heart disease reinforce the necessity for having young people look after their future health needs. The statistics outlined in Table 16–8 illustrate the scope of elementary and middle school children's chronic and communicable disease problems.[25]

COMMUNICABLE AND CHRONIC DISEASE

Table 16–8. Incidence of Chronic and Communicable Diseases Among Elementary and Middle School Children

Chronic Diseases	Communicable Diseases
50,000 children with eye disorders	300 annual cases of diphtheria
3 million children with severe hearing loss	39,000 reported cases of impetigo each year
10 percent with severe speech disorders	2,794 annual cases of tuberculosis
30,000 with cardiovascular problems	500,000 cases of gonorrhea each year
2,500 with diabetes	

Table 16–9. Suggested Grade Placement for Chronic and Communicable Disease Topics

Topic	Grade Placement						
	1	2	3	4	5	6	7–8
Modern concept of disease	*	*	*	*	*	**	***
Prevention and detection of disease	**	**	**	**	**	**	**
Communicable disease problems of elementary and middle school students	*	*	*	*	*	*	***
Chronic disease problems			*	*	*	**	***
Treatment of disease	*	*	*	*	*	*	**

Key: *** = major emphasis; ** = emphasis; * = touched upon or reviewed.

25. Warren E. Schaller and Alma Nemir, *The School Health Program*, 4th ed. (Philadelphia: W. B. Saunders Co., 1975), pp. 57–336.

As discussed in chapter 1 the prevention of disease requires an epidemiological approach. Rather than study the signs and symptoms of a long list of specific diseases, students need to grasp the ecological, personal, and genetic factors involved in chronic and communicable diseases. Those diseases studied in detail such as venereal disease and mononucleosis can serve as models for understanding the sources of infection, the spread of disease, and the body defenses. The safe use of medications, the dangers of self-diagnosis, and the knowledge of when to seek medical attention should be emphasized.

SCOPE AND KEY QUESTIONS OF COMMUNICABLE AND CHRONIC DISEASE

A MODERN CONCEPT OF DISEASE

How can disease be defined?

What is the difference between chronic disease and communicable disease?

What are the factors involved in the chain of infection?

What is the germ theory of disease?

How does disease spread?

Why is there an increase in chronic disease?

What is the scope of our modern chronic and communicable disease problem?

What are the types of pathogens and other disease-causing agents?

What is epidemiology?

What is meant by *infectious, contagious, pandemic, endemic,* and *epidemic*?

What are the body defenses against disease?

What is the role of heredity in disease?

What are the host, agent, and environmental factors in disease?

PREVENTION AND DETECTION OF DISEASE

How can you protect the health of others?

How has your life been affected by a chronic or communicable disease?

What are the principles of disease control?

What are the signs and symptoms of illness?

How can the chain of infection be broken?

What is the role of genetics in disease causation?

What are the seven danger signals of cancer?

What are the signs and symptoms of the major chronic diseases?

What factors contribute to your resistance or susceptibility to disease?

What is the role of the epidemiologist in disease prevention and control?

What kinds of decisions should we make in order to prevent heart disease and cancer?

Why do people avoid seeking treatment when they recognize serious symptoms of chronic or communicable disease?

How are you responsible for the health of others?

COMMUNICABLE DISEASE PROBLEMS OF ELEMENTARY AND MIDDLE SCHOOL STUDENTS

What are the causes, symptoms, and long-range effects of the following diseases: (1) mumps, (2) measles, (3) mononucleosis, (4) rheumatic fever, (5) hepatitis, (6) pneumonia, (7) gonorrhea, and (8) syphilis?

How would you describe the causes, prevention, and treatment of the common cold?

Why are worldwide diseases such as malaria, typhus, yellow fever, and schistosomiasis becoming increasingly important?

How do you contribute to the spread of disease and to your susceptibility to disease?

How does personal cleanliness influence the spread of disease?

CHRONIC DISEASE PROBLEMS

What are the major chronic diseases?

How often are young people victims of a chronic disease?

What kinds of chronic diseases do young people have?

What are some of the causes, characteristics, and prevention of the major chronic diseases?

How can you reduce the risks of having a major chronic disease?

Which disease do you dread the most?

How can people deal with a disabling or fatal disease?

TREATMENT OF DISEASE

When should medical treatment be sought?

What are the dangers of self-treatment and self-diagnosis?

How would you describe the safe way to use medications?

What is meant by the fact that all drugs have side effects?

Why do some people seem to recover from illness against impossible odds and others succumb so easily?

How can adolescents seek medical attention for venereal disease without anyone finding out?

Why is it considered unsafe to take several different kinds of medications at the same time?

How much of a chance do you have to survive cancer?

What are some of the modern advances in the treatment of the major chronic and communicable diseases?

Why is early detection critical in the treatment of any disease?

What are your feelings about euthanasia, about debilitating surgery to prolong life a few months or years, and about a crippling disease?

How can medical science create medical problems?

What should you do when you are not feeling well?

The key for suggested grade level use of the following teaching strategies is explained on page 327.

A MODERN CONCEPT OF DISEASE

Have students compile lists of key words and definitions for chronic and communicable diseases.

Have students prepare reports on such topics as old theories of disease; famous pioneers in medicine; infamous epidemics and why they occurred; and other topics related to the causes and spread of disease.   I   U

Bulletin boards can be centered on such themes as the chain of infection, factors concerning man, host and environment, schematic diagram of the spread of disease, diseases trans-

TEACHING STRATEGIES IN COMMUNICABLE AND CHRONIC DISEASE

mitted from animal to man, food handling and disease, defenses of the body, and other topics within the epidemiology of disease. P I U

Discussions involving small groups or the whole class can concern such topics as these:

What causes chronic disease and communicable disease?

How does the body resist disease?

What is the role of environment in disease?

Who is the most susceptible to disease?

What are the different types of pathogens and other disease-causing agents?

Why do epidemics occur?

Describe the chain of infection

How does disease spread from one person to another? P I U

Guest speakers from the local public health department can effectively reinforce the concepts of how disease spreads and how it can be controlled. P I U

PREVENTION AND DETECTION OF DISEASE

Bulletin board: Center displays around such issues as rules for protecting others through proper use of handkerchiefs, covering the mouth when sneezing, not sharing food with another, and cleanliness in disease. Charts can be developed on the kinds of chronic and communicable diseases people have, and themes can be generated around topics such as the kinds of environmental factors that influence occurrence of such diseases as lung cancer, heart disease, high blood pressure, poisoning, food-related diseases, and other conditions. P I U

Demonstrations: A number of demonstrations can be undertaken to illustrate cleanliness, the presence of germs, and how to protect other persons from one's germs.

Have students handle common table salt and then wash their hands. If they lick their fingers, they will still detect a salty taste. Discuss the importance of cleanliness in controlling the growth of microorganisms.

To illustrate the presence of germs have students inoculate petri dishes with swabs from various areas of the body; by coughing or sneezing into the dish; by having an insect walk through the dish; by shaking dust from around the room or from clothing into the dish. Place the dishes in a warm area and observe the growth of bacteria for several days. Always include a sterile control dish for purposes of comparison. I U

The importance of careful food handling can be illustrated by boiling peeled potatoes and then placing them in sterile containers. Inoculate some of the potatoes with microorganisms by handling them with dirty utensils or hands. Place in a warm place and observe. Again use a sterile control. In addi-

tion leave one of the containers uncovered to illustrate the
number of organisms in the air.   P I U

Have students ask their parents about the kinds of chronic disorders such as heart disease, diabetes, and rheumatic fever
that have occurred on both sides of the family. Also ask about
the longevity of parents and grandparents. Students should
then analyze this data and determine their susceptibility to
these disorders and their longevity potential. Note that life-
style, diet, and stress play significant roles in their longevity
potential.   U

Discussions in the area of prevention and detection could be
done on the following topics:
    Role of cleanliness in the spread of disease
    How to protect others from one's disease
    The signs and symptoms of illness (general)
    The danger signals of heart disease, cancer, diabetes,
       and other illnesses
    The role of microorganisms in disease
    Useful roles of microorganisms
    Safe food-handling and home-canning procedures
    Animal diseases that can be transmitted to human beings
    Safety with animals
    The role of stress and fatigue in disease
    The personal decisions needed to avoid chronic disease
       problems   P I U

Teaching-learning stations can be utilized in the following areas:
the general signs of illness, symptoms of specific disorders,
how to protect yourself and others from disease, the spread
of disease, and the defenses of the body against disease.
Each station should contain appropriate slides, filmstrips,
study guides, and other materials for the students.   I U

COMMUNICABLE AND CHRONIC DISEASE PROBLEMS

Value discussions can be utilized to have students explore their
feelings concerning aging, death, dying, euthanasia, physical
handicaps, terminal illnesses, and other factors at the opposite end of the birth and health cycles.

Buzz groups: This activity works well for this topic. Some of the
appropriate topics might include the following:
    How to explain death to younger brothers and sisters
    Personal experiences with the death or critical illness of
       a loved one
    How to react or talk to a severely ill or dying person
    What is expected of us at funerals or wakes   I U

Student reports and individual study projects can be combined
with oral reports to the class, bulletin boards, displays, charts,
and written reports. Topics can include the following:
    Environmental problems and disease
    Worldwide diseases

Poverty and disease
Childhood diseases   I   U

Discussions: Plan class discussions on such topics as the following:
  How has disease affected your life?
  What is venereal disease? How can venereal disease be pre-
    vented?
  What can you do if you have a venereal disease?
  What are the signs and causes of specific chronic and com-
    municable diseases?
  Which diseases do you consider the most dangerous?
  How can one avoid chronic diseases?   I   U

A wide variety of guest speakers can be utilized in the areas of
  chronic and communicable disease. Speakers can be invited
  from the American Cancer Society, American Heart Association, mental health associations, public health disease
  control personnel, and venereal disease caseworkers.   I   U

Because so many terms and symptoms are part of communicable
  and chronic disease lessons, any number of classroom games
  can be developed. This activity not only provides a break
  from normal classroom routine, but also provides the opportunity to review the key words in this unit.   I   U

The material also lends itself well to problem solving. For example, such problems as first aid for someone having a seizure
  and other temporary care for the sick can provide some important experiences. Discussion of human relations aspects
  of dealing with seriously ill or dying individuals can also be
  useful.   P   I   U

TREATMENT OF DISEASE

Acquaint students with the various medical facilities within the
  community through field trips. Include agencies dealing
  with low-cost medical services such as neighborhood health
  centers and the public health department.   P   I   U

Through the use of student special interest projects and reports
  have the class investigate the opportunities for health careers. Include consideration of the training required for these
  occupations.   U

Discussions: Utilize classroom discussion techniques for such
  topics as these:
      When to seek medical attention
      The cost of medical services
      The dangers of self-treatment and self-diagnosis
      Why some patients survive seemingly against impossi-
        ble odds while others give up
      Why individuals should seek prompt medical attention
        for venereal disease, cancer signs, and the important
        symptoms of the more dangerous diseases
      The safe use of medications and prescription drugs

Problems in the use of prescription drugs such as side
effects, individual tolerance levels, allergic reactions, and quality control.   P I U

Have students role play visits to the doctor's office, to the school
nursery, to the emergency room, and to a quack doctor.   P I

Have displays and bulletin board themes illustrating modern medical advances and careers. Some guidelines for when to seek
medical attention can also be posted.   P I U

Hold a show and tell session in which students can relate their
own experiences with a chronic or communicable disease,
with a trip to the emergency ward, with an operation, and
with a stay in a hospital room.   P I

Have student reports on modern medical advances, milestones
in the treatment of disease, and future predictions for the
treatment of disease.   I U

References

Accident Facts. Chicago: National Safety Council, 1974.

Alevizos, Gus, Walsh, Robert, and Aherne, Phil., eds. *Socioeconomic Issues of Health*. Chicago: American Medical Association, 1973.

American Dental Association. *Survey of Needs for Dental Care*. Chicago: American Dental Association, 1965.

Anderson, C. L. *Health Principles and Practice*. 5th ed. St. Louis: C. V. Mosby, Co., 1972.

Bauer, Marjorie. "Skin Diseases and the Adolescent." *Journal of School Health* 5 (1970): 236–238.

Comfort, Alex. "Eat Less, Live Longer." *New Scientist* 53 (1972): 689.

Commoner, Barry. *Science and Survival*. New York: Ballantine Books, 1973.

Dubos, René. *So Human An Animal*. New York: Charles Scribner's Sons, 1968.

Friedman, Lawrence A. "Impact of Teacher-Student Dental Health Education." *Journal of School Health* 44 (1974): 140–143. March, 1974.

Green, J. C. "Dental Health Needs of the Nation." *Journal of American Dental Association* 84 (1972): 1073–1075.

Kime, Robert E. *Health: A Consumer's Dilemma*. Belmont, Calif.: Wadsworth Publishing Co., 1970.

Masters, Donald H. "The Classroom Teacher . . . Effective Dental Health Education." *Journal of School Health* 42 (1972): 257–261.

Mayer, Jean. *Health*. New York: D. Van Nostrand Co., 1974.

National Clearinghouse for Alcohol Information of the National Institute on Alcohol Abuse and Alcoholism. "Second Special Report Updates Alcohol Knowledge." *NIAAA Information and Feature Service*, 20 Octo-
ber 1974.

Schaller, Warren E., and Nemir, Alma. *The School Health Program*, 4th ed. Philadelphia: W. B. Saunders Co., 1975.

Scherp, Henry W. "Dental Caries: Prospects for Prevention." *Science* 173 (1971): 1199–1205.

School Safety 5 (1969): 26.

Stolpe, J. R., Mechlenberg, R. E., and Lathrop, R. L. "The Effectiveness of an Educational Program on Oral Health in Schools for Improving the Application of Knowledge." *Journal of Public Health Dentistry* 31 (1971): 30.

Toffler, Alvin. *Future Shock*. New York: Random House, 1970, Bantam Books, Inc., 1971.

U.S., Department of Agriculture. *Dietary Levels in the United States, Spring, 1965*. Washington, D.C.: Government Printing Office, 1968.

U.S., Department of Health, Education, and Welfare. *Eye Examination Findings Among Children in the United States,* DHEW Publication, no. 721057. Washington, D.C.: Government Printing Office, 1972.

U.S., Department of Health, Education, and Welfare. *The Health of Children*. Washington, D.C.: Government Printing Office, 1970.

Winick, Myron. "Childhood Obesity." *Nutrition Today* 9 (1974): 6–12.

Chapter 17
EVALUATING THE SCHOOL HEALTH PROGRAM

Why should schools be held accountable for their product?

What is the difference between measurement and evaluation?

Why should schools have appropriate evaluative techniques to accurately assess health education, health services, and healthful school environment?

What new problems are now facing school evaluators?

In recent years educational evaluation has generated a large amount of interest among politicians, teachers, school administrators, parents, and other concerned persons. Some of this interest has stemmed from the accountability movement at federal and state levels which has filtered down to the community level and into the educational system. Citizens are now asking questions concerning the effectiveness of the educational programs, while school administrators are being asked to make policy decisions, allocate resources, and modify or develop programs based upon more objective measures. Teachers today may well find themselves in an era of educational accountability. Many professional educators believe that educational accountability systems offer immense promise for improving the quality of the educational system.

Since the education profession must be concerned with the proper role of evaluation, educators will need detailed facts and supportive data for the decision-making process. Concrete data are necessary in all areas from educational programs to facilities and budgetary matters.

Before the evaluative aspects of the school health program are discussed, it is helpful to distinguish between certain fundamental concepts and terms. A widespread misconception of evaluation is that it is synonymous with measurement. Measurement consists of an assessment of the current status of a phenomenon in a particular manner. Basically, as the term implies, measurement involves counting or enumerating so that one can describe how large or how small something is. Thus, we can determine the health knowledge or attitude scores of students on an examination, the number of injuries to school students, and any other quantitative measurement that might be useful in the school health program. Evaluation is a much broader term that consists of assessments of merit regarding educational phenomena in which one determines the relative worth of whatever is being evaluated.[1] In evaluation the results of different measurements are used to arrive at value judgments. For example: How effective is the health instruction program? Is the school health service program worthwhile?

An evaluation of the school health program is useful in determining the needs, assessing the strengths and weaknesses, and improving the various areas that comprise the total health program.

Oberteuffer and associates suggest certain basic principles of program evaluation that should serve as guidelines for those concerned with the evaluative process.

1. Evaluation should be continuous and concurrent with program activities.
2. It should embrace all the important functions of the school health program including instruction, services, and activities.
3. It should be concerned with outcomes, process, and structure.
4. Evaluation should be cooperative. All who are affected by the evaluation should participate. This includes administrators, teachers, pupils, parents, physicians, nurses, hygienists, nutritionists, and community representatives.
5. Evaluation should be focused upon the important values that underlie the health program of the school. Those values are best expressed in terms of program objectives and goals stated during the program planning period.
6. A long-range evaluation program should be planned so that no one year would involve a complete study of every aspect of school health education.
7. Data gathering and record keeping should be performed to aid in the evaluation of the functions of school health education and not as ends in themselves.[2]

EVALUATION OF SCHOOL HEALTH EDUCATION

Evaluative techniques employed in health education may be of either a subjective or an objective nature. Subjective techniques include various procedures such as observations, checklists, anecdotal records, questionnaires, surveys, interviews, self-appraisals, discussions, and informal autobiographies. Usually subjective evaluation is employed to assess health attitudes and practices. Objective evaluative techniques refer to objective-type paper-and-pencil tests that yield quantitative data. Teacher-made tests and standardized tests are examples of techniques falling into the objective category. While these techniques may also be employed to determine health attitudes and practices, their main value appears to be in determining the cognitive skills that students have obtained.[3]

School health education attempts to provide learning experiences for the purpose of influencing knowledge, attitudes, and practices relating to

1. W. James Popham, *Evaluating Instruction* (Englewood Cliffs, N. J.: Prentice-Hall, 1973), p. 10.
2. Delbert Oberteuffer, Orvis Harrelson, and Marion Pollock, *School Health Education* (New York: Harper & Row, 1972), p. 418.
3. John Fodor and Gus Dalis, *Health Instruction: Theory and Application* (Philadelphia: Lea & Febiger, 1974), p. 111.

individual and community health. Consequently, program evaluation should be concerned with all three aspects and involve many different evaluative techniques to provide data in order to determine how well the program is meeting the objectives.

OBSERVATIONS

Observations may often provide clues concerning a child's attitudes and health practices. For example, after teaching a unit on communicable diseases and stressing the need to protect the health of others, the teacher may observe that more children now cover their mouth or nose when coughing or sneezing. Other examples might include the observation that Mary's visual problem was corrected through the acquisition of glasses or that John now crosses the street with the traffic light after a unit on pedestrian safety. Many opportunities exist during the day in the classroom, on the playground, and on field trips to observe the health attitudes and practices of children.

CHECKLISTS, QUESTIONNAIRES, AND SURVEYS

Checklists, questionnaires, and surveys may also provide information on a wide range of topics relating to knowledge, attitudes, and behavior. These techniques might be employed by the teacher to determine a child's attitudes concerning nutrition, safety practices, health practices, and so on. Likewise they may also be employed to determine knowledge with respect to community health resources and other health related areas.

ANECDOTAL RECORDS

Anecdotal records are short summaries of some incident of significant behavior that is observed. They may provide information about classroom behavior as well as about behavior observed on the playground or in the cafeteria or other facets of school life. One of the major problems in obtaining evidence on behavior is that of obtaining a valid anecdotal report. Anecdotes should not include any reference by the teacher as to why the behavior occurred. An anecdote should only describe the observed behavior of a student. Records of this type have come under criticism for being time-consuming if teachers were to fill out a report for every child in the classroom. Perhaps their major contribution is in their utilization for children with specific personality or behavioral problems. Ideally, in this situation they would provide additional clues for the teacher, nurse, counselor, and others concerned to see how the child behaves in different situations. Positive anecdotal records are as important as negative ones. Unfortunately, some teachers record only the undesirable or antisocial behavior of their pupils.

INTERVIEWS

Interviews with students, parents, nurses, counselors, teachers, and other school personnel may provide the teacher with clues as to why certain attitudinal or behavioral changes may have occurred in children.

SELF-APPRAISAL AND PUPIL EVALUATION

Techniques of this type may be of value in determining knowledge gains and/or attitudinal and behavior change. Students might appraise their nutritional intake, safety practices, and health habits. Pupil evaluation might include comments by the students on what they have learned after a given unit of instruction.

Subjective techniques employed by themselves would probably be of slight value to the classroom teacher. However, the selection of several subjective techniques combined with more objective data can provide insight into the cognitive, attitudinal, and behavioral changes occurring within children.

OBJECTIVE TECHNIQUES

TEACHER-MADE TESTS

The teacher-prepared test is the most common technique employed for assessing pupil knowledge. Since a test generally represents a sample of all the possible questions that might be asked, it is imperative that the test constitute a fair and representative sample of questions to assess pupil performance. Before developing a test, teachers should understand the purpose the test is to serve, what skills and content areas are to be measured, and what their relative weights are to be. The major benefit of preparing one's own test is that in the very process of writing questions one is forced to define teaching objectives in terms of specific skills and understandings.

Generally, test items are classified as either subjective (essay) or objective. Essays allow pupils to express their answers in their own words; however, the quality of the answer must be judged subjectively by the teacher. The written essay if properly developed should require pupils to present evidence, to evaluate, to analyze, and to solve problems that require a higher level of critical thinking than merely recognizing a correct answer on an objective test. While essays have been criticized for not being reliable with respect to variation of assigned grades by the same teacher from day to day, they can be useful in measuring outcomes that some objective tests may not be able to achieve.

OBJECTIVE TESTS

Objective tests usually restrict students' answers to brief phrases or words and can be scored by anyone having the correct responses. Objective-type questions can be developed as completion items in which the pupil *supplies* the response or as true-false, multiple-choice, and matching items in which pupils *select* a response from among several presented.

Completion items   The short answer or completion item is characterized by the presence of a blank in which the student supplies the answer to the question or solution to the problem called for in the directions. Since the student is required to write the answer, the emphasis is upon recall rather than upon recognition. The major problem in writing completion items is to develop questions that have a single correct response. Teachers are often quite surprised to discover the variety of correct responses that may appear to questions that they had conceived as having only one answer. For example a question such as: Heat exhaustion is less serious than _____ may provoke a variety of answers even though the teacher wanted "heatstroke" as the correct response. However, a recall item such as; In _____ immunity the body produces its own antibodies, has only one correct answer which is "active." Completion items are relatively easy to construct; however, if used excessively, they may result in overemphasis on memorization. In addition they are generally inappropriate for measuring understanding, application, interpretation, and other complex learning outcomes.

True-False items   This type of item consists of a statement to be judged true or false or a question which is to be answered yes or no. It is useful when the desired outcomes are either to determine the truth or falsity of a statement, to distinguish between fact and opinion, or to discriminate between appropriate and inappropriate responses. Disadvantages of true-false questions include the following: (1) guessing is encouraged since there is a fifty-fifty chance of selecting the right response; (2) ambiguities, unimportant details, and irrelevant clues may be added to the question; and (3) many important concepts, objectives, and inferences cannot be expressed in statements that are universally true.

Multiple-choice items   Although the multiple-choice item does not lend itself to measuring a pupil's ability to organize ideas, it is generally considered to be the most versatile and reliable objective type of test item. Advantages of the multiple-choice item include the following: (1) it offers a wide sampling of content in a relatively short period of time; (2) it establishes a forced-choice situation which requires that the pupil demonstrate the specific ability called for by each item; (3) the guessing factor is considerably reduced, particularly if four or five responses are provided; and (4) it can be objectively scored. Following is an example of multiple-choice items for testing for health knowledge.[4]

Directions: Select the letter of the best answer and place it in the space provided.

1. _____ Alcohol is oxidized in the (a) blood (b) liver (c) stomach (d) lungs (e) kidney.

2. _____ An example of an official health agency is the: (a) American Heart Association (b) National Safety Council (c) National Institute on Alcohol Abuse and Alcoholism (d) National Association for Mental Health (e) American Cancer Society.

3. _____ The denial of one's own weakness by shifting a problem or the blame for a situation to other persons is called: (a) regression (b) identification (c) projection (d) egocentrism (e) repression.

4. _____ The leading cause of death in the United States is: (a) cancer (b) heart disease (c) accidents (d) influenza (e) pneumonia.

5. _____ The federal agency concerned with the safety of all new drugs is the: (a) Federal Trade Commission (b) Food and Drug Administration (c) Better Business Bureau (d) American Medical Association (e) Department of Commerce.

Matching items   Although easily constructed and objectively scored, matching items cannot be used as effectively as multiple-choice items for measuring understanding. This type of item consists of a list of premises and a list of responses. The student is directed to match one of the responses to each of the premises. The simple matching exercise is chiefly used for identification of names, terminology, structure, function, and similar

4. Sample questions are from a seventh grade test.

associations. The major disadvantage of this type of test item is the fact that the major emphasis is placed on the mere memorization of factual material. Ideally, the matching lists should be kept short so that they can be easily handled by the student. Some teachers may compose a test having as many as 25 items in each list. Thus if a pupil is to compare each of 25 premises with each of the 25 responses, he is required to make a total of 625 comparisons. Obviously, not only is this too tedious a task to impose upon the student, but it also sacrifices the economy of the testing time. Generally, matching questions should be limited to about 10 items. The following is an example of matching test items used in testing for health knowledge.[5]

Directions: On the line at the left of each item in Column A write the number of the matching item selected from Column B.

Column A	Column B	
___ phobia	1. Freud	5. projection
___ psychoses	2. obsessive-compulsive	6. Maslow
___ neuroses	behavior	7. Jung
___ psychoanalytical theory	3. extreme fear	8. suicide
___ hierarchy of needs	4. schizophrenia	

STANDARDIZED TESTS

Numerous standardized tests have been developed for assessing health knowledge, attitudes, and behavior. An excellent review of evaluation instruments available in health education for the elementary teacher is found in a published bibliography developed by Solleder.[6] A major value of standardized tests is that they have been developed by specialists so that the general quality of questions is high. Furthermore, they have been subjected to careful statistical analysis in order to control for difficulty and discrimination. Also, norms are available to compare the performance of pupils with the performance of other pupils with known characteristics. Disadvantages of standardized tests include the following: (1) they may not always relate to specific objectives formulated for a particular group of pupils; (2) some tests may be obsolete since advances in the health sciences occur at a rapid pace; and (3) it is doubtful that these instruments really measure attitudes or practices; more likely they measure knowledge of the attitude or practice desired.[7] Finally, many times it is difficult to find a test that covers only a single unit of study, and thus teachers are forced to develop their own tests.

EVALUATING SCHOOL HEALTH SERVICES AND SCHOOL ENVIRONMENT

Both of these areas are generally more easily evaluated than health education since several checklists for this purpose are available. Questions relating to such items as frequency of health examinations, dental inspections, and screening tests; activities of personnel involved; follow-up counseling procedures; prevention and control of communicable disease; emergency and first-aid provisions; equipment; and records are generally included on most forms to assess the quality of school health services. Checklists involving the

5. Sample questions are from an eighth grade test.
6. Marian Solleder, *Evaluation Instruments in Health Education* (Washington, D. C.: American Association for Health, Physical Education, and Recreation, 1969).
7. Fodor and Dalis, *Health Instruction,* p. 113.

area of healthful school living generally have questions with respect to the school site, water supply, waste disposal, fire protection, ventilation, heating, lighting, seating, sanitary facilities, lunchroom service, play facilities, school safety program, and emotional climate within the school. Anderson has developed an excellent scale for evaluating the quality of healthful school living.[8] Other forms such as that published by the California State Department of Education are available for evaluating the entire elementary school health program including administration, health instruction, health services, and healthful school environment.[9] A copy of this instrument is provided in Appendix B.

Since some prepared instruments may not be applicable to all schools, it may be more convenient for most evaluation committees to examine several of the available instruments and determine what items they feel would fit their particular situation.

A LOOK AT THE FUTURE: PROSPECTS AND PROBLEMS IN EVALUATION

Evaluators have become much more sophisticated in their understanding and application of appropriate research methods, in statistical analysis, and in the development and refinement of various evaluative techniques that may be employed in the evaluative process. However, most experts would agree that the major focus will now have to center on the impact that programs and services have on students as well as on the economic costs to the tax-paying community. Evans points out some of the newer problems that education evaluators must now be concerned with.[10]

1. As educational research and evaluation have proliferated, the people and institutions who are the objects of these studies have come to express their resistance to these procedures. This has been observed particularly with respect to minorities and poverty groups.

2. The increased sensitivity to evaluation studies on the part of some school administrators has created reluctance to participate in such studies for fear of what might happen to their programs if the evaluation produces negative findings.

3. Evaluations increasingly encounter unrealistic expectations on the part of policymakers with respect to the speed at which evaluations should be completed.

4. Due to possible public debate over the validity of certain evaluation methods and results, evaluators may be placed in the position of defending their evaluations and their suitability as a basis for policy decisions.

SUMMARY

Today, the general public is more knowledgeable about education than at any other point in history. They are asking such basic questions as How do you know your program is effective? and What is the most economical approach? Educators must be able to provide answers to these questions in this era of accountability. We cannot sit back and wait for evaluation to happen while industry spends millions on research and development for new and improved products. Seldom has education made more than a token effort

8. C. L. Anderson, *School Health Practice*, 5th ed. (St. Louis: C. V. Mosby Co., 1972).

9. "Criteria for Evaluating the Elementary School Health Program," (Sacramento: California State Department of Education, 1962).

10. John Evans, "Evaluating Education Programs: Are We Getting Anywhere?" *Educational Review*, September 1974, p. 11.

to improve its product. Recently, business and industry have steadily moved into educational product development in many curriculum areas including health education. If educators do not begin to evaluate their own programs, others might assume the responsibility to fill the void. This fact alone should motivate educators to gain the necessary expertise in evaluation. Stake very aptly states that "evaluation audiences do believe that to understand education one needs to understand what people expect from educaion. As long as that is true, evaluators have an obligation to make a careful search for objectives, standards, and other judgment data."[11]

Discussion Questions

1. Justify your position with respect to educational accountability to the public.
2. Distinguish between the terms *measurement* and *evaluation*.
3. Discuss the various types of subjective techniques that may be utilized to assess health knowledge, attitudes, and behavior. What are their advantages? their disadvantages?
4. What are some advantages and disadvantages of test questions involving completion, true-false, multiple-choice, and matching items?
5. Of what value are standardized tests to a classroom teacher?
6. What basic principles of program evaluation might serve as guidelines for the evaluative process?
7. What areas are generally evaluated in the school environment?
8. What areas are evaluated in health services?
9. Discuss some of the new problems that evaluators must now be concerned with.

References

Anderson, C. L. *School Health Practice.* 5th ed. St. Louis: C. V. Mosby Co., 1972.

Evans, John. "Evaluating Educational Programs: Are We Getting Anywhere?" *Educational Review,* September 1974, pp. 7–12.

Fodor, John, and Dalis, Gus. *Health Instruction: Theory and Application.* Philadelphia: Lea & Febiger, 1974.

Oberteuffer, Delbert, Harrelson, Orvis, and Pollock, Marion. *School Health Education,* New York: Harper & Row, 1972.

Popham, W. James. *Evaluating Instruction.* Englewood Cliffs, N.J.: Prentice-Hall, 1973.

Solleder, Marion. *Evaluation Instruments in Health Education.* Washington, D.C.: American Association for Health, Physical Education, and Recreation, 1969.

Stake, Robert. "Objectives, Priorities, and Other Judgment Data." *Review of Educational Research* 40, no. 2 (1970): 181–205.

11. Robert Stake, "Objectives, Priorities, and Other Judgment Data," *Review of Educational Research* 40, no. 2 (1970): 205.

Appendix A

WALL
CHART:
COMMUNICABLE
DISEASE
INFORMATION

COMMUNICABLE DISEASE INFORMATION
DEPARTMENT OF PUBLIC HEALTH

DISEASE	EARLY SIGNS AND SYMPTOMS	RASH (Skin Manifestations)	INCUBATION PERIOD	METHOD OF TRANSMISSION	CONTROL OF CASES	
					Isolation (Quarantine)	Exclusion From School
CHICKENPOX	Skin eruption associated with fever.	Occurrence early, thickest on trunk, with successive crops of red, raised dots, which turn into fluid-filled blisters and then dry up to form scabs.	Two-three weeks, commonly thirteen-seventeen days.	From person to person. Through articles freshly soiled by discharges from skin and mucous membranes of patient.	For not less than six days after the appearance of eruption.	Yes, until end of isolation.
DIPHTHERIA	Sore throat with gray-white patches. Moderate fever. Croupy cough.	None.	Two-five days, occasionally longer	From person to person. Through articles freshly soiled by discharges from nose and throat of case or carrier. Through milk contaminated by case or carrier.	Until two successive cultures from both nose and throat, taken not less than 24 hours apart, are negative for diphtheria bacilli.**	Yes, until end of isolation.
GERMAN MEASLES	Rash, slight swelling of glands on back of neck.	Small, pinkish-red blotches, beginning behind ears and on face.	Fourteen to twenty-one days.	From person to person. Through articles freshly soiled by discharges from nose and throat of patient.	Not required, except that contact between cases and women in early pregnancy should be strictly avoided. If close contacts include a woman in early pregnancy she may receive prophylactic immune globulin at the direction of her physician.	Recommended for 5 days after appearance of rash.
MEASLES	Starts like a cold with fever, watery eyes and nose, sometimes sneezing and slight cough.	Occurs third to fifth day after onset of fever, composed of groups of dull red blotches on face which spread downward on body.	Ten to fourteen days.	Same as above.	Until seven days after the appearance of the rash.	Yes, until end of isolation.
MUMPS	Fever, nausea, pain and swelling about jaws.	None.	Twelve-twenty-six days, commonly eighteen days.	Same as above.	Not less than 2 days after swelling subsides.	Yes, until end of isolation.
Meningococcal MENINGITIS (Cerebro-Spinal Fever)	Sudden onset with fever, headache, vomiting, sometimes convulsions followed by higher fever and stiff neck and back.	Frequently a red, pin-point like rash is seen in the disease.	Two to ten days. Commonly three-four days.	From person to person. Through articles freshly soiled by discharges from nose and throat of case or carrier.	Until twenty-four hours after start of chemotherapy.	Yes, until end of isolation.
POLIOMYELITIS	Headache, nausea, vomiting, muscle soreness or stiffness, stiff neck, fever, nasal voice and difficulty in swallowing, with regurgitation of liquids through the nose.	None.	Commonly seven to twelve days.	Not definitely known but probably by close contact with case or carrier, their nose and throat discharges and feces.	None required. Isolation is of little value because spread of infection is greatest preceding onset of the disease.	Yes, until end of acute phase of the disease.
SCARLET FEVER and STREPTOCOCCAL SORE THROAT	Sudden onset, with fever, vomiting, sore throat and development of rash and "strawberry tongue."	Bright red, pin-point dots, appearing first on neck and upper chest. (These may be absent.) Streptococcal sore throat is scarlet fever infection without a rash.	One-three days, rarely longer.	From person to person. Through articles freshly soiled by discharges of patient. Through milk contaminated by case or carrier.	Isolation required, but may be terminated after 24 hours treatment with antibiotics, provided treatment is continued for a minimum of ten days and the nose, throat, glands and ears are normal on inspection.	Yes, until end of isolation.
WHOOPING COUGH (PERTUSSIS)	Starts with symptoms of a cold; characteristic "whoop" develops in cough. Coughing frequently occurs in spasms and accompanied by vomiting.	None.	Ten days, commonly seven days.	From person to person. Through articles soiled by discharges from throat of patient.	Minimum of three weeks after appearance of paroxysmal cough. May have liberty of home and yard provided he does not come into contact with other children.	Yes, until end of isolation.

SCHEDULE OF IMMUNIZATION*

DISEASE	PREFERRED AGE INITIAL DOSE	IMMUNIZING ANTIGEN	BOOSTER DOSE
DIPHTHERIA TETANUS and PERTUSSIS	2-3 months of age	A.P. Diphtheria and Tetanus toxoids and Pertussis vaccine	0.5 cc. 1 year later
TETANUS and DIPHTHERIA (Adult use)	Age 6 years and over	A.P. Tetanus and Diphtheria toxoids combined, adult use	0.5 cc. 6 mo.-1 year later & every 8-10 years thereafter
POLIOMYELITIS	2-3 months of age	Trivalent Oral (Sabin)	See "Recommended Procedures for Immunization" (No. 5.002)

*For latest information on immunizations, contact your physician or the local medical society.

KEEP THE SCHOOLS OPEN AND DISEASE OUT!

Closing schools as a means of controlling epidemics of measles, whooping cough, scarlet fever, mumps, diphtheria, and other common communicable diseases should be considered as a last resort to be used only when thorough application of all other measures fails. As a control method, it is clumsy and unsatisfactory, for it fails to control and results in the loss of school time and money. The modern method of careful, daily inspection of infected schools, isolation of sick children and quarantine of contacts, is both effective and economical.

The immediate reporting to the local health officer of all cases of communicable diseases will greatly reduce the opportunities for the spread of these diseases.

CONTROL OF CONTACTS		SPECIAL FEATURES
Adults	Children	
No restrictions.	No restrictions. May attend school.	Mild disease. Seldom any after-effects. May be severe in adults.
All home contacts, who continue to live on premises, quarantined for duration of disease and must submit nose and throat cultures. If one culture from nose and one from throat are free from diphtheria bacilli, immune contacts may live off premises and carry on regular work. *See wage earner provision.		Diphtheria can only be controlled by maintaining a high level of immunity in the population. (Carriers are usually the source). Immunization recommended for adults. See "Recommended Procedures for Immunization," Circular No. 5.002.
No restrictions. If contacts include a woman in early pregnancy, she should consult with her physician.	No restrictions. May attend school.	A very mild disease with no after effects (except in early pregnancy when complications in fetus may occur). May be confused with scarlet fever or measles. Early and correct diagnosis important; prophylactic use of immune serum globulin immediately upon recognition of exposure in a pregnant woman may be considered.
No restrictions.	No restrictions. Immune serum globulin can be used to prevent or modify disease, according to year of age and condition of general health at time of exposure. See special directive No. 206-A.	A highly contagious disease, most serious in pre-school children. Urge that all infants be immunized with live measles vaccine. See "Recommended Procedures for Immunization," Circular No. 5.002.
No restrictions.	No restrictions. May attend school.	Infectious early. May cause complications in adults. Recommendations for use of live mumps vaccine, see package insert.
No restrictions.		Contacts must be placed under close medical supervision which may include drug prophylaxis.
No restrictions. It is recommended that children with direct contact to a case be kept under medical surveillance for two weeks from date of last exposure. Voluntary limitation of physical activity to reduce severity of disease if it should develop is also recommended. Adult home contacts, who are engaged in the production of milk and milk products on the premises in which a case is isolated, may continue such production provided that all milk and milk products are sent directly to a pasteurizing plant.		Use of live poliomyelitis vaccine is recommended. See "Recommended Procedures for Immunization," Circular No. 5.002.
**No restrictions, except on food handlers.		Chemotherapeutic agents are recommended because of possibility of complications.
None.	Exclusion of non-immune children from school and public gatherings for 14 days after last exposure to a household or similar case.	Most dangerous to pre-school children. Immunization in infancy against whooping cough is urged. See "Recommended Procedures for Immunization," Circular No. 5.002.

*The wage earner, who has submitted a nose and throat culture negative for diphtheria bacilli, may be permitted to continue his work provided he is over 16 years of age, has no direct contact with the patient and is not a food handler, school teacher or employee around a school or other place where there are children, and provided also that permission is granted in writing by the local health authority. This privilege is granted solely for the purpose of permitting the wage earner to continue his occupation and he shall not enter any other premises not in line with his employment. If he violates these restrictions, he shall be placed under quarantine, unless he moves to another address and continues to live there during the quarantine period. It should be understood that this is not a blanket privilege for a wage earner, and that permission for this type of modified quarantine will be rescinded by the Illinois Department of Public Health if local health authority does not insist on proper isolation of patient.
**For details see "Rules and Regulations for the Control of Communicable Diseases."

RINGWORM OF THE SCALP

Ringworm of the scalp occurs in children, is highly contagious and becomes epidemic in schools. It begins as a small, rounded, elevated, scaly, grayish patch on the hairy scalp. Affected hairs are dry, brittle and usually broken. Eventually the hair is lost, leaving bald patches. Itching is usually mild. Infected children should be excluded from schools and other public places until healing has taken place. All towels, washcloths, toilet articles, etc. should be disinfected. When one or more cases occur in a school, all children should receive a careful examination of the scalp with the use of filtered ultra-violet light. Pets, particularly kittens, should be inspected under filtered ultra-violet light as they may be carriers of ringworm. Proper treatment should be provided for each case discovered.

PEDICULOSIS OR LICE

Lice are small, light gray insects, which lay eggs or "nits" in the hair, especially at the nape of the neck and about the ears. Symptoms are itching and irritation of the scalp. Close inspection will reveal the insects moving about the head and "nits" fastened securely to the base of the hairs. The condition, though easily cured, is highly contagious, and when found in a school room, the infected child should be excluded. The hair of all the other children should be inspected.

SCABIES OR ITCH

A highly infectious eruption caused by a mite and found most frequently between the fingers and on the forearms, but may involve the entire body. Ordinarily, it takes the form of small, scattered red spots, among which there may be some watery or pus-filled small blisters. Marked itching is typical of the disease, which is chronic unless treated. The infected child should be excluded from school and should be kept away from others until cured. Whenever the disease occurs, all members of the family should be inspected for it.

Appendix B
CRITERIA
FOR
EVALUATING
THE
ELEMENTARY
SCHOOL
HEALTH
PROGRAM

Criteria for Evaluating the Elementary School Health Program provides school personnel with a tool to use in making an evaluation of the school health program. The results of such an evaluation reveal the strengths and weaknesses of the program. Where weaknesses are revealed, the school health committee may act to bring all the available forces into action for the express purpose of securing strength in the program where weaknesses exist and for planning ways all other phases of the program may be kept strong.

The criteria for evaluating the school health program were developed by a committee of the California Fitness Project and School Health Education Evaluative Study, Los Angeles area, that worked three years under the general chairmanship of Edward B. Johns, Professor of Health Education, University of California, Los Angeles. Separate sets of criteria were developed for the elementary school, the secondary school, and the junior college. Each set of criteria was field-tested in a sampling of schools throughout the state as well as reviewed by a group of curriculum specialists and school health personnel. C. Carson Conrad, Chief of the Bureau of Health Education, Physical Education, and Recreation, California State Department of Education, is Co-ordinator for the California Fitness Project.

The members of the subcommittee responsible for developing the *Criteria for Evaluating the Elementary School Health Program* were Grace Axelson, Colleen Boehm, Isabel Casares, Viola Hudson, Katherine Martin, teachers, and Helen Doak, Anna Schwartz, James Black, Reta Ryan, supervisors and directors, Alhambra City Elementary School District; Jo Beckwith, Gladys Bell, Julian Bradford, Grace Garrettson, Mary Grim, Rhoda Grubb, Ann Learman, Anita Link, Yvette Rawlinson, Erna Reis, teachers, Raye Fowler, Anna Ryan, Pearl Wendt, school nurses, Howard Harmon, Arvle Dedmon, supervisors and directors, Whittier Elementary School District; Elma Plappert, Los Angeles County Tuberculosis and Health Association; Aubrey W. Calvett, Field Representative, California State Department of Education, and Ethel T. Bell, University of California, Los Angeles, who served as consultants to the group; and Sylvia Yellen, Consultant in Health Education, Alhambra City Elementary School District, and Mary Ellen Johns, Director of Health, Whittier Elementary School District, who served as co-chairmen of the committee. Edward B. Johns, University of California, Los Angeles, was Co-ordinator of the School Health Criteria Project and also a consultant. Patricia Hill, Consultant in Health Education, California State Department of Education, was a consultant on the School Health Criteria Project and prepared the material for publication.

The criteria in each set are organized into four divisions:

I—Administration, II—Health Instruction, III—Health Services, and IV—Healthful School Environment. The criteria are expressed in terms of desirable practices and presented in the left column. The evaluation should be made by a representative group of the faculty, including administrators, teachers, health service personnel, and others. The results should express judgments that are approved by the evaluation committee as a whole.

Provision is made for the quality of each *provision* or *practice* stated in the criteria to be judged on a four-point scale: *excellent, good, fair, poor*. If the provision is not made, the practice is not followed; or if the quality is fair or poor, there is space for listing changes needed. At the top of each section, space is provided for recording recommended steps to be taken in relation to the changes needed. Care should be taken to make recommendations that will not have an adverse effect on provisions or practices already judged excellent or good.

Published by the California State Department of Education, Sacramento, 1962. Roy E. Simpson, Superintendent of Public Instruction

SUGGESTED PROCEDURE FOR USING THE CRITERIA FOR EVALUATING THE ELEMENTARY SCHOOL HEALTH PROGRAM

1. Determine the membership of study group to evaluate the program.
2. Determine the need for consultant help.
3. Study thoroughly the criteria and the provisions for making the desired evaluations.
4. Determine whether the program meets each criterion.
5. If the criterion is met, determine the quality of the provision or practice according to the following scale: *Excellent*—near perfection; *Good*—satisfactory; *Fair*—slightly less than satisfactory; *Poor*—unsatisfactory.
6. If the criterion is not met—that is, the provision not made or the practice not followed—indicate by a check in the appropriate column.
7. Compile a list of the changes needed and determine how the changes can be secured to best advantage.
8. Set up a priority for accomplishing the changes.
9. Develop recommendations for making the needed change and record in appropriate space at the top of each section.
10. Submit the recommendations to the administration for action.

Criteria for Evaluating the Elementary School Health Program

Criteria	Quality of Provision or Practice					Changes Needed
	Excellent (near per- fection)	Good (satis- factory)	Fair (slightly less than satis- factory)	Poor (unsatis- factory)	Provision not Made or Practice not Followed	
I. ADMINISTRATION						
A. The policies of the district's governing board provide for a school health program designed to help all pupils achieve the degree of health their potentialities permit through health instruction, health services, a healthful school environment—essentials of the program.	Recommended steps to be taken:					
1. The policies provide for a comprehensive and well-planned program of health instruction.						
2. The policies provide for essential health services.						
3. The policies provide for the maintenance of a healthful school environment.						
B. A written statement of the school district's point of view regarding the kind and quality of the school health program is available.	Recommended steps to be taken:					
1. The statement of point of view makes apparent the direction to be taken in providing health services.						
2. The statement of point of view makes apparent the direction to be taken in the program of health instruction.						
3. The statement of point of view makes apparent the direction to be taken in providing and maintaining a healthful school environment.						

C. Responsibility for planning, developing, and administering the district's school health program is delegated by the governing board of the district to the district superintendent of schools.

Recommended steps to be taken:

1. A health committee with a membership that includes school personnel, representatives of community health services, and representatives of the other important segments of the community is assigned advisory responsibilities for the district's school health program.

2. The superintendent has defined the duties of each person who has responsibility for providing health services.

3. The superintendent has defined the duties of each person who has responsibility for health instruction.

4. The superintendent has defined the duties of each person who has responsibility for the promotion and maintenance of a healthful school environment.

5. The superintendent has defined for the principal his responsibility for the school health program.

6. The superintendent and the principal have defined for the teachers and other members of the school staff their responsibilities for the school health program.

D. The principal of the school has outlined the practices that are employed in operating the school health program.

Recommended steps to be taken:

Criteria for Evaluating the Elementary School Health Program—cont.

Criteria	Quality of Provision or Practice					Changes Needed
	Excellent (near perfection)	Good (satisfactory)	Fair (slightly less than satisfactory)	Poor (unsatisfactory)	Provision not Made or Practice not Followed	
1. A health council or committee with a membership that includes an administrator, teachers, health personnel, and, when possible, counselors, custodians, and school lunch personnel is assigned advisory responsibilities for the school health program.						
2. Each member of the staff is informed regarding the health services the district provides.						
3. Each member of the staff is informed regarding the health instruction offered by the school.						
4. Each member of the staff is informed regarding the prescribed procedures for first aid and emergency care.						
5. Each member of the staff is informed regarding the provisions that are made for developing and maintaining a healthful school environment.						
6. Responsibility for the leadership needed to make the school health program function efficiently is assigned to a member of the school staff who has special preparation in health education.						
7. Procedures are established for members of the staff to report improvements in health instruction.						
8. Procedures are established for members of the staff to report changes needed in the health services provided the school.						
9. Procedures are established for members of the staff to report improvements needed in the school environment.						

10. Procedures are established for members of the staff to report changes needed in the prescribed procedures for first aid and emergency care.

E. Clerical help, equipment, and supplies, in keeping with the pupil population, are provided for the health services program.

Recommended steps to be taken:

1. Clerical help is provided health service personnel to assist with record keeping.

2. Audiometers and vision screening equipment, preferably lighted Snellen cabinets, are available as needed.

3. All equipment used in health services is maintained in working condition.

4. Essential equipment such as cabinets for supplies, cots, and scales are available in the school.

5. Essential supplies such as those used in first aid, communicable disease control, health appraisal activities, and record keeping are available in the school.

F. Health personnel are adequate in number and specialization to provide needed services.

Recommended steps to be taken:

1. School nurses are available in a ratio of one nurse for each 1,000 to 1,400 pupils. (Distances traveled to visit homes and type of terrain should be considered in determining the desired ratio.)

2. Physicians are available for consultation and advice.

EVALUATING THE ELEMENTARY SCHOOL
HEALTH PROGRAM

Criteria for Evaluating the Elementary School Health Program—cont.

Criteria	Quality of Provision or Practice					Changes Needed
	Excellent (near perfection)	Good (satisfactory)	Fair (slightly less than satisfactory)	Poor (unsatisfactory)	Provision not Made or Practice not Followed	
3. Dentists are available for consultation and advice.						
4. Health service personnel serving the school are regularly credentialed.						
G. The professional library and the school library are well supplied with health materials.	Recommended steps to be taken:					
1. The professional library contains up-to-date books, courses of study, and periodicals on health.						
2. The materials in the professional library cover all phases of the school health program.						
3. The school library contains up-to-date books and periodicals on health.						
4. The books and periodicals in the school library are within the pupils' range of reading ability.						
5. The books and periodicals in the school library are adequate in number for the school population.						
H. Each classroom is supplied with the materials needed for use in health instruction.	Recommended steps to be taken:					
1. The classrooms for each grade are supplied with the basic textbooks in health that are supplied by the state.						

2. Each classroom is supplied with health materials, in addition to the state-adopted textbooks, that cover each phase of health.

3. The scope of the materials in each classroom is sufficient to provide for all the pupils, from the slowest to the fastest learner.

I. The in-service education program for school personnel provides for health instruction to have the same emphasis as other areas of instruction.

Recommended steps to be taken:

1. Sessions are devoted to presentation of current factual information about health.

2. Methods of health teaching to obtain changes in pupils, attitudes and practices are discussed and suggestions for improvements in instruction are presented.

3. Evaluation of the school health program is discussed and suggestions for program improvements are presented.

J. The in-service education program for school personnel provides for study of the school health services.

Recommended steps to be taken:

1. The services provided by health personnel are reviewed in relation to their purpose.

2. The procedures employed in providing health services are reviewed.

3. Health services are studied in relation to all other phases of the school program.

EVALUATING THE ELEMENTARY SCHOOL
HEALTH PROGRAM

389

Criteria for Evaluating the Elementary School Health Program—cont.

Criteria	Quality of Provision or Practice					Changes Needed
	Excellent (near perfection)	Good (satisfactory)	Fair (slightly less than satisfactory)	Poor (unsatisfactory)	Provision not Made or Practice not Followed	

II. HEALTH INSTRUCTION

A. A course of study for health, a course of study and a teacher's guide or a combination course of study and teacher's guide is provided by the school district or the office of the county superintendent of schools for use in the school.

Recommended steps to be taken:

1. A course of study and a teacher's guide for health are available in the school.

2. A combination course of study and teacher's guide is available in the school.

3. The course of study provides for a developmental program of instruction.

4. The teacher's guide outlines the teaching procedures suggested for the various types of learning activities.

5. The course of study or teacher's guide contains provision for instruction to be adapted to pupils' health needs.

B. The course of study contains statements of the purposes of health instruction and the objectives to be sought; an outline of the contents that shows both scope and sequence; units of instruction, lists of materials and sources of materials, and recommended means and procedures for evaluating pupils' progress.

Recommended steps to be taken:

1. The course of study in health provides for a complete program of health instruction.

2. The objectives are stated to provide for the following:
   a. Learning essential health information.

   b. Developing desirable health attitudes.

   c. Acquiring good health practices.

   d. Learning to think critically on health problems.

   e. Developing the ability to make reasoned judg-
      ments regarding ways health problems may be
      solved.

3. The scope of the content for the total program includes the following:
   a. Structure and function of the body.

   b. Food and nutrition.

   c. Physical activity and play.

   d. Rest, sleep, and relaxation.

   e. Mental health.

   f. Family health.

   g. Dental health.

   h. Disease prevention.

   i. Habit-forming substances.

EVALUATING THE ELEMENTARY SCHOOL
HEALTH PROGRAM

Criteria for Evaluating the Elementary School Health Program—cont.

Criteria	Quality of Provision or Practice					Changes Needed
	Excellent (near perfection)	Good (satisfactory)	Fair (slightly less than satisfactory)	Poor (unsatisfactory)	Provision not Made or Practice not Followed	
j. Safety and first aid.						
k. Consumer health.						
l. Community health.						
4. The sequence in which the content is introduced and developed is outlined for the total program.						
5. The scope of the content for each grade is outlined.						
6. The sequence in which the content is introduced and developed is outlined for each grade.						
7. The basic program of health instruction is developed through the use of units devoted primarily to health.						
8. Health instruction is enriched by making it a correlated phase of units in other subjects such as science, social studies, and homemaking.						
9. Pupils' interests and needs are utilized as motivation for learning.						
10. Health instruction is adapted to the pupils' abilities by employing the following methods, separately or in combinations: a. Problem solving.						

b. Discussion.

c. Demonstration.

d. Reading.

e. Recitation.

f. Research.

g. Construction.

h. Experimentation.

i. Group activities.

11. Instruction is adapted to the age level and repeated as necessary to ensure the maintenance of previous learnings—mere repetition is avoided.

12. Instruction is enriched through the use of the up-to-date information that is made available by official and voluntary health agencies and professional associations.

13. Instruction is enriched by the use of up-to-date audiovisual materials such as films and film strips, charts and pictures, and radio and television programs.

14. Pupils' progress is subjected to continuous evaluation.

15. Reteaching is provided as needed according to evaluation results.

EVALUATING THE ELEMENTARY SCHOOL
HEALTH PROGRAM

Criteria for Evaluating the Elementary School Health Program—cont.

	Quality of Provision or Practice					Changes Needed
Criteria	Excellent (near per-fection)	Good (satis-factory)	Fair (slightly less than satis-factory)	Poor (unsatis-factory)	Provision not Made or Practice not Followed	

III. HEALTH SERVICES

A. A health services guide is provided by the school district or by the office of the county superintendent of schools.

Recommended steps to be taken:

1. A health services guide provided by the school district or the office of the county superintendent of schools is available in the school.

2. The guide contains the objectives for health services.

3. The guide outlines the procedures employed in providing health services.

4. The guide contains suggested ways health services can be adapted to meet special needs of individuals and of the total school population.

B. A health service committee, preferably a subcommittee of the health council or committee, has advisory responsibility for health services.

Recommended steps to be taken:

1. The health services committee has a membership representative of the school administration, teachers, school health personnel, counselors, and speech therapists.

2. The health services committee has the advice of physicians, dentists, and other health specialists in the community as needed.

C. Health services are provided in accordance with the provisions of the guide, provided, however, that the advice of the health services committee is an important consideration in decisions regarding adaptations that are required to meet special needs of individuals and of the total school population.

Recommended steps to be taken:

1. Health services are provided in accordance with the provisions outlined in the health guide.

2. The health services are evaluated periodically.

D. The school health services are of sufficient scope to provide school personnel the information and assistance needed to determine status of, protect, and promote the health of pupils.

Recommended steps to be taken:

1. Guidance and assistance are provided in securing an appraisal of each pupil's health status.

2. Guidance and assistance are provided in securing appraisals of the health of school personnel.

3. School personnel, pupils, and parents are counseled regarding the results of health appraisals and ways to protect and promote one's health.

4. Guidance in securing corrections of remedial defects is provided parents.

5. Guidance and assistance are provided in the identification of pupils with unobservable handicaps who may need special educational opportunities.

6. Procedures designed to help prevent and control disease are established.

7. First aid for the injured and emergency care for cases of sudden illness are provided.

EVALUATING THE ELEMENTARY SCHOOL
HEALTH PROGRAM

Criteria for Evaluating the Elementary School Health Program—cont.

Criteria	Quality of Provision or Practice				Changes Needed
	Excellent (near perfection)	Good (satisfactory)	Fair (slightly less than satisfactory)	Poor (unsatisfactory)	Provision not Made or Practice not Followed
8. School health services are coordinated with those provided by professional health agencies in the community.					
9. Health personnel help to develop and promote sound health practices among pupils, parents, and school personnel.					
10. Health personnel help teachers to utilize community health resources—physicians and dentists, the public health department, voluntary health agencies, and others—to enrich the school program of health instruction.					
E. School health personnel encourage and guide teacher observation of pupils' health characteristics and accept referrals of pupils whose characteristics are unlike those of the well child.	Recommended steps to be taken:				
1. Teachers are encouraged to be constantly alert to observe pupil characteristics that deviate from those of the well child.					
2. Nurse-teacher conferences are conducted to provide teachers with help regarding pupil characteristics that may indicate conditions of health that should have special attention.					
3. Procedures are established for teachers to refer to the school nurse pupils whose health appears to deviate from that of the well child.					

F. School personnel inform and advise parents regarding medical examinations their children should have and assist in making provision for the medical examinations as necessary.

Recommended steps to be taken:

1. Parents are advised to have medical examinations for their children prior to school entrance.

2. Parents are encouraged to have their children given at least one medical examination during the years they are in elementary school.

3. Parents are informed when their child's behavior in school indicates less than normal health and encouraged to secure for him a medical examinations.

4. Parents are encouraged to be present when their children are given medical examinations.

5. Provision is made for pupils to have medical examinations as required by existing conditions. (Preferably this provision is made in cooperation with the local medical society.)

6. Procedures are established for the transmission of the results of medical examinations from physicians to the school.

7. The forms used for the transmission of medical examination findings are approved by school personnel and the local medical society.

8. The results of medical examinations are recorded on the pupils' health records.

9. Procedures are established for the cumulative health record to follow the pupil from grade to grade and school to school.

EVALUATING THE ELEMENTARY SCHOOL
HEALTH PROGRAM

Criteria for Evaluating the Elementary School Health Program—cont.

Criteria	Quality of Provision or Practice					Changes Needed
	Excellent (near perfection)	Good (satisfactory)	Fair (slightly less than satisfactory)	Poor (unsatisfactory)	Provision not Made or Practice not Followed	
G. School personnel inform parents of the importance of eye examinations for children prior to school entrance, maintain a vision-screening program, and inform and advise parents regarding eye conditions of their children that require the attention of a specialist.	Recommended steps to be taken:					
1. Parents are advised to have their children's eyes examined by a specialist prior to school entrance.						
2. Teachers are encouraged to be constantly alert to signs of visual difficulty being experienced by a pupil.						
3. During children's first year in school the Snellen Test is administered to each one who did not have a professional eye examination prior to his entrance to school.						
4. The Snellen Test is administered at least once each two years to each pupil in the total school population.						
5. A color test is administered to each pupil while he is in the elementary grades.						
6. The Snellen Test and the color test are administered by a teacher qualified for the work (has successfully completed a one-unit college course in vision screening or had six hours of instruction in vision screening given by a supervisor of health) or by a school nurse.						

7. Pupils below the third grade who fail to read the 20/40 line with either eye and those in the third grade and above who fail to read the 20/30 line with either eye are retested by the school nurse.

8. The parents of children who fail in the retest (the same standards are required on the retest as are required on the first or screening test) are informed of the findings and advised to have their children's eyes examined by a specialist.

9. The results of vision-screening tests administered by the schools are recorded on pupils' health records.

10. Parents are encouraged to request the specialists who examine their children's eyes to report the examination results to the school.

11. The results of examinations by specialists are recorded on the pupils' health records.

H. School health personnel provide for all pupils to have group hearing tests at regular intervals, individual tests for pupils discovered with hearing difficulties; inform and advise parents regarding their children's need for examinations by ear specialists; and recommend classroom adjustments for children with hearing difficulties.

Recommended steps to be taken:

1. A group pure tone audiometer test is administered annually to all pupils below grade four to determine their hearing acuity.

2. A group pure tone audiometer test is administered at least once each two years to all pupils in grades four and above to determine their hearing acuity.

3. Pupils who are identified by the group pure tone audiometer test as having hearing losses of 20 decibels or more in any two sound frequencies or one of 30 decibels or more in a single frequency are given individual pure tone audiometer tests.

EVALUATING THE ELEMENTARY SCHOOL
HEALTH PROGRAM

Criteria for Evaluating the Elementary School Health Program—cont.

Criteria	Quality of Provision or Practice					Changes Needed
	Excellent (near perfection)	Good (satisfactory)	Fair (slightly less than satisfactory)	Poor (unsatisfactory)	Provision not Made or Practice not Followed	
4. Pupils new to the school are given a pure tone audiometer test if their health records do not contain the results of recently administered hearing tests.						
5. Individual pure tone audiometer tests are given all pupils whose school performance may be indicative of hearing loss. (Defective speech, school retardation, inability to follow oral directions, emotional responses, undesirable behavior.)						
6. Both group and individual pure tone audiometer tests are administered by individuals who are properly certificated.						
7. The parents of children who have hearing losses of 20 or more decibels in any two sound frequencies or 30 or more decibels in a single frequency are informed of their children's difficulties and advised regarding the importance of having their children's ears examined by an otologist.						
8. Pupils with hearing difficulties are seated for classroom instruction so that the effects of the hearing difficulties are held to the possible minimum.						
9. The results of hearing tests administered by the schools are recorded on pupils' health records.						
I. Health services provide for parents to be informed regarding their children's need for regular dental examinations beginning prior to the children's entrance to school, and for parents of children who have defective dental conditions to be informed regarding the undesirable effects of the conditions and advised regarding essential treatment.	Recommended steps to be taken:					

1. Parents are informed of the importance of having their children's teeth examined and given the care needed prior to the children's entry to school.

2. Parents are encouraged to have their children's teeth examined by a dentist at least once each year, more often if recommended by the dentist.

3. Pupils are encouraged to report immediately cavities or other conditions of the teeth that disturb them

4. Poor conditions of the teeth observed by school nurses and teachers are reported to the pupil's parents along with recommendations for the required dental care.

5. Parents of pupils with dental conditions that are apparently causing speech difficulties are advised to secure dental help for their children.

6. Parents of pupils with dental conditions that are apparently causing emotional upset are advised to secure dental help for their children.

7. Pupils with dental emergencies such as fractured teeth and traumatic injuries to jaws are immediately referred to a dentist.

8. Arrangements are made for the schools to participate in communitywide dental activities.

9. A dental care card developed cooperatively by school personnel and members of the dental society is used by dentists to report to the school results of examination and dental work in process or completed.

10. The results of dental examinations and other information provided by dentists are recorded on the children's health records.

J. Pupils' growth characteristics are observed to determine deviations in growth patterns that merit special attention.

Recommended steps to be taken:

Criteria for Evaluating the Elementary School Health Program—cont.

Criteria	Quality of Provision or Practice					Changes Needed
	Excellent (near per-fection)	Good (satis-factory)	Fair (slightly less than satis-factory)	Poor (unsatis-factory)	Provision not Made or Practice not Followed	
1. Pupils are weighed at the beginning of each semester and their weights are recorded on growth charts in their health records.						
2. Pupils' heights are measured at the beginning of each semester and their heights are recorded on growth charts in their health records.						
3. Gross deviations in pupils' growth patterns are discussed with the pupils' parents and recommendations are made for securing medical help.						
4. Pupils are observed for posture that deviates from normal and the deviations noted are recorded on the pupils' health records.						
5. Parents of children with posture difficulties are advised to secure medical help for their children.						
6. Recommendations are made for modifications in the physical education program that are needed for pupils whose growth characteristics require special consideration.						
K. Follow-up procedures are taken as necessary—begin when pupils with health difficulties are identified and conclude when the health difficulties have been corrected or their effects minimized.	Recommended steps to be taken:					
1. The school nurse confers with teachers regarding pupils in their classrooms who have been identified as having health problems.						

2. The school nurse confers with parents regarding the health problems of their children and advises them regarding steps to be taken.

3. The school nurse visits the home of each pupil with a health problem as necessary to encourage the parents to secure the required help for the child.

4. When a pupil's health problem has been corrected, his classroom teacher is so informed.

5. The health record of each pupil with an identified health problem contains essential information regarding progress made in correcting or minimizing the problem.

L. Health counseling and guidance is provided.

Recommended steps to be taken:

1. School health personnel counsel pupils regarding their health problems.

2. School health personnel counsel teachers regarding their health problems.

3. Case conferences are held as needed to secure the necessary adjustments in the educational programs of pupils with health problems.

4. Case conferences are held to assist pupils with special health problems to make the best possible personal and social adjustments.

5. The nurse holds conferences with parents to discuss the health of their children and how the children's adjustment to the school program is being affected.

Criteria for Evaluating the Elementary School Health Program—cont.

Criteria	Quality of Provision or Practice				Changes Needed
	Excellent (near perfection)	Good (satisfactory)	Fair (slightly less than satisfactory)	Poor (unsatisfactory)	Provision not Made or Practice not Followed

Criteria					
6. Information regarding counseling provided and results obtained is recorded on the pupils' health records.					
M. Provisions are made for supplying teachers with health information concerning handicapped pupils and for recommending cases for whom home teaching may be necessary.	Recommended steps to be taken:				
1. The nurse provides each teacher the health information about each physically handicapped child that is needed to make the required adaptations in the classroom and in instruction.					
2. The nurse assists in recommending cases for whom home teaching may be necessary.					
N. The health service program includes provisions for the prevention and control of communicable diseases.	Recommended steps to be taken:				
1. Parents of preschool children are advised by the school to protect their children as early as possible against communicable diseases for which immunization is available.					

2. School personnel cooperate with representatives of the local health department in planning community immunization programs that are to be available to pupils.

3. The school cooperates with local health agencies in conducting a tuberculosis case-finding program for pupils and school personnel.

4. School health personnel report to the local health department the cases of diseases specified by the department.

5. Parents are notified of in-school exposures to communicable diseases other than common colds.

6. Pupils suspected of having communicable diseases are isolated while they are waiting to be removed from school.

O. The health service program provides emergency service for injury and sudden illness and for disasters.

Recommended steps to be taken:

1. Written policies and procedures for first aid and emergency care are provided to all school personnel.

2. The policies and procedures pertaining to first aid emergency care are approved by the local medical society or the health department.

3. First aid is administered promptly to injured or ill pupils.

4. Phone numbers of parents and of physicians to call in emergencies are on file for each pupil.

5. Parents are notified immediately in instances of serious injury or illness.

Criteria for Evaluating the Elementary School Health Program—cont.

Criteria	Quality of Provision or Practice					Changes Needed
	Excellent (near perfection)	Good (satisfactory)	Fair (slightly less than satisfactory)	Poor (unsatisfactory)	Provision not Made or Practice not Followed	
6. Teachers are prepared to render first aid.						
7. Periodic reviews of up-to-date first-aid procedures are provided for all school personnel.						
8. First-aid kits are available in each classroom and in the principal's office.						
9. The contents of first-aid kits are replaced as required to maintain complete complements.						
10. The school nurse periodically inspects first-aid kits and replenishes the supplies.						
11. First-aid equipment, such as stretchers and blankets, is stored in readily accessible places.						

IV. HEALTHFUL SCHOOL ENVIRONMENT

A. The school environment is protected by employing personnel whose health is good, requiring all personnel to have regular health examinations, and providing measures that encourage good health practices.

Recommended steps to be taken:

1. Preemployment medical examinations are required of all personnel.						
2. Periodic medical examinations are required of all personnel.						

3. All school personnel are required to have an intra-dermal tuberculin test or a chest Xray prior to employment, every two years thereafter.

4. A specified amount of sick leave with pay may be earned annually by all school personnel.

5. The work load is distributed equitably among personnel.

6. Counseling and guidance are provided school personnel as needed.

7. Medical insurance plans are available to all personnel.

8. School personnel are encouraged to remain away from school when they have symptoms of communicable diseases.

9. Teachers set good examples of healthful living.

B. A wholesome emotional climate prevails and essential provisions are made for its maintenance.

Recommended steps to be taken:

1. The morale of teachers is at a high level as indicated by the following conditions:
   a. The teachers are relaxed and free from tensions.
   b. The teachers have confidence in themselves and in their pupils.
   c. The teachers are happy and sincere in their work.

2. The following provisions are made for the maintenance of staff morale at a high level:
   a. Leaves of absence without pay are granted for specified purposes.

Criteria for Evaluating the Elementary School Health Program—cont.

	Quality of Provision or Practice					
Criteria	Excellent (near perfection)	Good (satisfactory)	Fair (slightly less than satisfactory)	Poor (unsatisfactory)	Provision not Made or Practice not Followed	Changes Needed
b. Sabbatical leaves for study or travel are granted certificated personnel in accordance with written policies of the district.						
c. Communication is maintained between the administration and teaching personnel.						
d. A teamwork approach is utilized in the prevention and solving of staff problems.						
3. The following provisions are employed to create classroom environments that are conducive to learning:						
a. The teachers adapt learning experiences to each child's developmental pattern of growth and needs.						
b. The daily program provides for a balance of quiet and active experiences.						
c. Opportunities are provided for each child to release tension by participating in various types of aesthetic and physical activities.						
d. Teachers discuss required behavior standards with pupils.						
e. Pupils share responsibility for securing desired classroom behavior.						
f. Discipline procedures are fair and consistent.						
g. The teacher-pupil ratio permits the individualization of instruction to the extent required for maximum learning.						

Appendix B

h. The classrooms are clean and orderly.

i. The pupils share responsibility for the care of materials in the classroom.

j. The grading procedures are fair.

k. The grading procedures are understood by all concerned.

4. Pupils are given the following types of opportunities to develop as self-directing individuals:
   a. To share responsibility for solving social problems such as those caused by littering the school grounds and pupils who are unwilling to cooperate in school activities.

   b. To assume leadership responsibility through participation in classroom and student government activities.

   c. To plan and organize school activities under teacher supervision.

5. Teachers are helped by the principal and special school personnel—the school psychologists, counselors, curriculum consultants, and others—to solve problems that arise in their classes.

6. School personnel and parents are encouraged in the following ways to work cooperatively in solving the problems that are causing pupils to make less than maximum use of their abilities:
   a. Essential provisions are made for teacher-parent conferences.

   b. Parents are invited to visit the school to discuss the problems of their children.

   c. Parents are kept informed regarding the educational program that is offered—the objectives and teaching methods.

Criteria for Evaluating the Elementary School Health Program—cont.

Criteria	Quality of Provision or Practice					Changes Needed
	Excellent (near per-fection)	Good (satis-factory)	Fair (slightly less than satis-factory)	Poor (unsatis-factory)	Provision not Made or Practice not Followed	
C. The school food services are conducted so that each pupil has opportunity to have a wholesome and nutri-tionally adequate lunch in an environment that is plea-sant and sanitary, and pupils are helped to learn the importance of good eating habits, eating well-balanced meals, using good table manners.	Recommended steps to be taken:					
1. A Type A lunch, a lunch that meets the nutritional standards of the Type A lunch, or both are served daily.						
2. Candy and sweetened beverages not ordinarily served with meals are not available in the school.						
3. Pupils' nutritional practices are observed and in-struction is given to secure improvements needed.						
4. The school food service program is supervised by persons qualified to advise on nutritive values and sanitary practices.						
5. An in-service education program in food prepara-tion and handling is conducted for food service personnel cooperatively by the school and the local health department.						
6. Food service procedures meet the standards set by the local health department.						
7. Lunchroom and kitchen facilities meet the standards set by the local health department.						
8. Lunchroom and kitchen facilities are periodically inspected by sanitarians from the local health de-partment.						

D. The health service unit provides the required space for each type of activity conducted in the unit and is properly equipped with built-in facilities.

Recommended steps to be taken:

1. A sink with hot and cold running water located for convenient use.

2. A toilet room equipped with a toilet and washbasin with hot and cold running water.

3. An enclosed area for isolating pupils who are ill.

4. The necessary space and conditions required for administering vision-screening tests.

5. An area that is relatively free of disturbing noises for administering hearing tests (or a mobile unit).

6. Office space.

7. An enclosed area for conferences with pupils, parents, and teachers.

E. The school site meets the standards that are established for schools as set forth in the California Administrative Code, Title 5.

Recommended steps to be taken:

1. The size of the elementary school site meets the recommendations set forth in Title 5 of the California Administrative Code. (Five net usable acres plus one additional acre for each 100 pupils of predicted ultimate enrollment, plus one additional acre for each 100 or major fraction of the number of seventh and eighth grade pupils for the predicted ultimate maximum enrollment.)

Criteria for Evaluating the Elementary School Health Program—cont.

Criteria	Quality of Provision or Practice				Changes Needed
	Excellent (near per-fection)	Good (satis-factory)	Fair (slightly less than satis-factory)	Poor (unsatis-factory)	Provision not Made or Practice not Followed
2. The school is centrally located in the geographic area served.					
3. The area in which the school is located is relatively free of disturbing noises, noxious odors, and other distractions.					
4. Water drains rapidly from outdoor areas.					
F. A planned procedure is followed to detect and correct possible unsafe conditions of buildings, grounds, and equipment.	Recommended steps to be taken:				
1. School personnel are constantly alert to observe buildings, grounds, and equipment for possible hazardous conditions.					
2. Hazardous conditions are corrected immediately after they have been reported.					
3. Regular inspections of the school plant are made by specialists such as firemen and public health sanitarians.					
4. Written reports of the results of the inspections are presented to the school health council, the admin-istration, and the school board.					

Recommended steps to be taken:

G. The buildings and play areas are designed to provide for the successful operation of the school program and kept in good condition.

1. Regular inspections of the school plant are conducted by administrative personnel to ensure proper maintenance.

2. The buildings are located so as to permit flexibility in the use of outdoor areas.

3. All walkways connecting buildings and classrooms have roofs.

4. All doors providing exits from buildings are equipped with panic bars.

5. Ceilings and walls of classrooms and inside corridors are constructed with sound-absorbing materials.

6. Areas or rooms in which noise-producing activities such as band practice and playing games take place are located at points where noises are likely to be least disturbing to classes held in other areas.

7. The enrollments in classes assigned to rooms are not in excess of the number of pupils for which the rooms were originally planned.

8. The height of classroom furniture is sufficiently varied to provide comfortable working conditions for pupils of various sizes.

9. The play areas are fenced for the safety of the pupils.

10. The surfaces under play apparatus are of a desirable type.

Criteria for Evaluating the Elementary School Health Program—cont.

Criteria	Quality of Provision or Practice					Changes Needed
	Excellent (near perfection)	Good (satis-factory)	Fair (slightly less than satis-factory)	Poor (unsatis-factory)	Provision not Made or Practice not Followed	
11. Driveways are located where hazards to pupils are kept to a minimum.						
H. Essential provisions have been made to secure in each classroom the conditions needed for eye comfort.	Recommended steps to be taken:					
1. The lighting in classrooms is soft, even, properly distributed, and sufficiently bright for eye comfort.						
2. The desks and tables are arranged so that the working surfaces are free from glare.						
3. Chalkboards, furniture, and other fixtures have non-glossy finishes.						
4. The interior walls and ceilings are painted light colors and have dull finishes.						
5. The colors of the walls, ceilings, and chalkboards are conducive to eye comfort.						
I. The classrooms and the library are heated and ventilated as required to provide good working conditions for teachers and pupils.	Recommended steps to be taken:					
1. Room temperature is maintained at a comfortable level (68°–70° F).						
2. Each room contains a thermometer that is installed on a wall about 4 feet above the floor.						

3. The ventilating system provides 15 cubic feet of fresh outdoor air per person per minute in classrooms and libraries.

4. Air movement in occupied areas is controlled to the extent that there are no noticeable drafts.

5. Windows that may be opened for ventilation are equipped with deflectors or ventilators.

J. Drinking fountains in the building and on the school grounds are sufficient in number, of desirable design, of proper height, and conveniently located.

Recommended steps to be taken:

1. An adequate number of drinking fountains are available (one for each 75 pupils and at least one on each floor of a multistoried building).

2. The drinking fountains are of a design approved by the local health department.

3. The drinking fountains are of a height suitable for use by children.

4. The drinking fountains are conveniently located for pupil use.

5. The water supply is regularly inspected by health department personnel.

K. The handwashing and toilet facilities are sufficient in number and well kept.

Recommended steps to be taken:

1. The toilet rooms are readily accessible from classrooms and play areas.

Criteria for Evaluating the Elementary School Health Program—cont.

Criteria	Quality of Provision or Practice					Changes Needed
	Excellent (near perfection)	Good (satisfactory)	Fair (slightly less than satisfactory)	Poor (unsatisfactory)	Provision not Made or Practice not Followed	
2. Each toilet room contains at least one washbasin equipped with hot and cold running water for every 50 pupils using the room.						
3. An adequate number of toilets for girls are available (one for each 30 girls).						
4. An adequate number of toilets and urinals are available for boys (one for each 60 boys, one urinal for each 30 boys).						
5. The heights of the toilets are proper for the age groups that use them.						
6. Washbasins are installed at proper heights for the age groups that use them.						
7. A supply of liquid or powdered soap is available near each washbasin.						
8. Paper towels are available near each washbasin.						
9. The supply of toilet paper and hand towels is replenished each day at specified intervals.						
10. The toilet rooms and fixtures are kept clean.						
L. Fire prevention equipment is conveniently located and inspected at regular intervals.						

Recommended steps to be taken:

1. All school personnel know the location of fire signal switches in the school and of fire alarm boxes near the school.

2. Manually operated fire signals are installed in convenient and prominent locations.

3. Fire extinguishers are of a type approved by the local fire department and are inspected at regular intervals by fire officials.

4. Fire extinguishers are placed in locations recommended by fire officials.

M. The procedures to be followed in the case of various types of disasters are known by all school personnel and pupils.

Recommended steps to be taken:

1. Written procedures to be followed in times of disaster are displayed in prominent places throughout the school.

2. School personnel and pupils have practiced and know the procedure to be followed in case of a fire, an earthquake, or other disaster.

3. Fire drills are held monthly.

4. Drills for disasters other than might be caused by fire are held at specified intervals throughout the school year.

Appendix C
SOURCES OF FREE AND INEXPENSIVE HEALTH AND SAFETY EDUCATION MATERIALS

Alcohol and Drugs

Abbott Laboratories
Dept. 383, Abbott Park
North Chicago, Ill.   60064

Aetna Life and Casualty
Educational Resources
Audio-Visual Services
151 Farmington Avenue
Hartford, Conn.   06115

American Medical Association
Bureau of Health Education
535 North Dearborn Street
Chicago, Ill.   60610

Ciba Pharmaceutical Products, Inc.
Division of Ciba-Geigy Corp.
556 Morris Avenue
Summit, N. J.   07901

Connecticut General Life Insurance Co.
Advertising and Public Relations-319
Hartford, Conn.   06115

John Hancock Mutual Life Insurance Co.
Manager, Community Relations
200 Berkeley Street
Boston, Mass.   02117

Licensed Beverage Industries, Inc.
Division of Educational Studies
485 Lexington Avenue
New York, N. Y.   10017

Mental Health Materials Center
419 Park Avenue South
New York, N. Y.   10016

Metropolitan Life Insurance Co.
Health and Welfare Division
1 Madison Avenue
New York, N. Y. 10010

National Association for Mental Health
43 West 61st Street
New York, N. Y.   10019

National Congress of Parents and Teachers
700 North Rush Street
Chicago, Ill.   60611

National Institute on Alcohol Abuse
and Alcoholism
National Institute of Mental Health
5600 Fishers Lane
Rockville, Md. 20852

National Institute of Drug Abuse
Dept. HEW
11400 Rockville Pike
Rockville, Md.   20852

National Institute of Mental Health
5600 Fishers Lane
Rockville, Md.   20852

National Safety Council
School and College Dept.
425 North Michigan Avenue
Chicago, Ill.   60611

Pharmaceutical Manufacturers Association
Public Relations Division
1155 Fifteenth Street, N.W.
Washington, D. C. 20005

Public Affairs Committee, Inc.
38 Park Avenue South
New York, N. Y.   10016

U.S. Department of Health, Education,
and Welfare
Food and Drug Administration
5600 Fishers Lane
Rockville, Md.   20852

Chronic Disorders

Aetna Life and Casualty
Educational Resources
Audio-Visual Services
151 Farmington Avenue
Hartford, Conn.   06115

Allergy Foundation of America
801 Second Avenue
New York, N. Y.   10017

American Cancer Society
Vice-President for Public Education
219 East 42nd Street
New York, N. Y.   10017
(contact local office)

American Diabetes Association
1 West 48th Street
New York, N. Y.   10020

American Heart Association
Inquiries Section
44 East 23rd Street
New York, N. Y.   10010
(consult local office)

American Lung Association
1740 Broadway
New York, N. Y.   10019

American Medical Association
Bureau of Health Education
535 North Dearborn Street
Chicago, Ill.   60610

Arthritis Foundation
GPO Box 2525
New York, N. Y.   10036

Association for the Aid of Crippled
Children
Division of Publications
345 East 46th Street
New York, N. Y.   10017

Connecticut General Life Insurance Co.
Advertising and Public Relations-319
Hartford, Conn.   06115

Epilepsy Foundation of America
1828 L Street, N.W., Suite 406
Washington, D. C.   20036

Foundation for Research and Education
in Sickle Cell Disease, Inc.
423 West 120th Street
New York, N. Y.   10027

John Hancock Mutual Life Insurance Co.
Manager, Community Relations
200 Berkeley Street
Boston, Mass.   02117

Muscular Dystrophy Association of
America, Inc.
Community Services
810 Seventh Avenue
New York, N. Y.   10019

National Cystic Fibrosis Research
Foundation
60 East 44th Street
New York, N. Y.   10017

National Epilepsy League, Inc.
116 South Michigan Avenue
Chicago, Illinois   60603

National Foundation
1275 Mamaroneck Avenue
White Plains, N. Y.   10605

National Institute of Allergy and
Infectious Diseases
Office of Information
Bethesda, Md.   20014

National Institute of Child Health
and Human Development
Office of Information
U.S. Public Health Service
9000 Rockville Pike
Bethesda, Md.   20014

National Kidney Foundaiton
116 East 27th Street
New York, N. Y.   10010

National Multiple Sclerosis Society
Public Relations Dept.
257 Park Avenue South
New York, N. Y.   10010

National Tay-Sachs and Allied Diseases
Public and Professional Information
122 East 42nd Street
New York, N. Y.   10017

Public Affairs Committee, Inc.
381 Park Avenue South
New York, N. Y.   10016

United Cerebral Palsy Association
66 East 34th Street
New York, N. Y.   10016

Communicable Diseases

American Medical Association
Bureau of Health Education
535 North Dearborn Street
Chicago, Ill.   60610

American Social Health Association
1740 Broadway
New York, N. Y.   10019

Center for Disease Control/CEMA
1600 Clifton Road, N.E.
Atlanta, Ga.   30333

Connecticut General Life Insurance Co.
Advertising and Public Relations-319
Hartford, Conn.   06115

John Hancock Mutual Life Insurance Co.
Manager, Community Relations
200 Berkeley Street
Boston, Mass.   02117

Metropolitan Life Insurance Co.
Health and Welfare Division
1 Madison Avenue
New York, N. Y.   10010

National Center for Disease Control
Department HEW
1600 Clifton Road N.E.
Atlanta, Ga.   30333

National Foundation
1275 Mamaroneck Avenue
White Plains, N. Y.   10605

National Institute of Allergy and
Infectious Diseases
Office of Information
Bethesda, Md.   20014

National Institute of Child Health
and Human Development
Office of Information
U.S. Public Health Service
9000 Rockville Pike
Bethesda, Md.   20014

Public Affairs Committee, Inc.
381 Park Avenue South
New York, N. Y.   10016

Public Health Service
Environmental Health Service
U.S. Dept. HEW
Rockville, Md.   20852

World Health Organization
Office of Public Information
1501 New Hampshire Avenue, N.W.
Washington, D. C.   20006

Consumer Health/Quackery

American Dental Association
Bureau of Dental Health Education
211 East Chicago Avenue
Chicago, Ill.   60611

American Hospital Association
840 North Lake Shore Drive
Chicago, Ill.   60611

American Medical Association
Bureau of Health Education
535 North Dearborn Street
Chicago, Ill.   60610

Arthritis Foundation
GPO Box 2525
New York, N. Y.   10036

Consumers Union of United States, Inc.
256 Washington Street
Mount Vernon, N. Y.   10550

Public Affairs Committee, Inc.
381 Park Avenue South
New York, N. Y.   10016

U.S. Department of Health, Education,
and Welfare
Food and Drug Administration
5600 Fishers Lane
Rockville, Md.   20852

Dental Health

American Dental Association
Bureau of Dental Health Education
211 East Chicago Avenue
Chicago, Ill.   60611

American Dietetic Association
1 West 48th Street
New York, N. Y.   10020

Connecticut General Life Insurance Co.
Advertising and Public Relations-319
Hartford, Conn.   06115

National Dairy Council
111 North Canal Street
Chicago, Ill.   60606

National Institute of Child Health
and Human Development
Office of Information
U.S. Public Health Service
9000 Rockville Pike
Bethesda, Md.   20014

National Institute of Dental Research
Information Officer
U.S. Public Health Service
Bethesda, Md.   20014

Public Affairs Committee, Inc.
381 Park Avenue South
New York, N. Y.   10016

Public Health Service
Environmental Health Service
U.S. Department HEW
Rockville, Md.   20852

U.S. Department of Agriculture
Agricultural Research Service
Washington, D. C.   20250

World Health Organization
Office of Public Information
1501 New Hampshire Avenue, N.W.
Washington, D. C.   20006

Enivronmental Health

American Automobile Association
Pennsylvania Avenue at 17th Street, N.W.
Washington, D. C.   20006

American Cancer Society
Vice-President for Public Education
219 East 42nd Street
New York, N. Y.   10017
(contact local office)

American Lung Associaiton
1740 Broadway
New York, N. Y.   10019

Public Affairs Committee, Inc.
381 Park Avenue South
New York, N. Y.   10016

Family Life and Sex Education

American Institute of Family Relations
5287 Sunset Boulevard
Los Angeles, Calif.   90027

American Medical Association
Bureau of Health Education
535 North Dearborn Street
Chicago, Ill.   60610

International Cellucotton Products, Inc.
919 North Michigan Avenue
Chicago, Ill.   60611

Kimberly-Clark Corp.
Life Cycle Center
P.O. Box 20001
Neenah, Wis.   54956

Mental Health Materials Center
419 Park Avenue South
New York, N. Y.   10016

National Association for Mental Health
43 West 61st Street
New York, N. Y.   10019

National Congress of Parents and Teachers
700 North Rush Street
Chicago, Ill.   60611

National Council on Family Relations
1219 University Avenue, S.E.
Minneapolis, Minn.   55414

National Institute of Child Health
and Human Development
Office of Information
U.S. Public Health Service
9000 Rockville Pike
Bethesda, Md.   20014

National Institute of Mental Health
5600 Fishers Lane
Rockville, Md.   20852

Personal Products Corporation
c/o Association Sterling, Inc.
P.O. Box 117
Ridgefield, N. J.   07657

Public Affairs Committee, Inc.
381 Park Avenue South
New York, N. Y.   10016

Sex Information and Education Council
of the United States
Publications Office
1855 Broadway
New York, N. Y.   10023

Tampax Incorporated
Department HI
Educational Director
5 Dakota Drive
Lake Success, N. Y.   11040

Food and Nutrition

American Dental Association
Bureau of Dental Health Education
211 East Chicago Avenue
Chicago, Ill.   60611

American Dietetic Association
620 North Michigan Avenue
Chicago, Ill.   60611

American Dry Milk Institute, Inc.
130 North Franklin Street
Chicago, Ill.   60606

American Heart Association
Inquiries Section
44 East 23rd Street
New York, N. Y.   10010
(consult local office)

American Institute of Baking
Consumer Service Dept.
400 East Ontario Street
Chicago, Ill.   60611

American Meat Institute
59 East Van Buren Street
Chicago, Ill.   60605

Borden Company
Consumer Services
350 Madison Avenue
New York, N. Y.   10011

Cereal Institute, Inc.
135 South LaSalle Street
Chicago, Ill.   60603

Florida Citrus Commission
Production Dept.
Lakeland, Fla.   33801

General Foods Corp.
General Foods Kitchens
250 North Street
White Plains, N. Y.   10625

General Mills, Inc.
Public Relations Dept.
9200 Wayzata Boulevard
Minneapolis, Minn.   55426

Kellogg Company
Dept. of Home Economics Services
Battle Creek, Mich.   49016

National Dairy Council
111 North Canal Street
Chicago, Ill.   60606

Nutrition Foundation, Inc.
99 Park Avenue
New York, N. Y.   10016

Public Affairs Committee, Inc.
381 Park Avenue South
New York, N. Y.   10016

United Fresh Fruit and Vegetable
Association
77 14th Street, N.W.
Washington, D. C.   20005

U.S. Department of Agriculture
Agricultural Research Service
Washington, D. C.   20250

U.S. Department of Health, Education,
and Welfare
Food and Drug Administration
5600 Fishers Lane
Rockville, Md.   20852

Wheat Flour Institute
Supervisor of Distribution
14 East Jackson Boulevard
Chicago, Ill.   60604

General Health

American Medical Association
Bureau of Health Education
535 North Dearborn Street
Chicago, Ill.   60610

Cleveland Health Museum
8911 Euclid Avenue
Cleveland, Ohio   44106

Connecticut General Life Insurance Co.
Advertising and Public Relations-319
Hartford, Conn.   06115

John Hancock Mutual Life Insurance Co.
Manager, Community Relations
200 Berkeley Street
Boston, Mass.   02117

Kemper Insurance
Advertising and Public Relations Dept.
110 Tenth Avenue
Fulton, Ill.   61252

Liberty Mutual Insurance Co.
Public Relations Dept.
175 Berkeley Street
Boston, Mass.   02117

Metropolitan Life Insurance Co.
Health and Welfare Division
1 Madison Avenue
New York, N. Y.   10010

Prudential Insurance Company of America
Public Relations Dept.
Prudential Plaza
Newark, N. J.   07101

Public Affairs Committee, Inc.
381 Park Avenue South
New York, N. Y.   10016

Travelers Insurance Companies
Marketing Services
One Tower Square
Hartford, Conn.   06115

Health Careers

American Cancer Society
Vice-President for Public Education
219 East 42nd Street
New York, N. Y.   10017
(contact local office)

American Dietetic Association
620 North Michigan Avenue
Chicago, Ill.   60611

American Lung Association
1740 Broadway
New York, N. Y.   10019

American Medical Association
Bureau of Health Education
535 North Dearborn Street
Chicago, Ill.   60610

American National Red Cross
17th and D Streets, N.W.
Washington, D. C.   20006

American Osteopathic Association
Editorial Dept.
212 East Ohio Street
Chicago, Ill.   60611

National Health Council
1740 Broadway
New York, N. Y.   10019

Public Affairs Committee, Inc.
381 Park Avenue South
New York, N. Y.   10016

Mental Health

American Institute of Family Relations
5287 Sunset Boulevard
Los Angeles, Calif.   90027

Child Study Association of America,
Wel-Met, Inc.
50 Madison Avenue
New York, N. Y.

John Hancock Mutual Life Insurance Co.
Manager, Community Relations
200 Berkeley Street
Boston, Mass.   02117

Mental Health Materials Center
419 Park Avenue South
New York, N. Y.   10016

National Association for Mental Health
43 West 61st Street
New York, N. Y.   10019

National Council on Family Relations
1219 University Avenue, S.E.
Minneapolis, Minn.   55414

National Institute of Child Health
and Human Development
Office of Information
U.S. Public Health Service
9000 Rockville Pike
Bethesda, Md.   20014

National Institute of Mental Health
5600 Fishers Lane
Rockville, Md.   20852

Public Affairs Committee, Inc.
381 Park Avenue South
New York, N. Y.   10016

Personal Hygiene

American Medical Association
Bureau of Health Education
535 North Dearborn Street
Chicago, Ill.   60610

American Podiatry Association
20 Chevy Chase Circle, N.W.
Washington, D. C.   20010

International Cellucotton Products, Inc.
919 North Michigan Avenue
Chicago, Ill.   60611

Kimberly-Clark Corp.
Life Cycle Center
P.O. Box 20001
Neenah, Wisc.   54956

Lever Brothers Co.
Public Relations Division
Consumer Education Dept.
390 Park Avenue
New York, N. Y.   10022

Personal Products Corporation
c/o Association Sterling, Inc.
P.O. Box 117
Ridgefield, N. J.   07657

Procter and Gamble
Public Relations Dept.
P.O. Box 599
Cincinnati, Ohio   45201

Tampax Incorporated
Department HI
Educational Director
5 Dakota Drive
Lake Success, N. Y.   11040

Safety and First Aid

Aetna Life and Casualty
Educational Resources
Audio-Visual Services
151 Farmington Avenue
Hartford, Conn.   06115

American Automobile Association
Pennsylvania Avenue at 17th Street, N.W.
Washington, D. C.   20006

American Fire Insurance Companies
80 Maiden Lane
New York, N. Y.   10007

American Insurance Association
Engineering and Safety Service
85 John Street
New York, N. Y.   10038

American Medical Association
Bureau of Health Education
535 North Dearborn Street
Chicago, Ill.   60610

American National Red Cross
17th and D Streets, N.W.
Washington, D. C.   20006

Bicycle Institute of America
122 East 42nd Street
New York, N. Y.   10017

Connecticut General Life Insurance Co.
Advertising and Public Relations-319
Hartford, Conn.   06115

Institute of Makers of Explosives
420 Lexington Avenue
New York, N. Y.   10017

Institute for Safer Living
American Mutual Liability Insurance Co.
Wakefield, Mass.   01880

Johnson and Johnson
501 George Street
New Brunswick, N. J.   08901

Kemper Insurance
Advertising and Public Relations Dept.
110 Tenth Avenue
Fulton, Ill.   61252

Metropolitan Life Insurance Co.
Health and Welfare Division
1 Madison Avenue
New York, N. Y.   10010

National Fire Protection Association
470 Atlantic Avenue
Boston, Mass.   02210

National Safety Council
School and College Dept.
425 North Michigan Avenue
Chicago, Ill.   60611

National Society for the Prevention
of Blindness
79 Madison Avenue
New York, N. Y.   10016

Pharmaceutical Manufacturers Association
Public Relations Division
1155 Fifteenth Street, N.W.
Washington, D. C.   20005

Travelers Insurance Companies
Marketing Services
One Tower Square
Hartford, Conn.   06115

The Senses

American Foundation for the Blind
15 West 16th Street
New York, N. Y.   10011

American Medical Association
Bureau of Health Education
535 North Dearborn Street
Chicago, Ill.   60610

American Optometric Association
Public Information Division
700 Chippewa Street
St. Louis, Mo.   63119

Better Vision Institute, Inc.
230 Park Avenue
New York, N. Y.   10017

National Safety Council
School and College Dept.
425 North Michigan Avenue
Chicago, Ill.   60611

Public Affairs Committee, Inc.
381 Park Avenue South
New York, N. Y.   10016

Smoking and Health

American Cancer Society
Vice-President for Public Education
219 East 42nd Street
New York, N. Y.   10017
(contact local office)

American Dental Association
Bureau of Dental Health Education
211 East Chicago Avenue
Chicago, Ill.   60611

American Heart Association
Inquiries Section
44 East 23rd Street
New York, N. Y.   10010
(consult local office)

American Lung Association
1740 Broadway
New York, N. Y.   10019

American Medical Association
Bureau of Health Education
535 North Dearborn Street
Chicago, Ill.   60610

Metropolitan Life Insurance Co.
Health and Welfare Division
1 Madison Avenue
New York, N. Y.   10010

National Clearinghouse for Smoking
and Health
U.S. Public Health Service
5600 Fishers Lane
Rockville, Md.   20852

National Congress of Parents and Teachers
700 North Rush Street
Chicago, Ill.   60611

Public Affairs Committee, Inc.
381 Park Avenue South
New York, N. Y.   10016

INDEX